CONFLICTS OF INTEREST IN CLINICAL PRACTICE AND RESEARCH

CONFLICTS OF INTEREST IN CLINICAL PRACTICE AND RESEARCH

Edited by

Roy G. Spece, Jr., J.D.
Professor of Law
The University of Arizona
College of Law

David S. Shimm, M.D., F.A.C.P.
Associate Professor of Radiation Oncology
The University of Arizona
College of Medicine

Allen E. Buchanan
Granger Professor of Business Ethics (School of Business)
Professor of Philosophy
Professor of Medical Ethics (Medical School)
University of Wisconsin, Madison

New York   Oxford
OXFORD UNIVERSITY PRESS
1996

Oxford University Press

Oxford   New York
Athens   Auckland   Bangkok   Bombay
Calcutta   Cape Town   Dar es Salaam   Delhi
Florence   Hong Kong   Istanbul   Karachi
Kuala Lumpur   Madras   Madrid   Melbourne
Mexico City   Nairobi   Paris   Singapore
Taipei   Tokyo   Toronto

and associated companies in
Berlin   Ibadan

Library of Congress Cataloging-in-Publication Data
Conflicts of interest in clinical practice and research /
edited by Roy G. Spece, Jr., David S. Shimm, Allen E. Buchanan.
p. cm. Includes index.
ISBN 0-19-508024-6
1. Medical ethics.   2. Conflict of interests.
I. Spece, Roy G., 1948–
II. Shimm, David S.   III. Buchanan, Allen E., 1948–
[DNLM: 1. Conflict of Interest.   2. Ethics, Medical.
3. Referral and Consultation.
4. Health Maintenance Organizations.
5. Research
W 50 C7485 1995] R724.C627 1995 174'.2—dc20
DNLM / DLC for Library of Congress   94-42514

1 3 5 7 9 8 6 4 2

Printed in the United States of America
on acid-free paper

To our parents:

Mollie A. and Roy G. Spece, Sr.

Cynia and Melvin G. Shimm

and to
Allen Buchanan's brother,
Steve N. Buchanan

Foreword

Concern about conflicts of interest in clinical practice and biomedical research has heightened during the past two decades, mainly in response to the increasing role of commerce in medicine and the many kinds of financial arrangements that have evolved. Opinions differ about the wisdom of encouraging market forces in health care, but not about the importance of preserving the integrity and trustworthiness of physicians and scientists, whatever the circumstances. All agree that patients need to be able to rely on the commitment of their physicians, just as society needs to rely on the objectivity and good intentions of its medical scientists. Hence the growing concern that the financial interests of physicians and researchers in the new health care market may conflict with their professional responsibilities. Much of this volume attempts to provide a description and analysis of this problem in all its still growing manifestations and complexities—a much needed task never before undertaken with such thoroughness. But conflicts of interest in medicine are not only economic in origin. Tensions between professional duties and personal interests are ubiquitous, and they do not always involve money. These too are carefully identified and explicated. And in the process, readers gain information and insights not easily to be found elsewhere.

The editors and their contributors have expanded our notions of conflict of interest in medicine. In doing so, they have in effect defined a new field of study, one that involves many disciplines and affects all of society. They have not filled in all the details or resolved all the problems—they could not be expected to—but they have made an impressive start. Future studies will build on the foundations laid here. Although we cannot predict what the next generation of analysts and policy makers will be thinking, we can be sure they will have to deal with the facts and ideas so thoughtfully discussed here.

Arnold S. Relman, M.D.
Editor-in-Chief Emeritus
New England Journal of Medicine
Professor Emeritus, Medicine and
of Social Medicine, Harvard Medical School
Sr. Physician, Brigham & Women's Hospital

Preface

Like many multidisciplinary projects, this book originated fortuitously. In the course of writing a pair of papers on the legal and ethical issues raised by *per capita* funding of industry-sponsored clinical trials[1] two of the editors (RGS & DSS) searched unsuccessfully for a book on conflicts of interest faced by clinicians. We felt that this represented a gap in the literature that needed to be filled. With the assistance of the third editor (AEB), an outline and potential contributors were identified, and the book proceeded on to its present form.

Because physicians are not trained to look for conflicts of interest, they often find themselves enmeshed in them without recognizing the problem. It is our intent to provide physicians and others interested in health care and public policy with a framework for recognizing conflicts of interest (the *sine qua non* for managing them), and tools for resolving them.

This is a challenging time to address conflicts of interest because they are and will continue to be affected by reforms in the health care industry. Nevertheless, major issues addressed herein will endure regardless of any imaginable change in our health care system. For example, conflicts of interest can only be identified in the context of the proper role of physicians vis-a-vis patients, specific third parties, and society in general. To a large extent, these concepts are bound up with the questions: What does it mean to be a professional? What constitutes a proper physician-patient relationship?

Changes in our health care system may alter the answers to these (and related) questions, and, in turn, redefine conflicts of interest. However, the conceptual and empirical work herein can guide examination of such modifications. Similarly, health care reform may rechannel, but will never eliminate, the inevitable tensions among certain interests of providers, patients, and third party payer(s). Even with change to a strict salary system, say, physicians may be tempted to further their own interests—for example, in conserving free time or energy—at the expense of patients' or payers' interests in limiting health care expenditures. Finally the issue of disclosure versus prohibition in dealing with conflicts of interest will endure with any conceivable change in our health care system.

The book is divided into four sections. The first addresses conflicts of interest from a theoretical perspective, and draws heavily from the legal profession, which has devoted substantial effort to identifying and resolving conflicts of interest. The second section addresses two issues that loom large in the current health care environment—physician ownership of ancillary businesses (self-referral), and incentives to limit care in the interest of cost containment. Here, a number of authorities, with often contrasting viewpoints, address these concrete situations, applying the principles outlined in the first section. The third section addresses the conflicts of interest generated by the involvement of the pharmaceutical industry in clinical research, in formal and informal medical education, and, thereby, in clinical practice. The response of the clotting factor concentrate fractionators to the threat of hepatitis and, then, HIV contamination of their products is used as a case study. The final section addresses conflicts of interest in research, a topic that has generally been skirted in discussions of human subjects experimentation.

Although the contributors to this work come from many disciplines, we have attempted to unify and simplify citation forms. We have used a legal source, the Blue Book: A Uniform System of Citation (15th ed. 1991), as a starting point, deviating somewhat to accommodate authors from other disciplines. For example, we have placed legal and medical articles as well as books and newspaper pieces in the following format: [first and last name of author (without middle initial)], [name of article], [volume] [journal or newspaper or book] [page] [(date)].

Tucson, Arizona   *R. G .S.*

Tucson, Arizona   *D. S. S.*

Madison, Wisconsin   *A. E. B.*

November, 1995

---

1. David Shimm and Roy Spece, Industry Reimbursement for Entering Patients into Clinical Trials: Legal and Ethical Issues, 115 *Ann Intern Med.* 148 (1991); David Shimm and Roy Spece, Conflict of Interest and Informed Consent in Industry Sponsored Clinical Trials, 12 J. Legal Med. 477 (1991).

Contents

Contributors

Baruch Brody, Ph.D.
Leon Jaworski Professor of
  Biomedical Ethics
  and Director of the Center for
  Ethics, Medicine, and Public Issues
College of Medicine
Baylor University
Houston, Texas

Allen E. Buchanan, Ph.D.
Granger Professor of Business Ethics
  School of Business
  Professor of Philosophy, and
  Professor Medical Ethics
  Medical School
University of Wisconsin
Madison, Wisconsin

Michele Y. Burpeau-Di Gregorio,
  Ph.D.
Director, Continuing Medical Education
College of Medicine
The University of Arizona
Tucson, Arizona

E. L. Erde, Ph.D.
Professor of Family Practice
University of Medicine
  and Dentistry of New Jersey
School of Osteopathic Medicine
Stratford, New Jersey

Leslie Francis, Ph.D., J.D.
Professor, College of Law
Associate Professor of Philosophy
University of Utah
Salt Lake City, Utah

Mark A. Hall, J.D.
Professor of Law and Public Health
School of Law and Bowman Gray
  School of Medicine
Wake Forest University
Winston-Salem, North Carolina

Geoffrey C. Hazard, Jr., LL.B.
Sterling Professor of Law
Yale Law School
Yale University
New Haven, Connecticut

Edward J. Huth, M.D.
Editor, Online Journal of
  Current Clinical Trials
Editor Emeritus, Annals of
  Internal Medicine
Bryn Mawr, Pennsylvania

Thomas L. Kurt, M.D.
Clinical Professor of Medicine
University of Texas
  Southwestern Medical Center
  and former Regional Medical Officer,
  Southwest Region, FDA
Dallas, Texas

Jay Katz, M.D.
Elizabeth K. Dollard Professor of
  Law, Medicine and Psychiatry
Yale Law School
Yale University
New Haven, Connecticut

Jean M. Mitchell, Ph.D.
Associate Professor,
  Graduate Public Policy Program
  and Department of Family and
  Community Medicine
Georgetown University
Washington, D.C.

Nancy J. Moore, J.D.
Professor, School of Law
Rutgers University
Camden, New Jersey

E. Haavi Morreim
Associate Professor,
  Department of Human Values
  and Ethics
College of Medicine
University of Tennessee
Memphis, Tennessee

Marc A. Rodwin. J.D., Ph.D.
Associate Professor,
  School of Public and
  Environmental Affairs
Indiana University
Bloomington, Indiana

David S. Shimm, M.D., F.A.C.P.
Associate Professor,
  Department of Radiation Oncology

and Clinical Assistant Professor,
  Department of Internal Medicine
College of Medicine
The University of Arizona
Tucson, Arizona

Roy G. Spece, Jr., J.D.
Professor, College of Law
The University of Arizona
Tucson, Arizona

Charles W. Wolfram, LL.B.
Charles Frank Reavis Sr. Professor
  of Law
Cornell Law School
Cornell University
Ithaca, New York

Part I

Conflicts of Interest: A Conceptual Overview

1

Introduction

David S. Shimm and Roy G. Spece, Jr.

As medical technology advances and health care consumes an ever-increasing portion of our gross national product, the goals of health care quality, accessibility, equity, and efficiency come into deeper conflict with each other and with competing social interests. Health care currently consumes about 14 percent of our gross domestic product,[1] partially as a result of a 1000 percent medical inflation rate between 1960 and 1990 (four times the general rate of inflation).[2] Technologies such as screening for and treatment of genetic diseases portend further "advances"—in choices, costs, and conflicts. Despite our technical progress, as of 1993 approximately 37 million U.S. residents had neither public subsidy, personal means, nor private insurance providing access to health care.[3]

In this milieu, health care providers have been given conflicting messages: You are running a business and must compete so as to hold down the costs of medical care, but you must rise above the marketplace and fulfill extraordinary obligations to your patients and society.

In part, these conflicting messages—and the patchwork of laws, regulations, and institutions that convey them—reflect a societal ambivalence between concern about rising health care costs on the one hand and, on the other, a deep seated belief that health care is a unique need that must be adequately met for

1

all residents of the United States. The Clinton administration unsuccessfully embarked on a significant government initiative—to broaden access to health care but at the same time limit costs—that reflects these competing attitudes.[4] From the late 1980s on, moreover, new and proposed federal and state laws and regulations as well as medical society pronouncements have addressed conflicts of interest in medical practice and research. This focus on conflicts of interest reflects the part of our social conscience that insists that physicians should have extraordinary devotion to their patients. Conversely, the same period of time has brought government rules and private initiatives—most of which are captured by the term "managed care"—explicitly designed to force or encourage medical personnel to make trade-offs among the quality, accessibility, equity, and costs of health care. They deliberately create conflicts of interest. (Medical personnel have always faced such conflicts, but until now, they have been less prevalent and apparent). These government rules and private initiatives that deliberately create conflicts of interest reflect the part of our social conscience that demands control of medical costs and regard for societal interests other than medical care.

Although conflicts of interest in medicine have caused great concern, the issue has been neglected by scholars. This book is therefore devoted to the study of conflicts of interest from the perspective of authors trained in several disciplines: law, medicine, philosophy, business, health care policy, and economics. Each part of the text—except Part III, which consists of a single "bridge" chapter—begins with an introductory chapter that briefly summarizes the themes of the following chapters in the set. In this introductory chapter, however, before specifically addressing the themes discussed later in Part I, we will briefly review the history and meaning of "conflicts of interest."

History and Meaning of Conflicts of Interest

Law

Although conflict of interest has a substantial legal pedigree, it has been relatively ignored by philosophers and medical providers. Arguably, it originated in fiduciary law. A fiduciary is, roughly, a person upon whom the law imposes special duties of utmost regard for the interests of another (generally to the exclusion of the interests of others or the fiduciary himself) who is dependent upon the fiduciary because of his superior expertise or position. Persons to whom fiduciary duties are owed are typically dependent on the superior expertise of their fiduciaries, in whom they can be expected to, and usually have to, place a great deal of trust.[5]

The concept of fiduciary duty grew out of the law of trusts. Trusts are legal devices by which one person (the trustor) conveys property to another (the trustee) for the exclusive benefit of a third person (the beneficiary). Trustees are required to act solely in the interests of beneficiaries, eschewing considerations of their own or third parties' interests. They cannot compete with the trust; they can enter into personal financial transactions with the trust only in limited circumstances, and after full disclosure and knowing, intelligent consent by the beneficiary; and they cannot receive any incidental benefits in connection with their work, but are limited to reasonable compensation for performing services required of them as trustees.

Courts closely police the actions of trustees for conflicts of interest, i.e., situations involving the risk that trustees will compromise the interests of beneficiaries in favor of trustees or third parties. For example, if a trustee enters into a forbidden transaction, the beneficiary can sue to declare the transaction void and receive back any consideration paid even if the trustee acted in good faith, the price was fair, and the beneficiary was not harmed.

Extraordinary or fiduciary duties attached to trustees have been extended, in very similar form, to other relationships, such as principal/agent and lawyer/client. An elaborate body of ethical codes, legal opinions, and disciplinary proceedings by courts and bar associations governs the ethical conduct of lawyers. A substantial amount of this apparatus deals with conflicts of interest. Similarly, nonprofit corporations are governed by state statutes that police corporate officials' conflicts of interest, federal and state statutes attend to conflicts of interest of financial institutions and their personnel, and federal and state statutes control government employees' conflicts of interest.

Medicine

No similar structure of procedural and substantive standards and enforcement mechanisms applies to physicians. The American Medical Association (AMA) does police certain conflicts of interest, but this control is largely theoretical. Only about half of the physicians in the United States belong to the AMA.[6] It has no procedures for investigating misconduct or monitoring compliance. Its strongest action is expulsion from membership, and this rarely occurs. It basically leaves enforcement of its guidelines and principles to state licensing boards, which are themselves understaffed and focus on only the most blatant instances of misconduct, such as practicing while under the influence of drugs.[7]

The AMA has had a code of ethics since 1846. Although physicians did not commonly use the term "conflict of interest" until the 1980s, early in the nineteenth century the AMA discouraged certain behaviors that some commentators today might characterize as conflicts of interest: fee splitting with referring physicians, acceptance of commissions from pharmacies and medical supply firms, owning pharmacies, dispensing or patenting medical products, and advertising.[8]

According to Rodwin, in the 1950s the AMA defined fee splitting more narrowly, passed judgment against those engaged in it less harshly and less frequently, and reinterpreted and redefined its Principles of Medical Ethics to eliminate rules against dispensing medical products, owning medical facilities, and entering into joint ventures with medical suppliers and providers.[9] Thereafter, the AMA continued to soften its stance against the entrepreneurial activities of physicians. After Ronald Reagan's election as president in 1980, the federal government favored market competition as a way to improve the efficiency of medical care delivery. In 1980, prohibitions against fee splitting and earning income other than for services performed were dropped from the AMA Principles of Medical Ethics.[10] At the same time, several practices emerged or accelerated—some indirectly encouraged by federal reimbursement policies— that enabled physicians to obtain nonpractice income without traditional fee splitting: (1) payments to and from medical suppliers and providers for referrals; (2) income from referring patients to facilities in which they had invested; (3) dispensing drugs, selling medical products, and performing services they prescribed; (4) hospital purchase of physicians' practices; (5) payments made by hospitals to recruit and otherwise win the allegiance of physicians; (6) gifts from medical suppliers; and (7) risk sharing in health maintenance organizations (HMOs) and hospitals.[11] (These methods are further discussed throughout this book, particularly by Rodwin in Chapter 9.) At the same time, the public and certain physicians became concerned with the growth of for-profit health care, what the *New England Journal of Medicine's* editor, Arnold Relman, called "The New Medical-Industrial Complex."[12] By the 1990s, Relman admitted that even nonprofit companies were being drawn into the conflicts of interest posed by the entrepreneurial spirit pervading the medical marketplace.[13]

The AMA's response was essentially to replace rules that used objective standards prohibiting certain transactions with vague proscriptions that allowed physicians to police themselves. For example, major AMA conflict of interest guidelines issued in 1986 advised physicians to resolve all conflicts of interest in favor of patients and to arrange for alternate care when their interests clashed with those of patients. It did not, however, develop criteria to define such situations or appropriate behavior.[14] In Chapter 8, Nancy Moore further traces the AMA's response, including its final grudging condemnation of self-referral because of public opinion and impending legislation that would generally prohibit the practice.

Philosophy

Philosophers, including bioethicists, have generally ignored conflicts of interests. For example, the Encyclopedia of Bioethics does not even have an entry on the topic. Yet medicine has changed to the extent that conflict of interest has become one of the dominant moral problems pervading medical practice. Moreover, future health care reform is inevitable, and, it is bound to change conflicts of interest. For example, if physicians all become dependent on a single payer (one prominent if not politically feasible reform proposal), that payer will likely continue to exert pressure ("managed care techniques") to limit utilization of care that might benefit individual patients. Indeed, a single payer might be able to apply greater pressure and thus present a greater conflict of interest between individual patients' needs for care and groups of patients' or society's desire to limit utilization by individuals.

Aside from the most obvious issues of fraud and self-referral, however, none of the health care reform programs currently being discussed explicitly addresses the conflicts of interest created by the forms of practice posited within the specific plan. As Susan Wolf has pointed out, scholars, regulators, and practitioners must attend to the several issues related to conflicts of interest posed by health care reform, including the following questions : (1) If universal access is adopted in theory, what obligations, if any, will physicians have to reach out to previously uncovered and perhaps less profitable and harder to communicate with patients? (2) What obligations, if any, will physicians have to advocate for coverage of products and services that might benefit individual patients but might otherwise burden predetermined budgets? (3) Must physicians disclose therapeutic options that are explicitly excluded from coverage under an applicable health care plan? and (4) What organizational or other ethics need to be developed to reflect the changing forms of medical practice?[15]

Development of an Analytical Framework

Developing an analytical framework for defining and analyzing conflicts of interest will help answer questions posed by the continuing refinement of the "medical–industrial complex." Erde develops such an analytical approach in Chapter 2, arguing that conflicts of interest cannot be captured by simple definitions, but must be recognized by certain clusters of attributes that coalesce in specific social settings. We embrace his analysis (with a few minor exceptions), as well as his best attempt to venture a general definition of conflicts of interest in the medical context: "[E]ither motives that caregivers have and/or situations in which we could reasonably think caregivers' responsibilities to observe, judge, and act according to the moral requirements of their role are or will be compromised, often to an unacceptable degree."

In addition to this working definition, we offer the following observations about conflicts of interests to keep in mind throughout the following chapters, which explain particular forms of conflicts of interest.

First, there is disagreement over what constitutes a conflict of interest. Not all situations or motives that connote choice or concern are conflicts of interest. For example, a personal dilemma about choosing between reading a book and working out does not constitute a conflict of interest. Similarly, the temptation to call in sick to enjoy a day off work does not mean that there is a conflict of interest. Two notions help distinguish simple choices and temptations from conflicts of interest. The first idea is that conflicts of interest exist in relation to the roles and duties attached to those roles.

The second concept that helps identify conflicts of interest is that they connote concern about choices beyond the usual temptations that all individuals face. What must be identified is some baseline of normal choice and temptation from which one can measure deviations that are sufficient to constitute conflicts of interest. Although we will not establish that baseline, one possibility is the concern about choices commonly present in the free market. This is troublesome in the medical setting because of the typical market failures that beset the medical industry: (1) government and private third-party payers pay for the vast majority of medical care; (2) physicians direct the purchase of care for patients, while patients do not have the information and expertise to monitor their physicians' prescriptions and referrals; (3) adequate information about quality and cost is often not readily available even to physicians; and (4) patients are vulnerable and often desperate to obtain care, regardless of its costs.

Much more work needs to be done to explore the proper baseline from which to judge deviations that are sufficient to constitute conflicts of interest. One point, however, is clear. Baselines are judged from different perspectives. What might be considered a conflict of interest from a strictly moral perspective can be viewed as an essential and nonproblematic part of a decision-making process from a public policy or legal perspective. For example, there is a consensus among bioethicists that, from a moral perspective, physicians have fiduciary obligations to their patients.[16] As might be expected from the above discussion of fiduciary duties, this means that physicians have extraordinary obligations to their patients beyond those expected in a typical contractual relationship. This includes making patients' best interests paramount and disregarding self-interest. From a legal perspective, however, physicians at most owe only certain aspects of fiduciary duties to their patients. For example, in many jurisdictions the obligation to disclose facts to patients for the purpose of informed consent is determined, under statute or common law, by the customary practices of physicians rather than by a standard of complete disclosure of what reasonable patients would want to know.[17] Determining when nondisclosure might pose a conflict of interest in these jurisdictions would differ from the moral and legal perspectives.

Finally, it is helpful to address a couple of fine distinctions when attempting to identify conflicts of interest. Some commentators distinguish between conflicts of interest and conflicts of loyalty or obligation (e.g., between teaching and working on a research project in collaboration with a private company). We consider the latter a subset of the former. We do distinguish between conflicts of interest and breaches of obligation. The former are situations and motives that connote the risk of breaching obligations. The latter are completed acts.

General Perspectives on Conflicts of Interest

At this point, we focus on the themes of the remaining chapters in Part I. Once again, in Chapter 2, Edmund Erde develops a perspective on conflicts of interest. He explains why a simple account—a conflict of interest is a clash between a professional's pecuniary interests and the interests of his client/patient—is inadequate. And, drawing on a linguistic method largely inspired by Ludwig Wittgenstein, he argues that no set of necessary and sufficient conditions can usefully define conflicts of interest. The best that can be done is to provide "a map of a family resemblance of cases and criteria rather than of a uniform idea."

Erde (1) separates the descriptive and performative (evaluative) aspects of the meaning of conflict of interest; (2) briefly traces the term's historical use; (3) discusses various authorities' views about the definition and importance of conflicts of interests; (4) establishes taxonomies of interests (ideals—e.g., a conception of a life worth living; practical interests—e.g., safety and time; and predilections—e.g., animosity and friendship) and of conflicts (including their relationship to moral dilemmas) that individuals face in reconciling their and other persons' conflicting interests; (5) emphasizes that conflicts can arise not only between the interests of physicians and patients, but also among those interests and interests of specific third parties and society generally; (6) explains the importance of "social role" in analyzing conflicts of interest; (7) observes that both motives and social arrangements can give rise to conflicts of interest; (8) deconstructs the notion of a distinction between "real" and "apparent" conflicts of interest; and (9) suggests a method for distinguishing between trustworthy and untrustworthy motives and social arrangements. Throughout the chapter, Erde discusses actual or hypothetical cases to illustrate his points. As part of his "map," he does offer a tentative definition of the descriptive aspects of conflict of interest.

In Chapter 3, we address the daunting problem that, while one cannot identify conflicts of interest without specifying the moral requirements of a role, it is equally true that one cannot determine the moral requirement of a role without moral judgments and, ultimately, ethical theory. Study of conflicts of interest thus drives one to ethical theory in the broad philosophical sense. In Chapter 3, therefore, we discuss some fundamentals of ethical theory, describe a type of ethical theory that can be used to discern the ethically expected behavior of physicians, discuss criteria to judge competing ethical theories, and identify some basic principles that bioethicists, to some degree, agree are helpful guides to decision-making.

Since ethical reasoning is not calculation but discovery, in Chapter 3 we discuss sources where one can begin to find the morally expected role of physicians: literature on the physician–patient relationship, pertinent legal pronouncements, and ethical codes and practice guidelines for physicians. We explain the strengths and weaknesses of these sources. For example, the literature on the physician–patient relationship—as is generally true of medical or bioethics writing—does not pay sufficient attention to the interests of specific third parties or society generally. The models described best in the literature— paternalistic, informative, interpretive, and deliberative—focus almost exclusively on obligations to patients. They are useful, nevertheless, to illuminate those obligations in specific situations we draw from the reported case law. We supplement these models with two that force attention to obligations toward third parties and society: the physician as good citizen and the physician as dual agent.

In Chapter 4, Geoffrey Hazard, Jr., argues that both legal and medical professionals tend to avoid the conflict between patient/client interests and those of third parties and society by emphasizing an almost exclusive fealty to clients. At the same time, he argues, society assumes that an essential attribute of professionalism is service to the community. He asserts that conflict of interest "is the central ethical problem of a profession, and indeed the problem that gives a profession its defining characteristic." He uses conflict of interest broadly to encompass what Erde and we would characterize, in many instances, as mere conflicting interests.

Hazard advances the understanding of conflicts of interest and professionalism by (1) describing a multidimensional conflict of interest structure common to the "classic professions" of law and medicine as well as other professions; (2) analyzing similarities and differences among these dimensions in medicine and law; and (3) examining forms of control of conflicts of interest and their limitations. Conflicts of interest are presented on three levels: professional versus client/patient, client versus specific third parties, and client versus society. The primary obligations of professionals on these respective levels are self-restraint, mediation, and imposition of restrain on the patient/client.

Forms used to control professional conflicts of interest are professional codes, statutes, and regulations. These are broken down into four regulatory techniques: (1) prophylactic rules or prohibitions; (2) disclosure or informed consent requirements; (3) reference to recognized professional practice standards; and (4) intraprofessional consultation or second opinion. As to limitations of the various control devices, prophylactic rules cannot be used to manage conflicts that must be tolerated for the benefits they entail; informed consent rules are limited by patient/clients' ability to understand and professionals' own uncertainty; professional rules that incorporate professional standards incorporate the same uncertainty, and hence beg the question; and the same problems are involved, to a lesser degree, in intraprofessional consultation. Regulatory techniques, therefore, cannot resolve certain fundamental aspects of conflicts of interest—trust has to be placed in professionals, who must respond with self-consciousness and personal discipline. Areas of particular concern to professionals are financial exploitation and psychological exploitation through the use of superior knowledge, the patient's anxiety, and the patient's fear of uncertainty (and the professional's masking of it) to control the relationship and its goals and outcomes. In mediation, professionals must be especially aware of loyalty to the patient/client and protection of confidential information.

Allen Buchanan's analysis in Chapter 5 follows nicely from Hazard's. Hazard argues: "By definition the function of a profession is to serve interests beyond that of the professional's own self-interests.... [T]o analyze the problems of a professional's conflicts of interest is to probe the essence of the profession itself." Buchanan's thesis is that (1) the medical profession, in a normative sense, is a socially constructed inequality that must be justified by a demonstration either (a) that its benefits exceed its costs and that there is no less costly, morally acceptable alternative way to obtain these benefits or (b) that it is the result of a fair and mutually advantageous contract with society; and (2) that there does not appear to be such a justification.

Buchanan first notes the increasing concern over conflicts of interest presented by the new conditions of medical practice in our country; that is, private interests and government are exerting pressure on physicians to limit or even underutilize services, while hospital administrators and physicians themselves are creating incentive structures designed to increase revenues even at the cost of overutilization of services. This is often expressed as a fear that physicians are becoming entrepreneurs out for a quick buck rather than professionals whom the public can trust. These concerns derive from three questionable assumptions that together constitute the "myth of professionalism": (1) it is bad to erode public trust in physicians; (2) the public cannot trust physicians unless they are considered professionals; and (3) there is a medical profession in this country "according to a conception of what a medical profession is that makes it desirable that there be such a profession." Buchanan's chapter is designed to bare and critically examine these three assumptions, which, he correctly observes, frame the debate about conflict of interest. A secondary purpose is to demonstrate that these three assumptions "seriously restrict the range of policy options for dealing with problems of conflict of interest in a context of increasing pressures for rationing and growing entrepreneurial activity... and [tend] to prevent us from dealing with—and indeed even adequately understanding—the problem of conflict of interest."

In the final chapter of Part I, Charles Wolfram ventures a fascinating comparative analysis of conflict of interest regulation in law and securities firms; briefly summarizes the major components of conflict of interest regulation in the legal field; compares the use of "screens" (barriers to certain contacts or communications among members of a firm) as tools of conflict regulation in law and securities firms; and concludes that the much greater tolerance of these devices in the securities field is explained not by a difference in the underlying relationships or conflicts in the two fields, but primarily by a greater "social" need for large size in securities firms.

Wolfram concludes that the message for those who venture comparative analyses is that one must pay scrupulous attention to the context of each field subject to comparison:

> For those focusing on conflict-of-interest issues in the medical profession, the lesson can be simply put: beware of suggestions that the medical profession borrow wholesale and uncritically concepts, devices, institutions, or other substantial features from other professions in dealing with conflicts of interest within the medical profession. Some such loans may, after careful analysis, be found to show a high likelihood of catching hold successfully in medicine; others will be found to be poor risks; still others will work only after substantial modification to fit particular needs. All such possibilities should be considered before accepting the interprofessional loan.

We conclude Part 1 with a postscript to Chapter 6 that compares the control of information flow in the legal and financial contexts studied by Wolfram to certain situations in medical practice in which similar attempts have been made to bridle conflicts of interest by invoking confidentiality. The purpose of this postscript is to further flesh out the meaning of conflicts of interest.

Notes

1. Bureau of National Affairs (BNA), 1 *Health Care Policy Report*, Special Supplement to Issue No. 27, September 13, 1993, Clinton Administration Description of President's Health Care Reform Plan, "American Health Security Act of 1993," at 2.
2. Mark Hall and Ira Ellman, *Health Care Law and Ethics in a Nutshell 3* (1990).
3. BNA, supra note 1, at 2.
4. BNA, supra note 1.
5. The description here of the legal origins of conflicts of interest and the medical profession's historical approach thereto draws heavily from Mark Rodwin's excellent book, *Medicine, Money & Morals: Physicians' Conflicts of Interest 181–183, 19–52* (1993).
6. Telephone interview with Jill Hirt of the AMA, Sept. 27, 1993 by David Shimm.
7. Rodwin, *supra* note 5, at 43, 44.
8. *Id.* at 22, 41.
9. *Id.* at 36.
10. *Id.* at 40.
11. *Id.* at 223.
12. Arnold Relman, The New Medical–Industrial Complex, 303 *N. Engl. J. Med.* 963–970 (1980).
13. Arnold Relman, Shattuck Lecture—The Health Care Industry: Where Is It Taking Us?, 335 *N. Engl. J. Med.* 854 (1991).
14. Rodwin, *supra* note 5, at 41—42.
15. Susan Wolf, Health Care Reform and the Future Ethics, 24 *Hast. Cent. Rep.* 28–39 (March–April 1994).
16. See, e.g., Tom Beauchamp and James F. Childress, *Principles of Biomedical Ethics* (4th ed., 1994).
17. Ruth Faden and Tom Beauchamp, *A History and Theory of Informed Consent 30–31, 120, 129, 131–132, 135–37, 139, 201, 305–306* (1986).

2

Conflicts of Interests in Medicine: A Philosophical and Ethical Morphology

Edmund L. Erde

This chapter is meant to guide the reader through the bewildering set of conflicting claims and commentaries that have been made about conflicts of interest (CIs).[1] Confusion about CIs is engendered by erroneous efforts to capture in all-inclusive definitions the remarkable variety of values and arrangements that contribute to CIs.

Conflicts of interest are so pervasive and varied that they defy unitary definition. Rather, one must understand the contexts in which the concept is used, its many facets, and its different functions. This can be done by taking an extensive inventory of cases that are naturally (or erroneously) called CIs and noting the point of the term. Doing so provides a family resemblance of cases and criteria rather than a strictly defined uniform idea. In this sense, dealing with CIs in professional life entails developing a "moral sense" of what is acceptable akin to the "clinical judgment" that guides practitioners in their daily practice.

To understand the functions of CIs, the most important distinction is between (1) descriptive or informative indicators and (2) other communication agendas that aim to have an effect on listeners, such as alerting them to a threat. Descriptive indicators can be understood in terms of two separate foci: *motives*, which are mental (*e.g.*, physicians' desires), and *social arrangements*, which are not (*e.g.*, payment schedules and arrangements). Nondescriptive agenda items enable speakers to perform rather different tasks so that, for example, listeners can heed a warning or assess an explanation. This is *performative meaning*, or a performative agenda. Regarding CIs, it occurs as speakers use the relevant terminology to accomplish their specific purposes in communicating in contexts that they understand very well. Thus, performative meaning is the effect speakers expect to achieve beyond merely informing their audience.

This chapter begins by presenting a simple, unified account of the notion of CI that is tied to economics. This is critiqued as artificially narrow, especially by laying out some conflicting claims and comments about CIs. Having rejected the idea of getting a useful definition, I sketch the method that seems to provide the best grasp of the meaning of terms. Then I analyze distinct aspects of CIs: first, interests and other sorts of values that clash in CIs; next, *conflicts* and the sorts of situations in which physicians either experience dilemmas or ought to but fail to do so; and finally, the logic and contribution of the idea of *holding a role*, and the implications for assessing the morality of physicians having and acting on their own personal interests. Contrary to much rhetoric, attending to his[2] own advantage is not equivalent to a physician's having a CI because the responsibilities attached to being a physician do not mandate forsaking all self-regard.[3] Finally, I suggest a way to test for the ethical (rather than legal) aspects of having a CI so that individuals can assess whether their situation and conduct are trustworthy.

The Artificially Narrow Account

Definition: CIs occur when and only when a physician strays or is tempted to stray from his role-mandated duties for the sake of his own economic benefit. A classic statement of such a definition is offered by the 1979 edition of *Black's Law Dictionary* (the first edition with an entry for CI). There CIs are identified only with monetary concerns since a CI is defined as " a clash between public interest and the private pecuniary interest of the individual concerned."

I call this the "artificially narrow account." What recommends it is that it accommodates the common contention that some large portion of medical services could be harmlessly omitted.[4] An example may strike some readers as counterintuitive because it shows that persons with better insurance get poorer care than those with little or no insurance. Because this is counterintuitive, it arrays the structure of a CI all the more. Persons with lung cancer and good insurance received more dangerous, less effective care than those who lacked insurance. This is apparently due to the high reimbursement attached to the more invasive approach.[5] The disparity is unjust not only because the more expensive approach imposes unnecessary costs and inconveniences, but also because it imposes significant risks and harms.

An example concerns primary care:[6] In some practices, patients who complain of having a sore throat are treated differently just on the basis of which form of coverage they have.[7] Fee-for-service patients get a rapid strep test that gives immediate results and can yield a small profit to the physician. Health maintenance organization (HMO) patients get throat cultures which minimize physicians' costs but take days to provide results. The disparity is unjust if the rapid strep test is better for the patient, the HMO promised best available care, and the only reason for the delay is to enhance the physician's net income. When these conditions pertain, we think of the physician's conduct as involving a CI and use the associated terminology to perform, for example, the act of indicting or explaining that conduct.

This account of CIs can also be inferred from a review of most of the literature about them. For example, Neil R. Luebke[8] opens a discussion of CIs with a history of the relevant language. He reports no use of the term prior to the 1930s and claims that its origins bore strictly on financial concerns. Emotions and ties other than pecuniary interests were explicitly ruled out at the beginning. Disagreeing with earlier philosophical analyses, Luebke contends that the meaning of CI conforms to its historical roots. He rejects nonfinancial values as constitutive of CIs, contending that CIs occur only when economic gain undermines trustworthiness.

I contend that Luebke's account is too simple[9]; the logic of the term extends beyond its origins and includes much that he rejects; for example, the phrase "best interests" alludes to much beyond pecuniary interests[10] (as does "interest groups"). I agree with Luebke that one main focus of CIs is on how trustworthiness is undermined. I disagree that CIs involve pecuniary interests alone. And, beyond descriptive indicators of CIs that I include and he would not, I think Luebke neglects performative agendas.

So, what is the contribution of the concept of interests to CI? To answer, note what the term helps speakers distinguish, as disclosed by its uses and applications in language games—which are well-understood transactional contexts in which speakers instruct, provoke, warn, and so on.

Are the interests to which CIs allude always economic, or could ideals or hankerings be included? Much is gained and lost with either choice. Two gains from requiring an economic aspect are efficiency and importance: it supplies a term we need frequently and reflects the current concern with costs.

But the need to allude to economic motives in association with CIs is met by a variety of other concepts, such as fraud or cheating. It is merely statistically true and etymologically warranted in the context of contemporary medicine that alleging a CI connotes economic motives. Although physician misconduct for economic gain is vast and depressing,[11] the tie to economics is not a necessary condition of the use of CI terminology. We need not change our language to apply CI to noneconomic values; they are part of CI's use already.

Preliminary Problems with the Artificially Narrow Account

For three reasons, the Artificially Narrow Account does not say enough: (1) many roles and subroles are involved in health care, (2) some have sought a classic definition to determine whether some peculiar arrangements are CIs, and (3) opinions conflict about how much moral concern should arise about CIs. These three points are worth discussing.

First, beyond physicians, many other practitioners in health care are involved in CIs. Nurses, administrators of hospitals and nursing homes, social workers, public health officers, scientists, and others must be taken into account to fully grasp CIs' nature. For example, French officials could be charged with a CI because they knowingly allowed HIV-tainted blood into the blood banking system by delaying approval of an American technique to test contaminated blood. They did this to protect a French laboratory that was far behind in its research and development, a laboratory whose prospects for competing in the marketplace they wanted to foster.[12] If this is a CI, then health officials have some CIs not open to private practitioners. One could certainly argue that this was a conflict of loyalties rather than a CI. Such a position would emphasize that the officials' motives were role-based rather than personally selfish. Yet their action seems subject to condemnation as a CI as well (perhaps because pecuniary interests were involved).

Even if we restrict our thinking to physicians, there is concern about what their responsibilities are when they hold a subrole, such as expert witness.[13] Thus, the first reason for rejecting the Artificially Narrow Account is that it severely oversimplifies the complexity and variety of CIs.[14] The second reason is that some theorists want more than the Simple Account offers. Bradford Gray, for example, wants a definition to settle whether incorporating trivial laboratory work into an office practice or physicians dispensing medication in rural settings should be considered CIs.[15] He feels that he does not understand the meaning of the term well enough to know whether it applies to these situations. At least he cannot use the simple account to categorize or assess the cases that bother him.

The third reason the Artificially Narrow Account is inadequate is that we want a formulation rich enough to settle some nagging conflicts (of opinion) about how seriously to take CIs. Amid all the provocative remarks, claims, and counterclaims (some sketched in the next section), a conceptual point is perhaps overlooked: that we may not use the language of CIs until we have a performative agenda (*e.g.*, to alarm) arising in response to noted descriptive conditions. If so, no simple account or definition will provide what Gray requests or settle the disagreements I shall pose. For, as with most ideas, invoking the relevant language depends on having a prior performative agenda.

Samples of the Provocative and Paradoxical

Each member of the following list of items and comments about CIs is both misleading and contains insight. Although none may be very troubling in isolation, as a set they signal fundamental concerns.

Item 1: James S. Todd, commenting on Medicaid fraud, writes, "Every physician-patient encounter is a conflict of interest. Every physician-payer encounter is also a conflict of interest."[16]

Items 2 and 3: Although they do not address each other, consider the debate latent in positions taken by Albert Jonsen and Joanne Lynn. Jonsen argues that there is an incessant tension between self-interest and altruism, and that CIs unavoidably suffuse medical practice, causing many professional and personal problems.[17] He sees medicine as dominated by self-interest and thinks that it weakens the entire foundation of the profession. He sees little solution but holds professionals to a standard of selflessness.

By contrast, Lynn[18] finds CIs of little concern. She contends that providing economic incentives to restrain the use of interventions conflicts *constructively* with virtuous physicians' empathy, which acts as a safety net. Although she knows they are common, CIs are of small concern to her.

Who is right, Jonsen or Lynn? Do CIs threaten quality care? Are all equally troubling? Should they always be decided in favor of the patient? Are there occasions in which enhancing a physician's professionally derived economic interests may take precedence over the best interests of her patients? Are there cases in which Jonsen's point of view should prevail and others in which Lynn's should? Is this a verbal quibble in that each has a different meaning in mind and there is no substantive dispute between them? Some of these questions will be addressed below.

Item 4: Writing about the duty to treat HIV-positive patients, Edmund D. Pellegrino argues that physicians reveal their true ethics in the way they balance their own interests against those of patients. Pellegrino contends that medicine imposes an obligation to efface self-interest on physicians and calls for more teaching in medical ethics to focus on this issue.[19]

Is Pellegrino right? Is it essential to the nature of medicine and of being a physician (in contrast to being a businessperson) that one be self-effacing? Is the duty a matter of degree? Is it absolute? How should we decide whether an act of self-denial is a duty or above and beyond duty? Are doctors obliged to be martyrs? This should be a nagging set of questions. Holding practitioners to the standard implied both here and by Jonsen might well severely deplete the supply of physicians. We expect physicians to conform to this standard, yet we know that it is not reasonable—a point intimately connected with the next item.

Item 5: Consider a physician who has an extensive enough partnership that he can teach, do research, take vacations, go to continuing medical education courses, give papers, and so on. Perhaps his patients suffer from the discontinuity of care as a result. He injures the patient only by behaving as the design and structures of the practice permit. He is not the patients' sole doctor, acting on his own interests. What injures them is *not a lapse of his trustworthiness.* Rather, it is his conforming to the design of his practice, a design that is publicly known, understood, and accepted. Does the doctor have a clear CI in designing his practice and life in this way? What would be gained by saying so—heightened awareness?

Items 1-5 show why one might be perplexed about what CIs are—about the contradictory claims and the paradoxical and provocative notions involved. One might also be confounded about what, if anything, ties all cases together—which can create a nagging desire to attempt to say what CIs really are. But I do not think a classic definition will work, nor, as the next section shows, do we need one.

A Comment on Method

Part of my intent is to show that, given the range of cases and the variety of claims and contentions about CIs, no useful and strict definition of CI exists. Nor is one needed. *Pace* Gray (and others), we do well enough sorting clear cases from unclear ones without such a definition. There is no chaos that a definition would fix, no tool we need that is nascent in one. This can only be confirmed by surveying the terrain of the concept and noting its landmarks. We find we need something different from what definitions could provide, something more.

The method I am employing is largely inspired by Ludwig Wittgenstein. Citing two of Wittgenstein's metaphors might illuminate his method: First, clarifying an idea is more like charting the relationships among the many overlapping fibers in a rope than, say, tracking a strand of thread that runs through the rope since no such strand exists. Second, the evolution of a concept is like that of a city: additions of houses, neighborhoods, streets, parks, and so on are neither perfectly predictable nor random and irrational. They are made for particular purposes that may not have been foreseen early on. Changes in terrain, available materials, and wealth will influence the city's pattern of growth.

Making additions to a city is analogous to adding to a language game. These are very well understood contexts for which society has provided tools by means of which speakers communicate within those contexts. The tools are words and phrases. Additions become necessary as society changes by revising its practices, goals, possibilities, and so on.[20]

A major thesis of this work is that two divergent aspects of meaning must be understood in order to appreciate the semantics of CIs: (1) the descriptive or structural aspect and (2) the performative aspect.[21]

Descriptive meaning reports the existence of structural elements of two types: It may report (a) actual motives of, say, physicians. This is the use in, for example, "The doctor was tempted to suggest an unnecessary operation to get the fee." Or it reports (b) *social arrangements*, such as fee schedules or reward systems. This is the use in, for example, "Kickbacks to doctors from company Z provide an incentive for them to use Z's pacemakers."

Thus the motives or social arrangements that constitute CIs might or might not lead to conduct that constitutes a breach of obligation. CIs are to be distinguished from acts of breach of obligation that they do or might cause. For example, in the pacemaker scenario, there is a CI inherent in the social arrangement. However, prescribing a pacemaker for a particular patient would constitute a breach of obligation only if the doctor believed that the specific pacemaker were inappropriate or inefficient for that patient.

The other aspect of meaning is performative. A variety of communication goals (beyond describing) are enabled by the language of CIs. These include (1) *warning* practitioners, patients, and administrators of temptations or other moral dangers, and (2) *insinuating*, *accusing*, or *condemning* physicians for particular failings. They can also include *explaining* why individual cases and general social designs go astray. Both sorts of meaning—(1) and (2)—must be studied to articulate the concept of CIs.

Instead of a definition of CIs, then, an account of a certain sort based on an extensive inventory is needed to explain the paradoxes and satisfy the desires mentioned above (if anything will). To provide it, I must explain the role CI language plays in our communication. This requires both identifying the descriptive indicators of the term and explaining something of the evolving tasks and contexts society has delimited that make having such a concept valuable (and evolving).

The method, in short, is based on this contention. To understand the logic of human ideas, one must understand the language games from which the ideas emerge and the uses to which the related language is put in those contexts. This requires great familiarity with—and acknowledgment of the roles of—sets of distinctions and beliefs. Thus, to grasp what they are, we must examine cases that are naturally called CIs and note the point of using the term. Doing so provides a map of a family resemblance of cases and criteria rather than a strictly defined, uniform idea.

Apply all this to Item 1 above—Todd's contention that every encounter with a patient and/or a payer is a CI. Todd's position is nonsense with an insight. The nonsense is manifest in thinking about what would happen were we to follow the recommendation implicit in his position: comments we consider important now would be trivial in that language, for accusing someone of having a CI would be saying something that goes without saying. And this would create havoc, since we would lose the ability to distinguish cases we feel are different enough to want to mark differently, given particular goals and contextual details. Thus, Todd proposes ultimate nonsense—ultimate loss of power to distinguish differences we care about.

However, Todd has an insight. He has identified often missed descriptive connections between cases we take to be different in kind: to wit, that being an ordinary doctor in an ordinary physician-patient relationship includes *potential* for the doctor to be tempted by personal motives to stray from role fidelity. To some extent, though, this is just another way of saying that doctors are human.

Todd's statement is a provocative way of indicating connections. Its intelligibility relies on our background knowledge that there is a difference in kind between potential intemperance and intemperate behavior. At the same time, its provocative nature, its destructive implications, and its insight all arise from a common source: proposing that the difference in kind be taken as only a difference in degree—equating CIs to ordinary relationships. Surely, ordinary relationships are structured in such a way that they contain some risk. Saying this may sometimes be illuminating, for it broadens our warrant to be cautious and even cynical. However, equating all cases, making them all conflictual, as Todd proposes, would destroy the usefulness of the CI vocabulary.

So, Todd's point is misleadingly put. It is much less alarming, much less paradoxical to say, as Baruch Brody does, "The existence of conflicting loyalties has always been a part of the patient-physician relation. Physicians have, in addition to their obligation to any individual patient, obligations to their other patients, to their families, to themselves, to their society, their religion, etc. Like everyone else, physicians live in a tangled web of conflicting obligations. They must learn how to balance these obligations rather than how to emphasize only one of them."[22] Brody's way of characterizing stresses on the doctor-patient relationship is, then, much more constructive than Todd's because, while both identify structures in the world, Brody's description is neither misleading nor provocative.

The juxtaposition of Brody's position to Todd's is an instance of the method I am using. A statement of it is this: To grasp an idea as fully as possible, one must make an inventory of the uses to which it is put in various contexts, as reflected in the contrasts among kinds of cases that its language allows us to describe. Making this inventory of cases and uses of terms is not easy. So much of the background of the cases and terms' uses must be articulated as to amount to sketching an aspect of culture. But having it will be worth the effort, yielding a rich grasp of the logic of human thought and community design.

To describe the contributions that the idea of CIs makes to contemporary American culture, then, I must distinguish its roles from those of other concepts and terms that might be associated or confused with it. To do so, I first focus on its semantic structure by contrasting CIs with conflicting interests and interests in conflict. The juxtaposition displays what each furnishes.

Types of Interests

What contribution does the notion of interests make to the notion of CIs? Part of the background for understanding both involves understanding motives, for CIs clearly involve concern about role holders' faithfulness in executing the duties of their role due to the motive of some sort of self-gain.

While some motives are personal—special to the person—others are universal—native to the human condition and invariant from person to person and context to context. As a society, we devised part of our concept of CIs to reflect concern about personal motives, interests, or values. For, as discussed above, we cannot use a term that always applies to every case with equal force, since such a term would be useless because pointless—its application would go without saying. Therefore, when we are focusing on motives, the concern is personal.[23]

The kinds of values that persons hold include ideals, a sense of what is practical, and predilections or gut-level inclinations.[24] Each shows how persons in general and professionals in particular can be motivated, and how each can generate CIs and conflicts that are not CIs.

Ideals

These are the values that provide a person with a sense of calling or meaning, and so should be thought of as intrinsic rather than instrumental.[25] They may derive from religious or professional indoctrination or from independent decisions after reflection. They are the locus of "moral" values—for example that one should (or should not) marry and raise a family, give to charity, or respect others.

In medicine broadly conceived, an ideal is to do research. This could lead to a CI within the role of being a physician. For example, a doctor's interest in fostering science may conflict with a patient's interest in being left alone, receiving established therapy, or hearing his physician's clinical opinion even if it is scientifically unwarranted.[26] Other ideals concern a life worth living.[27] Does a CI arise if a physician and patient hold different ideals about this, and the physician wants to act on her own notion[28] rather than respect the patient's?[29]

Practical Interests

These are the values that embody the person's sense of the worth of material elements involved in any trade-offs that must be made. Such elements are instrumental rather than intrinsic goods. Here, nothing of high principle is at stake. The bearers of such values are of many sorts. A physician has concern for her own time,[30] safety (*e.g.*, avoiding HIV infection), emotional resources (preventing burnout), and energy (hence convenience), among other things. Thus, under this rubric, many considerations—not just pecuniary ones—can generate CIs.

Practical interests might also lead physicians to breach the moral requirements of their role in ways that do not directly impact the care of their patients (a point neglected by the definition in the Simple Account). As professionals, physicians have a traditional duty to police their own profession.[31] However, physicians who discover fraud on the part of other physicians may decide not to report it due to the need to give depositions, appear in court or lose referrals from frightened or punitive colleagues. Hence, they breach duties of the role because of a personal interest that is practical, although we would not be likely to say that the person refrained from whistle blowing due to a CI. (What does this reluctance show about the concept?)

Referrals form a major portion of the concern with CIs.[32] Two examples that do not seem to be in the literature exemplify some nuances of this situation. First, a pediatrician formerly working in an outpatient clinic in New York City reported that without legal authority, his permission, or that of the patient's parent, sub-specialists from an associated hospital sent residents to review charts and demand referrals. The fees and increased access they got to "teaching material" made him suspect their claim to be doing quality assurance. Second, a cardiologist in private practice in the South reported that he would not, but his partners would, do procedures that lack clinical justification. They did the procedure because the patient's primary care physician sent the patient for the study rather than for consultation. To refuse to do it on the basis of the patient's history and physical examination would embarrass and alienate the sources of the referrals.

Another role conflict arises from practical interests when a physician takes care of a person with whom she sometimes works, such as a nurse. Suppose that the nurse frequently requests excuse notes for absences that the physician thinks are unrelated to disease, but the patient avows medical complaints when requesting them. The physician has a CI about writing the note because she is supposed to write the truth, but if she does, she reduces her ability to rely on the nurse at work. These are conflicting interests (rather than CIs) because the physician and patient have different goals. But it is also a CI in that what the patient wants conflicts with duties that society assigns to the role of being a physician. *This means that while CIs may focus on motives, they may also focus on social structures to the exclusion of motives.*

Predilections

These are dispositions to value something positively or negatively, for example, to prize it or despise it, trust it or fear it. They can be justified or prejudicial, rational or irrational, and can include tastes in activities such as hobbies and sexual preferences, as well as animosity and bonds such as friendship.

Revenge can be unconnected to practical interests and a source of CIs. It might motivate someone to leave the moral performance of his role in either of two ways. He might neglect its requirements, or he might be overly vigilant in prosecuting them. Regarding the latter, suppose that a doctor sits on a medical liability review board and a complaint arises involving a physician covered by an insurance company that once insured her. She might have a grudge against the company because it raised her rates and eventually became thoroughly unpleasant to deal with. Suppose, then, that she becomes offensively diligent in enforcing the rules against its customers. Knowing this would make it natural to allege that she has a CI in, say, assigning sanctions.[33]

At the opposite extreme, friendship or empathy can generate CIs. Take friendship. A physician allegedly wanted to protect a friend who had been in an automobile accident from being found to have alcohol in his blood. The physician was charged with having sent a sample of his own blood instead of the friend's to the police laboratory.[34] Another example: a psychiatrist might be tempted out of friendship (or being a feminist) to declare a hemophiliac incompetent because he hates women and rejects care from a female resident who requested a consultation so that she could override his rejection of her.[35]

Fear can also generate CIs. A doctor who fears death may have difficulty telling patients that they are dying. He may have an interest in avoiding the negative experience associated with disclosing the prognosis. That creates a CI *even if he tells the patient the prognosis. For in some cases, alleging that a CI occurred does not entail that the self-regarding motive won out. Nor does it presuppose that the patient has an interest in knowing his diagnosis. It may only require the belief that actual motives conflict with duties of the role.*[36]

This suggests that although CIs are sometimes poignant dilemmas, they need not be experienced as poignant or as dilemmas at all.[37] An interestingly subtle type of CI is apparent in cases discussed by Jerome P. Kassirer. He argues that decision-making is often structured so that physicians avoid particular risks. The first case involved a mentally ill woman who relapsed because her physicians did not want her to risk kidney damage from lithium. The second case involved a sixteen-year-old boy whose physicians refused him medical clearance to attend wilderness camp, although they considered him well enough to play sports vigorously and not to need treatment. The third case concerned a woman whose physician opposed her interest in delivering her baby at home because of difficulties with her first delivery due to the baby's head size. Kassirer declares that the physicians made these decisions out of both paternalism and self-interest. Of the latter, he alleges that the physicians are both protecting their consciences and reducing the risk of litigation even though the chances of dire outcome are small.[38]

Cases sometimes involve both practical interests and predilections. For example, patients may be placed in restraints so that the staff can get rest. Or a patient can get excuse notes or narcotics that are medically unwarranted because he is offensive to the physician, who wishes to reduce her exposure to the patient; a disruptive and offensive alcoholic patient in a waiting room full of patients will leave quickly if he gets what he wants.

Thus far, we have found that, though CIs are surprisingly pervasive and often associated with monetary interests, the Simple Account's exclusive focus on economic gain is too simple. Other sources of practical concern include time, safety, emotional resources, energy, prestige, license, and dedication to science. Motives arise from (1) ideals, (2) practical interests, and (3) predilections to determine or overdetermine a professional's action. We can use this framework to generate an analysis of the logical structure of dilemmas or more generally, interests that can conflict.[39]

Dilemmas: Kinds, Moral Status, and Sources

Dilemmas occur when values, rules, or principles that someone actually holds conflict with other values, rules, and principles that this person holds within a level or across levels. Hence, a dilemma can occur because ideals that bear on a given case seem to conflict with each other. Or a dilemma can arise because practical interests conflict with each other or with ideals or predilections. To organize the possibilities and to assess the moral status of conflicts, I offer the following three-part taxonomy of dilemmas.

Purely Nonmoral, Self-Regarding Dilemmas

These occur when one is focusing on one's own benefit or self-interest and there is a conflict about which of two objects of value (houses to buy, jobs to take) will best serve oneself. The choice will affect one's happiness greatly, but no duties are involved in the choice. Here one has a conflict but no CI.

Purely Moral, Others-Regarding Dilemmas

These occur when duties to other persons (or institutions) conflict with other duties. For example, a person has made promises and keeping one involves violating another, or a provider must decide which of several eligible patients will receive the one bed in the intensive care unit (ICU).[40] Dilemmas of this sort can also arise because one can be working in more than one kind of professional role at a time, such as physician, teacher, and researcher. In such circumstances, it may be unclear which duties should predominate.[41] Here one has a conflict and might have a CI (see the heading below entitled, *CIs Involving No Sense of Dilemma*).

Mixed Moral Dilemmas

These occur when serving the interests of or duty to another would injure an interest of one's own. For example, one may have accepted a job offer and then be offered something much more appealing, the acceptance of which would leave the first prospective employer in trouble. Although certain mixed moral dilemmas constitute CIs, this would not be one of them.

For physicians, this dilemma occurs when fulfilling a professional duty conflicts with satisfying a personal goal or interest.[42] This can constitute a classic CI. However, we must leave open the possibility that there may be mixed moral dilemmas in which one side represents legitimate self-regard conflicting with the legitimate and/or illegitimate interests of others (and maybe even duties to them).

The Idea of "Social Role" in the Concept of Conflicts of Interest

Much of the analysis of CIs draws on their compromising of the person's adherence to the responsibilities of his social role. Values construed as motives may undermine our faith in someone's executing the duties of his role, whether in the care of his own patients as individuals or as a member of a profession that is supposed to be self-policing. But what are the features of those roles that can suffer a CI?

A classic dilemma suggests an answer. In Aeschylus's *Agamemnon*, Agamemnon learned that he had to sacrifice his daughter, Iphigenia, to the gods. The expedition Agamemnon was leading had been suffering terribly as a result of being becalmed on the way to Troy. Many had starved already, and Agamemnon learned that, were he not to sacrifice her, everyone, including Iphigenia, would die.

Now change the case. Imagine that Agamemnon had a choice between saving his daughter and saving the bulk of the expedition. Its members could be concerned that Agamemnon had a CI as their leader, but it would be odd to suggest that his daughter could (as a matter of the rules of use of the expression) frame her concern in terms of a CI. There is an asymmetry here that indicates logical aspects of the concept of role as it bears on our understanding of CIs. This asymmetry suggests that only some roles can be involved in CIs. Which ones and why those?

It seems that the roles that could be involved would have the following features. (1) They are socially designed and elected, in contrast to those that seem natural and unavoidable. (2) They exist to serve the welfare or vital interests of others. (3) They involve discretion and judgment as part of the role holder's function. (4) Either the beneficiaries of the role holder's work or society in general must be able to trust the role holder simply because he holds the role.[43] The relationship between, say, the professional and his client crucially involves the professional's trustworthiness.

Disregard the actual social structures of ancient Greece, since it is *our* concept of CI that is being articulated. The first and fourth criteria are relevant. To us, it seems that Agamemnon could have declined to be the leader of the expedition, but it was impossible for him to decline to be his daughter's father. Her relationship with him does not make her adopt a commitment to trust him, whereas those under him do make such a commitment. In being obliged to kill Iphigenia, Agamemnon should have had a conflict as a father and even as a human being. But he would not be said to have had a conflict *of interest* as a father. He had it as a leader. Indeed, he had it as a leader whether he experienced it or not. But he had a conflict (not a CI) as a father only if he experienced a dilemma as such.[44]

This suggests that the idea of CI works differently from other sorts of conflicts. The grammar of our talk about conflicting opinions, desires, or loyalties implies that two or more items of the same sort conflict with each another. Sometimes this is our point in speaking of CIs in medicine—for example, that physicians who have a CI have two interests that conflict with each other, alleging a personal feeling of the physician or alleging that the physician's interests conflict with the patient's. But often we use the term to allude to social arrangements. We use it as a single, descriptive,[45] seemingly "hyphenated" term (conflict-of-interest) rather than as a report of a relation of two feelings conflicting with each other (*e.g.*, desires or interests). Or we use it to say that moral requirements of the role clash with other social arrangements in which the role holder finds herself. This leads to a deeper consideration of the implications of not sensing a dilemma.

CIs Involving No Sense of Dilemma

Essential to our task is understanding the contribution of the notion of "conflict" to the notion of CI. For example, is conflict best understood as the alternative to harmony? Speakers can mark their belief that an individual professional has an unsavory motivation by using the terms "conflict of motives" and "conflicting interests." Surely, "conflict of interests" marks these sorts of situations as well. But it also applies to situations in which general knowledge of human nature warrants the belief that the person's objectivity could plausibly be undermined *even without the person's feeling or knowing it*. Thus, to allude to an earlier example, physicians who manage their patients' sore throats according to the form of reimbursement may lack even an inkling of conflict or dilemma.

The absence of experiencing a dilemma points to some observations. Consider the case in which a physician is encouraged to lie in order to get a patient's mammogram paid for by an insurer. He "has to" lie because the insurer will pay for the test only if it is requested on the basis of clinical observations, not for preventive screening.[46]

We do not naturally think of this as being a CI, but should we? Motivated by his personal ideals, the physician is inclined to lie to an audience about something it has a right to know. If we declare that he has a CI, we still must grant that it is likely to be invisible to the doctor. It would be invisible because the moral core of his role involves acting and advocating for individual patients' welfare (Hippocratic *anthropolie*[47]). Moreover, in this case, the insurer's restrictions on physicians acting on the basis of that core ethic are repugnant and appear to be both ad hoc and economically motivated in such a way as to disregard patients' welfare. This means that the restrictions conflict with the ethos of medicine that is supposed to disregard cost.[48] Nevertheless, the payer has a right to know the reasons for the test, since it must know what it is paying for and whether the study is warranted when it is ordered; no one would contend that payers should pay by blind faith. The case of lying to the payer in order to have coverage for the mammogram shows that sometimes persons can be mistaken by not sensing that they have a dilemma or by not knowing what kind of dilemma it is. Sometimes, however, persons should not be said to have a dilemma just when they feel or sense one. For example, I have seen pediatricians haunted by whether they should feed an anencephalic baby who lacks a sucking reflex or whether they should put a baby with Potter's syndrome into an ICU (both syndromes are incompatible with life).

Thus, whether someone senses a dilemma is not a litmus test of the ethical nature of the situation. Ethical theory may originate because people have moral dilemmas, but once it starts, ethical theory goes beyond dilemma resolution to correct us both by occasional dilemma generation and by pseudo-dilemma deconstruction. In short, ethical theory can provide grounds for correcting persons in some circumstances because they sense a dilemma or in other circumstances because they do not.

This two-way ability to correct seems to be a major advantage of uniting under one term our concerns with (1) conflicts of motives and (2) worrisome situational structures that may or may not occasion a sense of conflict on the part of the professional and (3) how motives and situations may or may not influence behavior. Thus, a physician in an HMO might be so venal as to have no conflict since he has no inclination to fulfill a duty to a patient because he can gain (financially or otherwise) by contrary action. Or a physician might have no sense of conflict or dilemma when drug-seeking patients approach her for narcotics, lacking any medical indicators for them, because she is happy to be paid for simply fulfilling the request. This would represent both no conflict and a CI, since there is an opposition between personal economic gain and role duties to serve health and legitimate, health-related needs (or at least follow morally respectable legal prohibitions).

These cases are very important to our grasp of the concept of CI. For we would say of them that the physician acted from a CI even though he lacked any sense of conflict. This strengthens the argument that CIs constitute a family resemblance both to cases of motives and to causes (social structures) that undermine trust in clinicians. *And, as a further point about the meaning of the phrase, we can say that a CI can properly be mentioned even if the physician does not do wrong, that is, even if the CI does not mature into a breach of obligation.* For he may both resist temptation and, without having any temptation, be immersed in social structures that are compromising. Both of these are *part* of what we bring into focus by means of the concept of CI. And they are what Todd and Jonsen were misleadingly alluding to in Items 1, 2 and 3 above.

Some Uses of the Concept of CI in Context

Thus far, I have sketched some of the descriptive or structural elements that constitute CIs. But stopping here would omit a large part of what we must grasp to understand the term—the performative functions or agendas it serves in discourse.

To consider this aspect, I note that the use of the term varies significantly according to its temporal relation to the situation or action. For example, contemporary speakers of English use it in the past tense to allege either temptation (a mental occurrence) or actual (behavioral) wrongdoing. Two examples of this are as follows: (1) "Doctor Smith sold her interest in the equipment company to avoid a CI"—suggesting temptation or potential temptation, and (2) "Doctor Jones had a CI when she recommended that the patient get a pacemaker"—alleging wrongdoing. The alleged wrong might, for example, consist of recommending an unnecessary intervention to get a kickback from the manufacturer.

Addressing the temporal present by, for example, saying (3) "Dr. Brown has a CI" is a *warning* to the listener not to trust Dr. Brown or a warning to Brown not to trust himself, but neither use need allude to a feeling of conflict. Finally, focusing on the future and saying (4) "Dr. Green will have a CI" could constitute a warning to the general public to avoid her or to get a second opinion regarding her recommendations, or it could be a warning to Green to avoid the situation or to double-check her judgment and disposition in that context.

Past-tense uses include alleging or explaining. One might use it to explain why, for example, pacemaker implantation is disproportionately expensive[49] or why a physician refused to provide clearance for a teenager to go to a camp (Kassirer's example above).

That some CIs have no logical ties to motives implies that the distinction between *having a CI* and *having the appearance of a CI* is most likely to be bogus, radically overdrawn or misused, as I shall now show.[50] In some ways, the very suggestion of a distinction between apparent and real conflicts is nonsensical. The distinction's intelligibility depends upon the sense of asserting that sometimes a professional actually did or did not experience some conflict or dilemma. But, as I have shown, there need be no experience at all of having a dilemma in order for the attribution of a CI to make sense or be true of a conflict-free, happy, drug-selling doctor.

In other ways, the distinction between real and apparent CIs is overdrawn because those who say that professionals should avoid both conflicts and the appearance of conflicts fail to give appropriate weight to the general structural elements of roles and situations. They seem to think that only individuals can appear to have a CI, and thus that only individuals can avoid creating that appearance. Surely, in some conversational contexts, it is important to note that to be a physician in a given situation is ipso facto to have CI structures present because of something about the social structures. This provides the descriptive basis if one wants to explain or warn about some potential or past misconduct. But in other contexts, where the potential or past conduct is fine, it would be foolish because it is pointless, but also alarming and distracting, to mention an ipso facto CI.[51]

Finally, the distinction between real and apparent CIs is misused by those who suggest that disclosing the CI to the patient would be a partial remedy. This is a misuse of the distinction because all that disclosure can achieve is to make the appearance of conflict more evident. This then requires patients to be very distrustful and very assertive in largely implausible ways if they are to guard against being victims of the CI. The most that disclosure can accomplish is to put potential victims on their guard. It will not, however, resolve the CI or solve the problem. It will not destroy the descriptive accuracy of the structural allegation. At best, it might give potential victims a chance to avoid being taken in, but I hardly think that significant numbers of patients will, for example, refuse tests— even in a physician's lab—just because she has disclosed owning it. They might, to be sure, go to the doctor less often or seek a different doctor.[52]

This section has focused on the performative agenda behind the use of the language of CIs. Such use depends on structural or contextual relationships that form the descriptive basis of mentioning CIs. But these are too widespread to mention every time. There has to be another agenda, such as alleging, explaining, or warning, before mention of a CI would make sense or have a point.

The nature and pervasiveness of the structure means that this aspect of CIs cannot be prohibited. In part, this is because no one could be sure to be, and remain free of, both the motives and social structures that could make discussion of a CI useful. Rather, there can be mechanisms of scrutiny—analogous to hospitals' quality assurance and utilization review committees—that investigate circumstances that reach a level of visible warrant for concern. There can also be ways of reducing physicians' inclinations to give in to CIs (this will be mentioned again below).

Tolerable Self-Regard That Conflicts with Legitimate Patients' Interest

Physicians today find themselves in a terrible predicament. They are in a cultural trap created by mixed messages from a society that wants them to conform to three rival ethics: a professional ethic to serve the patient, a business ethic to thrive as entrepreneurs, and a communalist ethic that makes them responsible for the economic and medical health of the commons.[53]

The reality of the business ethic suggests that there must be moral limits to what we condemn when someone withholds the "best" treatment and does so for her own sake as part physician, part businessperson. The acceptable limits are reflected in three sorts of cases: (1) self-regarding actions that favor caregivers over patients and are *clearly unacceptable*; (2) cases in which it is dubious whether mentioning a CI has value, perhaps because the background conditions are humanly unavoidable and the incentives are trivial; and (3) cases in which having a practical interest is thoroughly proper, *whether there is or is not a CI*.[54] Discussions of type (1) are common. About (2) and (3), consider the following examples and issues.[55]

Does Dr. One, who is trained and competent to handle a particular problem, have a duty to refer a patient with that routine problem to Dr. Two, who some practitioners think is slightly better at handling the condition? As long as Dr. One's care meets the standard of care, it seems moralistic to say that he must refer patients to more skilled practitioners. And if Dr. Two is the best in the country, he does not have time, energy, facilities, and so on, to take care of every lesser doctor's cases. (Similar points could be made about reluctance to spend money to update equipment.)

Even when a physician is motivated by purely financial interests, not all conflicts or dilemmas would rightly be characterized as CIs. For not all financial interests need be venal or even inappropriate. Recall the different strep tests for HMO patients and fee-for-service patients. If the HMO contract is explicit about such discrepancies, and all have agreed to the physician's right to practice in this way, there is no inclination to allege a CI even though the rapid test would be better for the patient.

Now consider the case of a patient who requested a house call and, when the physician arrived, presented two other adults and a child for care. The physician believed that they lacked coverage and hoped to be seen at no additional charge. Here concern for income and time management are the legitimate interests of the physician, while trying to get the care without charge is an interest of the prospective patients. Depending on his ideals, this physician could at most have a conflict of etiquette or prudence, but not a CI.

Also, contemplate the legitimate economic interests of a physician conflicting with other legitimate interests of a patient. A twenty-year-old woman came to an office for the measles mumps and rubella (MMR) inoculation required by her college. She stated that she was pregnant and had not decided about carrying the pregnancy to term. Thus, the inoculation was out of the question since it might deform the fetus. Because the patient's father was in the waiting room and the patient did not want anyone—including her father—to know about the pregnancy, a question arose about how the physician should charge for the visit. How could he justly charge for the vaccination? The physician is entitled to be paid, and the father is entitled not to be charged for a service not delivered. The patient advocated charging her father without taking the shot. Her interest conflicted with the physician's economic interest and with his ideals about truth telling and keeping accurate records. Thus, important descriptive features of CIs are present. However, it would be very misleading to characterize the physician's dilemma as a CI, since this would insinuate (a performative) that the physician is tempted to be a corrupt fiduciary, and that does not apply.

Thus, it seems that many cases of self-regarding actions by a professional that are contrary to the interests of a patient are legitimate. The responsibilities of the role do not mandate forsaking all self-regard. It is not at all clear that a physician must accept all risks of exposure to HIV infection—for example, that she must put her ungloved hand into a patient's blood—if the doctor has an incidental wound of her own that is not fully healed.

Thus far, we have found that to have a CI is to be neither in a state of temptation nor in a dilemma, for although these might pertain, it is also true that neither must. Rather, to have a CI is to be in a situation in which one might plausibly be thought to do something immoral due to a motivation that might tempt most role holders (or this individual). The implication is that many persons of typical moral fiber would be likely to neglect the duties of their roles for the sake of their own values of any sort (not just economic, safety, friendship, etc.). One could be in that situation and never be tempted because one has no inclination to be good or because one winds up not feeling motivated to be bad! Nevertheless, the person would have to be said to have a CI.

Interestingly, the physicians in the following case changed from having no CI to having one. A group practice bought and ran a laboratory that was closing in its building. The group did this solely to prevent the inconvenience that the closing would mean to many patients, especially many older ones who would forego needed studies. After investing, the practitioners came to believe that they should profit at a rate that would match what their money would earn in a savings account. They evolved from ensuring that the laboratory had sufficient business to pay its way to ensuring that it had sufficient business to generate a profit. They evolved from an innocuous situation—a case that might or might not be described as a CI—into what could easily be considered a full-blown CI (which perhaps ought to be tolerated).

Some features of the following situation are so global and disheartening that we would not speak of it as a CI. Dr. L., a facial surgeon, is a scarce medical resource in his rural setting. He is on call for emergencies in two hospitals. Typically, his emergency patients have broken jaws, cheekbones, and orbits around the eyes. He characterizes his emergency patients as drunks or drug addicts who have often had their faces smashed by jealous husbands. Many are HIV positive. These patients do not have funds for his fee and/or to buy the antibiotics they must take for several months after their operation. Post discharge bacterial infections add greatly to Dr. L.'s work. Moreover, after every operation he finds blood under his glove, since he inevitably cuts himself with some of the wire he uses to fix a broken jaw.

The arrangement has even taken a sudden downturn because a trauma center has opened and many of the patients who would have come to him with funds and family or social support are now sent out of the area. He feels stuck with the riskiest, least remunerative, and socially most difficult patients from among whom had been a large mix of patients including a high proportion of better ones. If he decides to stop being available to the hospitals, because he does not like the risks and burdens in contrast to the rewards, is he acting out of a CI?

Assume that his characterization is reasonably accurate. This case illustrates that there are limits to energy, dedication, foregoing payment, and time spent that are morally owed as a function of holding a role. One could say that Dr. L.'s personal interests are *acceptably* in conflict with the demands of his role. This does not, however, mean that he is justified in dropping below the standard of care in individual cases. However, if Dr. L. is not involved in working on a patient and the arrangement with the hospitals conflicts with his legitimate desires, then (unless there is another source of obligation) he has no duty to continue to serve the hospitals. It is unclear whether Dr. L. has a CI in rejecting individual cases or in discontinuing his relationship with the hospitals. Such unclarity would seem to rest on the arguable assumption that there is a general duty to serve as a physician once trained, competent, and licensed. Using the language of CIs in this situation would be more of a distraction than a gain.

Finally, note some of the shape and limits of the notion of CIs regarding avoiding malpractice suits. Consider the case of a daughter who wanted to force dialysis on her mother and got leverage by threatening a malpractice suit if the medical team did not override her mother's competent refusal. This generated a CI, because the threat of a suit tempted the physicians to stray from their duty to their patient (even though a suit might have arisen no matter which way they had acted). But if, as in the next case, caregivers refuse to fall below the standard of care in order to avoid negligence, there is no clear CI even though there might be interests in conflict.

Mr. P. is a man in his late fifties. He is quadriplegic due to a C-2 fracture of the spine and is nearly completely dependent on a ventilator, and he also suffers from orthostatic hypotension. He resides in a nursing home that takes ventilator-dependent patients. He wants to live, and he wants to be weaned from the ventilator. His room is far from the nurses' station and quite out of the line of traffic, and his desired method of weaning is dangerous. He had been allowed to wean for one or two hours three times a day in an *unmonitored* setting—no alarms or nurse visualization. This was decided on the basis of a previous physician's order, but it breaks all the guidelines of the American Thoracic Society and places Mr. P. at great risk of stopping breathing with no one knowing, in part because he cannot even use a call button.

A new physician and a new program director begin to work at the facility at about the same time. They refuse to allow this situation to continue. The director explains to the administrators of the facility and to Mr. P. himself that there is great risk of inadvertent, otherwise avoidable death. They should consider themselves at great risk of malpractice liability in allowing him to continue to wean in this way. The director offers Mr. P. several options, including room changes and various technological options (some quite expensive for the institution) that reduce the risks to him. Mr. P. refuses all of them. He wants trach collar weaning in his room. The physician will not write orders for that form of weaning. The administrators and the team agree to refuse to do something tantamount to medical malpractice.

Someone (either Mr. P. or the administrators) initiate a consultation with the state department of health. Its investigation leads it to assert that the resident had a right to wean as he had in the past, even if that violated the standard of care. The previous physician's orders to wean as the patient wanted has, the state says, created a duty to continue to treat, even in an unsafe way. So Mr. P. is entitled to demand continued weaning in a manner dangerous to his life. He seems entitled to place the facility at risk of practicing substandard and otherwise unacceptable care. The agency orders the caregivers to treat the patient as indicated. The facility opts to risk taking a deficiency rather than run the malpractice risk and practice substandard care.

These last two cases show that avoiding allegations of negligence can cut two ways. It can mean (1) attempting to avoid a situation that has the descriptive features that merely signal legitimate interests in conflict or (2) acting to avoid allegations of negligence that can create a CI in the strong negative sense of genuine threats to or failures of trustworthiness, and thus fit some performative agendas that lead to the idea of CIs. In (2), it has the immoral cast that inclines the physician to violate the responsibilities of her role for her own sake. A paradigm of that is falsifying a record once a physician has reason to think that a malpractice suit has been filed against her.

A Definition Discussed and a Conflict Resolved

In spite of rejecting the possibility of defining, if a hankering for a short formula remains, the following "definition" *of the descriptive element* is plausible: CIs are either motives that caregivers have *and/or* situations in which we could reasonably think caregivers' responsibilities to observe, judge, and act according to the moral requirements of their role are or will be compromised to an unacceptable degree. This should be appreciated as pertaining to a family resemblance of criteria and cases that society wants to identify in labeling the concept.

The definition can be short and plausible only by trading on vagueness, ambiguities, and background assumptions. Nevertheless it indicates the texture of the concept along with some of its holes, it describes the reason for having the concept, and it characterizes the members of the concept's family to which speakers might allude in invoking the term.[56]

Even given its trading on vagueness, and so on, we can ask how right the definition is. Are there cases that fit it but do not seem to be CIs? What about cases that are of CIs that do not fit the definition? Do physicians who refuse to see patients for whom reimbursement is poor act from a CI?[57] They might not be violating the physician role with anyone because there is no doctor-patient relationship between individuals yet. If a physician is seeing what all of us would consider her fair share of Medicaid patients, it is not a violation of her role and not a CI to refuse to see another patient who will pay poorly.[58]

Nor is the fee-directed misconduct in the following case a clear instance of a CI: A physician who sent a bill that far surpasses usual and customary fees did not violate the caregiving duties of his role. He violated duties of the role only *after* providing the medical attention. That is, although this case fits the definition, it seem no more than an irritating borderline case.

Several features of this misconduct might prevent it from being a CI. First, there were adequate medical indications for the treatment. Second, consent was not sought on the basis of misleading information. Third, nothing in the professional acts was done either misleadingly or by force. Fourth, breaking faith with the precepts of medical science and/or truthfulness is an indicator of a CI, but no act of billing (whether excessive or even fraudulent) seems capable in itself of being considered a CI. Because the misconduct did not influence the care given and because the role is care oriented, billing behavior does not constitute acting out of the social definition of the role in such a way as to be a CI. (It may, of course, be wrong for other reasons and can be characterized as such in other terms.)

The discussion that justifies this definition suggests a way of reconciling the debate between Jonsen and Lynn mentioned earlier. Jonsen is worried about CIs that seem unavoidable and permeate the concerns of practitioners. He must be thinking of the motivational and structural foci of the concept of CI and must have in mind the sorts of mixed dilemmas in which the self-regarding option is immoral. Of these cases, it makes sense to take Jonsen's position and prescribe that professionals *generally* must refrain from acting on their own behalf. Lynn, by contrast, seems to have in mind those CIs that are descriptive but not motivating—that do not tempt virtuous physicians or do not tempt them much. These conflicting interests produce no experience of a dilemma that distracts from role duties, and so, of course, dedicated physicians deal with them very well, as she claims. For example, a treatment might be so appropriate that no virtuous physician would think of withholding it even in an HMO arrangement.

The innocuous CIs that Lynn has in mind could be mere social structures. If this is right, Jonsen and Lynn are talking past one another in focusing upon different members of the family resemblance of CIs and in jointly ignoring the performative agenda speakers have in invoking the language of CIs. Jonsen ignores the performative agenda by alleging that CIs are everywhere; Lynn ignores it by disregarding the *breadth* of appropriate concern. Further, they have an empirical disagreement about how much damage is being done. I would preserve the insight of each by recommending the following: Because persons naturally have practical and other interests, those we select to be physicians should have sufficient empathy and sense of calling to resist venality. Moreover, we ought to arrange social support for physicians so that their temptation is minimized and their empathy can remain high.

A Test for Trustworthiness

This resolution of the debate between Jonsen and Lynn will be more satisfactory if we can identify a test for determining when alarm pertains and when, if ever, motives and situations occasion self-regarding action that is morally tolerable. This will allow us to separate the many acts of self-regard that are acceptable from those that are not.

A plausible thought experiment is as follows: anthropomorphise each horn of the dilemma (motive or structural arrangement) so it can argue on its own behalf. Ask whether, in a free society, each horn's complaining publicly *about its being betrayed* yields coherent, long-term results.

For example, it would not be coherent for the business manager of a mixed group partnership to complain publicly that a primary care physician broke trust with the group by sending too few referrals for expensive procedures. There can be no publicly acceptable commitment to refer a quota of patients for costly procedures. Consumers would see such a commitment as illegitimate, and if patients had the choice to avoid such a practice, they would. Patients' avoidance would be defeating for the practice—making the public complaint a self-defeating, incoherent act.

The criterion of having a horn of a dilemma argue on its own behalf as though it were a person shows that practitioners' loyalty to their group practice is inappropriately (immorally) structured and hence a troubling CI if they have to refer a quota of patients to their partners. This implies that the trust relationship among members of the group can be structured morally only within the context of fulfilling trust to the patient first.

This, however, does not mean that a physician must serve all of a patient's interests. Capitulating to a patient's interest in having his care be free, for example, may be a betrayal of the legitimate trust of one's partners. Thus, when (and perhaps only when) each horn of the dilemma can coherently argue publicly for itself, the choice of that horn is morally pure.[59] It might be also acceptable to opt for a horn as the lesser of two evils. But remorse has a proper presence in the conscience of those who have to choose the lesser of two evil horns.

Conclusion

In summary, the analysis of CIs is highly complex. Taking all values in CIs to be economic makes all other sorts of values—ideals, other practical goals, and predilections—unavailable for study or use in explanations (or other performative agendas). Too much is lost by insisting that interests are always economic, suggesting that there is no other improper motive in medical practice. I have also reviewed the sorts of conflicts we encounter as dilemmas and as situations that ought to be experienced as dilemmas but are not. I have discussed the features that might characterize a role for a role holder to have a CI. And I have shown how one great advantage of the design of the concept is that it applies to motives and yet can be used performatively—for example, to condemn or warn role holders and beneficiaries about situations, as well as to insinuate, explain, and so on.

Our language includes tools that allude to many sorts of conflicts (of opinions, desires, loyalties, etc.). The meanings of these phrases indicate that an item of one sort (desires, for example) conflicts with another item *of the same sort*. CIs are different. In them, a motive might conflict with moral demands, or economic arrangements might conflict with moral demands. These are conflicts of two very different types in themselves, making the distinction between apparent and real CIs useful in some contexts—for example, to reduce alarm or to warn of extra candor. But it might also be misleading or even bogus. Finally, in spite of the moral requirements of the role(s) in question, not all behavior that favors the physician over the patient is wrong.

In medicine, the contrast between tragic dilemmas and CIs is worth maintaining, though that might not be so in, for example, law. CI terminology helps us indicate, for example, that we are alleging that a person violated a trust he could have kept but did not want to keep. His action is the product of a situation he should not have entered or a motive he should not have embraced. It is immoral, and the language of CI helps us label it thus. But what of the unavoidable need to resolve a tragic dilemma—one in which the actor must choose the lesser of two evils?

A person may have to violate the trust of one beneficiary on behalf of another because both cannot be honored (as in a purely moral dilemma). Then a CI would not be alleged, however one acts, unless there is some unusual conceptual or moral gain in so alleging. There might be such gain if, for example, the dilemma is tragic because the physician has a personal ideal (to do research) that conflicts with the social duty of fulfilling the trust of a fiduciary. Thus, some conflicts of ideals (loyalties) lend themselves to being called CIs (the French officials who allowed HIV-tainted blood to enter their nation's blood supply) and some do not.

I close with three misgivings about the quest to understand CIs for public policy purposes alone—for example, legislating against joint ventures or some sorts of referral arrangements. First, not everything can be covered by such regulations. A surgeon may want to serve her own economic interests or practice her technique and may slant her informed consent message so as to frighten a patient into accepting the procedure. A professional's power of persuasion is inherently so great that little can control her having her way.[60] This may ultimately justify "managed care" reviews, but I doubt that they could catch all (or even most) self-serving actions. Second, some CIs may be worth tolerating for patient convenience, such as having laboratory services within a medical practice.

Third, there is no way to eliminate the structural elements of CIs as that idea has come to be understood. Thus, Jonsen is right; the structure of CIs suffuses the professional lives of physicians. Lynn is also right; many practitioners handle those structures in ways that are perfectly fine and require no warning, explaining, insinuating, and so on.

The third point implies that since the descriptive elements cannot be eliminated, CIs cannot be completely forbidden.[61] What physicians will be able to do will remain, to a very large degree, a matter of conscience and conscientiousness. Thus, though public disclosure will not reduce CIs, the test sketched in *A Test for Trustworthiness* (see above) and related to public disclosure will help: imagine the action's having to defend itself publicly and ask whether patients will continue in the relationship freely. (This is not the same as forcing disclosure.) The thought experiment seems likely to indicate whether an acceptable interest of the practitioner conflicts with the fiduciary duties of her role.[62,63]

Notes

1. Geoffrey C. Hazard, Jr., in chapter four of this volume, writes as though the meanings (use, cases to which the language applies) are the same in law and other professions, especially medicine. I take issue with this conclusion. In medicine the language of conflict of interest is different from that of conflict of loyalties; evidently in law this is not so. This caution connects with the idea, developed later, that no univocal definition of CI is available or needed. Rather, CI applies to a family of cases, issues, and purposes and should be thought of as having a family resemblance. See *Types of Interests* in text for some articulation of the method I employ.

   In some ways, this chapter is more concrete than Hazard's through the examples discussed. In other ways it is more abstract, since it offers a look at the fine grain of such concepts as dilemma. I indicate some major comparisons and contrasts with Hazard's analysis in note 62.

2. To avoid the cumbersome "his or her," and so on, I use pronouns of either gender where grammar permits.

3. I expect that some readers will resist this conclusion because they have been persuaded by historical posturing and rhetoric. Others, no doubt, will affirm it as trivially obvious. These divergences alone make the conclusion interesting.

4. David Hadorn and Robert Brook, The Health Care Resource Allocation Debate: Defining Our Terms, 266 *JAMA* 3328 (1991).

5. E. R. Greenberg et al., Social and Economic Factors in the Choice of Lung Cancer Treatment, 318 *N. Engl. J. Med* 612 (1988).

6. I am not claiming that this describes a single range of seriousness of CIs, with those in primary care always less serious and those in tertiary care always more serious.

7. This example was provided by a resident.

8. Neil Luebke, Conflict Of Interest as a Moral Category, 6 *Bus. Prof. Ethics* 66 (1987). Luebke provided the history of the definition from *Black's Law Dictionary* that I cited above.

9. A comprehensive study that supports Luebke's historical claims is Albert Hirschman, *The Passions and the Interests: Political Arguments for Capitalism before Its Triumph* (1977). Hirschman tracks thinking about conflicts as far back as St. Augustine and reports that interests (in contrast to passions) were associated with expendable resources. Hirschman criticizes Adam Smith for having too narrow a focus on interests and, in effect, sides with me (107-108).

10. For an unreflective use of "interest" that shows this point, see Richard Momeyer, *Confronting Death* 100 (1988). There, writing of orthodox Jewish girls who were fated to become sexual objects of the Gestapo, Momeyer says that their headmistress argued that taking poison was "both in their interests and their obligation."

11. Prompting Edmund L. Erde, Economic Incentives for Ethical and Courteous Behavior in Medicine: A Proposal, 113 *Ann. Intern. Med* 790 (1990).

12. See Alan Riding, French Allowed AIDS-Tainted Blood, *New York Times* 7 (October 20, 1991). Whether to call this a CI could be controversial. See my discussion of CIs versus tragic dilemmas in the conclusion of this chapter.

13. See Christopher R. Barbrack, Beyond the Guessed Interests of the Child: The Role of the Expert Witness in Child Custody Cases, *Carrier Foundation Medical Education Letter* (May 1991), about being a paid expert witness regarding the best interests of a child in a custody dispute.

14. Nevertheless, the complex account I offer focuses on physicians and thus may miss nuances of the concept that society has come to tailor vis-a-vis other roles. For example, nurses' cir-

cumstance might influence how they compromise on duties to patients, and where and why they are subject to the language of CIs.

15. Bradford Gray, *The Profit Motive and Patient Care: Changing Accountability of Doctors and Hospitals* 199 (1991). Gray both calls for a definition and recants the call, saying we should distinguish "necessary" CIs from unnecessary ones (at 199). He conflates calling for a definition with evaluating arrangements.

16. James Todd, Professionalism at Its Worst, 266 *JAMA* 3338 (1991).

17. Albert Jonsen, Watching the Doctor, 308 *N. Engl. J. Med* 1531 (1983).

18. Joanne Lynn, Conflicts of Interest in Medical Decision-Making, 36 *J. Am. Geriatr. Soc.* 945 (1988).

19. Edmund D. Pellegrino, Editorial: Altruism, Self-Interest and Medical Ethics, 258 *JAMA* 1939 (1987).

20. Ludwig Wittgenstein, *Philosophical Investigations* 8, 32 (G. E. M. Anscombe, trans., 1953) (for the metaphors).

21. J. L. Austin, *How To Do things with Words* (J. O. Urmson ed.; 1965) is also a vital source of method. Many have elaborated Austin's approach. See, e.g., John Searle, *Speech Acts: An Essay in the Philosophy of Language* (1969). In this chapter, I use "performative" in a way that differs slightly from the classic sources, but only for simplicity's sake.

22. Baruch Brody, Special Ethical Issues in the Management of PVS Patients, 20 *Law, Medicine and Health Care* 113 (1992).

23. However, later I shall show that when the concern is so broad that it applies almost equally to all, we need not focus on the physician feeling a motive, but rather focus on the social arrangements as such.

24. But this set of distinctions is not meant to imply that what a person values must fit fully into just one or another of these.

25. Ideals are one sort of intrinsic value. One invests an object with intrinsic value if one prizes it for itself, while appreciating it as a means to something else invests it with instrumental value. Contrast admiring a work of art for its beauty (intrinsic value) with valuing it only because it covers a hole in a wall (instrumental value). See Alasdair MacIntyre, *After Virtue* 178ff (1981). Society may suffer from physicians having found activities (like operating) intrinsically valuable instead of valuable just as a means of helping patients and earning fees.

26. See Samuel Hellman and Deborah Hellman, Of Mice But Not Men—Problems of Randomized Clinical Studies, 324 *N. Engl. J. Med.* 1585 (1991). It is an account of how one must abandon the role of being a person's doctor in order to enroll her in a randomized clinical study that one is doing. For more on research, *see, e.g.*, David Shimm and Roy Spece, Industry Reimbursement for Entering Patients into Clinical Trials: Legal and Ethical Issues, 115 *Ann. Intern. Med.* 148 (1991).

27. Ezekiel Emanuel, A Communal Vision of Care for Incompetent Patients, 17 *Hastings Cent. Rep.* 15 (1987). Emanuel identifies five. They appear graduated in that if a patient meets the criteria for one level of life worth living, she automatically meets those below it. From lowest to highest, these are: vitalism (the view that any physical life is worth preserving), hedonistic (the view that if pleasure is more extensive than suffering, life is worth living), affective (the view that if the person can experience emotion, life is worth living), autonomy (the view that if the patient can exercise self-determination, life is worth living), and utilitarian (the view that if the person contributes more good to society than she drains away, life is worth living).

28. The case of Helga Wanglie may be an example of this. See, e.g., the several discussions in 21 *Hastings Cent. Rep.* 23 (1991).

29. Roy G Spece, Jr., asks, in effect, whether a CI would pertain if the physician held a view of a life worth living that was utterly commensurable with a homogeneous society's view and he

was acting on it, while the patient held a very different view. Spece's hypothetical has great value in indicating some of the influences of background social values on the meaning of conflict of interest. It indicates that trustworthiness to one's role may assume some conformity to general social values, not just to role-defined particulars.

30. See the critique of how psychotherapists manage appointment time in Daniel Goleman, Therapy: Critics Assail "Assembly-Line" Sessions, *New York Times* C1, C11 (April 17, 1984). If, as the old saw goes, time is money, this is less of a different practical interest than it first appears to be. Perhaps when professionals decline responsibility on the basis of lack of time they mean money, but they phrase it in a way that is more acceptable.

31. They owe this since they joined an institution that historically owed it as a duty through oaths and codes.

32. See Mark Siegler, Medical Consultations in the Context of the Physician-Patient Relationship, in *Responsibility in Health Care* 141 (George Agich ed., 1982).

30. I owe this example to Roy Spece, Jr.

34. *See* State: Doctor Faked Test to Aid Friend, *Philadelphia Inquirer* 2-BJ (November 19, 1991).

35. Thomas P. Hackett and Ned H. Cassem, *Massachusetts General Handbook of Psychiatry* 555ff (1978).

36. The language of CIs may be used to explain why the doctor took so long to get to the disclosure or did it so nervously, and so on.

37. We can say of an individual that she has a major dilemma she has to resolve within the week; we can say this even if she is asleep or working on a crossword puzzle. So, too, we can say of this or that person that he has a CI even if he is on vacation. There are also communication gains in being able to say that a corporation or organization has a CI even if no individual officer or employee experiences that CI.

38. Jerome Kassirer, Adding Insult to Injury: Usurping Patients' Prerogatives, 308 *N. Engl. J. Med.* 898 (1983).

39. An example of Lynn Payer's clarifies some differences between CIs and interests in conflict. Quoting Dr. Henk Lamerts, she projects the different numbers of sutures that might be used on a given wound by Spanish, Austrian, and Belgian physicians as two, six, and as many as possible, respectively. Dr. Lamerts says that the Spanish doctor is paid for the wound care alone, while the Belgian doctor is paid by the suture. This sounds as though a CI is involved, but a comment shows that it is merely differing interests: "Belgian culture values sutures, so they are put in. It's appreciated, so he gets paid for it." Lynn Payer, *Culture and Medicine: Varieties of Treatment in the United States, England, West Germany and France* 34 (1988).

40. For a criterion of a dilemma as purely moral and a way to test for it, See *A Test of Trustworthiness* in the text of this chapter.

41. Given the practical incentives to do research, there can be temptations that undermine the role of the investigator and the quality of the research done. Issues related to CIs for researchers include a general concern about universities. *See* Liz McMillen, Quest for Profits May Damage Basic Values of Universities, Harvard's Bok Warns, *The Chronicle of Higher Education* A1, A31 (April 24, 1991).

At the level of investigators, see David Kessler, Drug Promotion and Scientific Exchange: The Role of the Clinical Investigator, 325 *N. Engl. J. Med.* 201 (1991).

There is also the problem of finders' fees. *See* David Wheeler, Researchers Debate Ethics of Payments for Human Subjects, *The Chronicle of Higher Education* A7, A8, A9 (August 14, 1991). Also, see Shimm and Spece, supra note 26. And see the references that pertain to epidemiologic research in note 50 below.

See how reviewers' objectivity is called into question if they are paid by drug companies. See also concern about journals' power to supervise the quality of advertisements they accept, given the amount of money companies spend on ads in those journals, both in Michael Wilkes et al., Pharmaceutical Advertisements in Leading Medical Journals: Experts' Assessments, 116 *Ann Intern. Med.* 912 (1992).

This footnote exemplifies the "family resemblance" nature of CIs, since here we are mostly discussing researchers rather than physicians.

42. Acting to satisfy a personal interest is a strong mark of CIs, but it is neither a necessary nor a sufficient condition. Society's definition of the role of doctor tolerates acting on some self-regarding interests (see below).

43. This is overstated since, in much of society, we must have auditors and other kinds of overseers.

44. I am drawing on Martha C. Nussbaum's brilliant book, *The Fragility of Goodness: Luck and Ethics in Greek Tragedy and Philosophy* (1986). Nussbaum argues that Agamemnon's lack of suffering explains his condemnation by the chorus. Analogous points pertain to doctors.

45. I hope the reader sees that this section is a survey of descriptive meaning, as defined above.

46. Dennis Novack et al., Physicians' Attitudes Toward Using Deception to Resolve Difficult Ethical Problems, 261 *JAMA* 2980 (1989).

47. Ludwig Edelstein, The Professional Ethics of the Greek Physician, in *Ancient Medicine* 319-348 (Owsei Tempkin and C. Lilian Tempkin, eds., 1976).

48. Howard F. Stein, The Money Taboo in American Medicine, 7 *Med. Anthropol.* 1 (Fall 1983).

49. Allan Greenspan et al., Incidence of Unwarranted Implantation of Permanent Cardiac Pacemakers in a Large Medical Population, 318 *N. Engl. J. Med.* 158 (1988).

50. For examples of using this putative distinction or misusing it where it exists, see Gerald Turino et al., The Potential for Conflict of Interest of Members of the American Thoracic Society, 137 *Am. Rev. Respir.* Dis. 489 (1988). *Also, see* Tom L. Beauchamp, Ethical Guidelines for Epidemiologists, 44 (Suppl. I) *J. Clin. Epidemiol.* 151S (1991), and *Guidelines for Dealing with Faculty Conflicts of Commitment and Conflicts of Interest in Research*, adopted by the Executive Council of the Association of American Medical Colleges, February 22, 1990.

51. Perhaps some of these points apply to the idea of a potential CI as well.

52. For more ideas about disclosure (some of which I think wrong), see Dan Brock, Medicine and Business: An Unhealthy Mix?, 9 *Bus. Prof. Ethics J.* 21 (1990); Luebke, *supra* note 8; and Shimm and Spece, *supra* 26.

53. I am grateful to Mark Waymack of Loyola University (Chicago), who suggested the ideas about the three rival ethics in a letter of October 25, 1991.

54. Here structural elements of CIs would be present, as in all cases. But their weight is so light that mentioning danger, temptation, and so on would be inappropriate.

55. In effect, I am here showing that Pellegrino's call for self-effacing behavior (See *Samples of the Provacative and Paradoxical*, Item 4, in the text of this chapter.) might be horribly misleading; our understanding of the role of the physician requires neither financial nor physical martyrdom. Something seems muddled in his position.

56. We must, however, remember that a more adequate definition would allude to the performative agenda that speakers have in language games in which "conflict of interest" is a tool of communication.

57. *See,* e.g., Elizabeth Kolbert, New York's Medicaid Costs Surge, But Health Care for the Poor Lags, *New York Times* 1, 26 (April 14, 1991). She writes, "New York's reimbursement rates for private physicians are so low—in some categories they are second lowest after West Virginia's—that only 25 per cent of the state's doctors regularly treat Medicaid patients."

58. Note that here there is only an assumption that practitioners have a duty to treat Medicaid patients.

59. My thinking on this has been stimulated by that of Bernard Gert, especially in *The Moral Rules* (1975).
60. I am grateful to H. T. Engelhardt, Jr., for making this point vivid.
61. For criteria for deciding which CIs should be forbidden or eschewed, see Brock, *supra* note 52.
62. In contrast to Hazard's very helpful analysis in note 1, I think that "conflict of interest" has different rules of use in medicine than in professions, such as law. I am not sure that Hazard takes seriously enough the limits due to differences in economics that he notes on comparing them directly.

    In contrast to Luebke, supra at note 8, Hazard and I recognize that many values can generate CIs, not just economic ones. Hazard takes conflicting obligations to be part of the architecture of the concept, whereas I find that sometimes distinguishing conflicting loyalties from CIs may be important. For example, having duties to more than one patient and being unable to fulfill one without violating another is a dilemma but not a CI. To be sure, a physician's dedication to an ideal (*e.g.*, to do research) can sometimes be said to generate CIs.

    Hazard and I largely agree on the logic of practical interests in constituting CIs; however, he considers billing at an excessive rate a CI, while I reject that label (noting that it may be immoral for other reasons).

    Regarding what I call "predilections," Hazard's account and mine overlap extensively. His is especially helpful in explaining the professional's interest in defining and controlling the relationship with the client-patient. He considers this psychological exploitation. His points overlap with those of Kassirer, *supra* note 38, who states that to control uncertainty and potential malpractice litigation, physicians deprive patients of options important to them. Hazard indicates how this concern for control may lead both the practitioner and the patient to feel frustrated by elaborate explanations of diagnosis and treatment plans.

    Hazard shows how the descriptive indicators of CIs are not fully avoidable and that one must be concerned only about those that pose a "significant risk" of "material adverse effects." This is close to the position of Lynn, at note 18, but it shows Hazard's sensitivity to the role of performative agendas in giving accounts of meaning. That is what I aim to emphasize. In effect, we are saying that one should have a point to make, a goal to achieve when using the language of CIs. Potential candidates of performative meaning include warning, insinuating, explaining, and alleging. To use the descriptive indicators without clarity about the performative ones is conceptually and morally dangerous. It can mislead us about the shape and limits of duty, which includes the (limited) rights of professionals to pursue their ideals, practical interests, and predilections. Thus, Hazard is at least tacitly aware of the role of performative meaning in the use of language about CIs. However, he does not seem aware of the equivocation in the descriptive indicators: They can allude either to motives or to social structures.
63. I am grateful to Marvin Herring, Donald Light, Melody Ritt, and Anthony Serafini for comments on earlier drafts. I am especially grateful to Roy G. Spece, Jr., for many valuable comments.

3

Discovering the Ethical Requirements of Physicians' Roles in the Service of Conflicting Interests as Healers and as Citizens

David S. Shimm and Roy G. Spece, Jr.

Introduction

To avoid or properly manage conflicts of interest, physicians first must be able to recognize them. Erde argues in Chapter 2, however, that a set of necessary and sufficient conditions defining conflict of interest does not exist. Rather, the issue can be understood only by identifying certain attributes that, in particular combinations, constitute conflicts of interest in actual settings. Erde nevertheless offers a plausible general definition of what he calls the descriptive elements of conflicts of interest: "Either motives that caregivers have and/or situations in which we could reasonably think caregivers' responsibilities to observe, judge, and act according to the moral requirements of their role are compromised." He emphasizes that *conflicting interests* do not necessarily constitute *conflicts of interest*. Motives or situations that connote possible deviation from the ethical requirements of the physician's role are necessary to transform the former into the latter.

As indicated in Chapter 1, we have adopted Erde's analysis and his general definition of conflicts of interest. The purpose of this chapter is to probe various sources from which one can delineate the particular combinations of attributes or aspects of our culture that constitute conflicts of interest in specific health care settings.

The Pertinence of Ethical Theory

To identify a conflict of interest depends on the ethical requirements of a role, and the ethical requirements of a role depend on ethical judgments and, ultimately, ethical theory. Yet there are competing ethical judgments and especially ethical theories. To resolve these differences, one can refer to the professional codes like the American Medical Association's Code of Ethics. One can also refer to legal pronouncements characterizing certain conduct as a conflict of interest. As we will explore below, however, professional codes and legal pronouncements are incomplete and sometimes misleading sources of ethical information about conflicts of interest. We must therefore refer to ethical theory in the broad philosophical sense. Professionals determined to avoid or to manage conflicts of interest must understand the ethical standards that identify a conflict of interest in the first place.

This chapter will set forth some basic principles of ethical theory, describe a form of ethical theory that can guide physicians, discuss criteria to judge competing ethical theories (metaethical criteria), and identify some basic principles that bioethicists—even those who draw on different ethical theories—have judged as helpful to guide decision-making.

Although physicians cannot be expected to become philosophy professors, their responsibilities require that they conscientiously strive to apply coherent ethical principles and rules to do the right thing in each given situation. They must cultivate the disposition and abilities to distinguish ethical from factual questions and to attack both with vigor, discipline, logic, and sensitivity. Writings on ethical theory and its application to medicine are an obligatory source of information on the ethical requirements of the physician role and proper management of conflicts of interest in that role. Additional sources include (1) literature addressing the physician–patient relationship, (2) pertinent legal materials, and (3) ethical codes for physicians.[1]

Literature That Addresses the Physician–Patient Relationship

The literature examining the physician–patient relationship has described several models of this relationship that illustrate certain principles derived from, and central to, the ethical theories alluded to in *Some Basic Ethical Concepts* (below). These principles are beneficence, nonmaleficence, truth telling, autonomy, and justice. We will apply the models and the ethical principles that inform them to various clinical settings where physicians must face conflicting interests. However, literature on the physician–patient relationship generally ignores an important dimension of the physician role that Hazard describes in Chapter 4 as being essential to "professionalism": fealty to the interests of specific third parties and society generally (as well as to the interests of specific patients or clients).[2] The same criticism applies to the literature on biomedical ethical theories.[3] To deal with the problem of attention to third party and societal interests, we will propose two additional models of the physician role for analysis of situations in which interests of specific third parties or society generally might compete with the physician's or patient's interests: (1) the good-citizen model and (2) the dual agency model.

Ethical Codes

Although they offer insight into the physician role, physician ethical codes are also preoccupied with the physician–patient relationship to the exclusion of external obligations. There are several additional problems with ethical codes as a source of information about the physician role. First, they are promulgated by physicians, with an incentive to define the role to their benefit, a clear conflict of interest. A second and related point is that many of the historical roots of physician ethical codes can be traced to the Hippocratic Oath, which is part of a philosophy based on self-interest embraced by a minority sect of physicians over 2000 years ago.[4] This pedigree hardly connotes morality. Third, physicians have no special insight into the moral sentiments of society or training in ethical theory. They have the expertise to describe the facts on which ethical judgments in medical practice must be based, but even here, self-interest might cloud their judgment. Thus, they would not appear to have any special qualifications to formulate ethical codes. Fourth, most current ethical codes are so general and hortatory as to offer little practical guidance. Finally, ethical codes are promulgated by unelected and unrepresentative subgroups of physicians. Only a minority of physicians belong to the AMA,[5] the most influential medical body to promulgate a code of physician ethics. Indeed, as pointed out by Moore in Chapter 8, even various bodies within the AMA have disagreed on ethical standards concerning physicians' entrepreneurial activities. Nevertheless, ethical codes at least provide evidence of what some physicians consider to be their proper role in certain settings.

Legal Pronouncements

The law provides the fourth and final source of information about the physician role that we will examine. The law cannot directly teach us what is right; it is a common saw that law does not equal morality. Legal enforcement of morality might lead to greater wrong. For example, even if a person has an ethical duty to donate bone marrow necessary to save a relative, it might be a greater evil to coerce this contribution by law. Much law is, moreover, simply the expression of majority or special interest group preferences. The majority or special interest groups can act in their own interests to the detriment of less favored viewpoints. Certain constitutional checks aside, much law is founded, furthermore, on little more than the notion that we must continue past practices so that persons will be able to predict the consequences of their actions and behave accordingly. The large portions of law based on prejudice or routine are not promising sources of insight into the ethical requirements of the physician role.

Nonetheless, certain aspects of the law are a rich source of moral information about the physician role and about the reconciliation of values touched by medical practice and conflicts of interest within that practice. We will explore clinical practice and research contexts within which the law has either required, tolerated, or prohibited consideration of third-party or societal interests in addition to patients' direct interests, and we will compare various legal approaches to those resulting from applying different models of the physician–patient relationship.

Some Basic Ethical Concepts to Assist Physicians' Management of Conflicts of Interest[6]

The two major categories of ethical theories are consequentialist and nonconsequentialist. Consequentialist theories specify "good" and then define "right" actions as those maximizing that good. In contrast, nonconsequentialist theories rely on principles and rules that place constraints on our efforts to maximize the attainment of whatever ends we regard as good and even limit the range of ends it is ethically permissible to pursue. Nonconsequentialist theories take consequences into account but do not define the right as whatever maximizes some good, specified independently of considerations of rightness (or justice).

The best-known consequentialist theory is utilitarianism. It holds that the good is utility and the right is that which brings about the greatest net utility, with utility defined differently by various utilitarian schools. One common utilitarian theory identifies utility with "happiness." Others specify utility as "pleasure" or as simply the satisfaction of preferences. Some have criticized utilitarianism as sanctioning practices inconsistent with some of the most widely held and fundamental moral principles concerning fairness, just desserts, and equality of persons. For example, it could countenance random punishment of innocent persons if such a system were shown to deter crime and ultimately lead to a net gain in good. Some utilitarians have responded to this criticism by embracing "rule" rather than "act" utilitarianism. Rule utilitarianism calculates net value by examining the *expected consequences of rules or institutions* as opposed to the consequences of isolated acts. Act utilitarianism would justify random punishment, while rule utilitarianism would judge it as an institution or course of conduct and determine it to be counterproductive in the long run, since it would ultimately corrupt and terrorize society, thus creating a net loss.

There are many forms of nonconsequentialist theory. One form that has been very influential in contemporary normative ethics generally, and in biomedical ethics specifically, is contractarian theory. Contract theorists attempt to derive certain principles and rules (which establish certain rights and obligations, rather than focusing directly on consequences) to govern ethical decision-making from a hypothetical contract among members of society. Although these principles or rules may govern the basic structure of social institutions, they have implications for individual cases. This basic notion is open to the objection that one can manipulate the supposed contract to construct principles or rules that will justify nearly any action or institution. One response of particular relevance to someone interested in conflicts of interest is that, to avoid the possibility of persons designing the social contract to favor themselves, one can posit that the parties to the hypothetical contract be placed in a situation of impartiality. In Rawls' version of social contract theory, impartiality is ensured by the stipulation that the parties must reach agreement behind a "veil of ignorance" that denies them any information about their own particular interests and socioeconomic position that might bias their choice of principles.[7]

There exist metaethical criteria to judge the relative strength of competing ethical theories. Useful metaethical criteria have been listed by Beauchamp and Childress: the theory should (1) be "as clear as possible"; (2) be "internally coherent" and "consistent"; (3) be as "complete and comprehensive as possible" in listing moral principles and their implications"; (4) be as simple as possible; (5) "provide enough insight to help us understand the moral life" ("explanatory power"); (6) "give us grounds for justified belief" and "have the power to criticize defective beliefs, no matter how widely accepted" ("justificatory power"); (7) be able to produce "judgments that were not in the original data base of particular and general considered judgments on which the theory was constructed" ("output power"); and (8) not have "requirements" so demanding that they probably cannot be satisfied by or could be satisfied by only a few extraordinary persons or communities.[8] No theory will be found without objection on some ground. The task is to choose the best course.[9]

Beauchamp and Childress have used contract theory to construct an ethical decision-making process relevant to physicians. They distinguish among principles, rules, and judgments that can be derived from an overarching contract theory. Principles are the broad descriptions of values or clusters of values derived from an ethical theory to guide ethical decision-making. Rules are derived from principles and apply to a specific context. Finally, judgments are specific decisions made in the setting of individual cases.

Beauchamp and Childress' principles are (1) respect for autonomy, (2) nonmaleficence, (3) beneficence, and (4) justice. "Respect for autonomy" requires "treating agents so as to allow or to enable them to" act when their actions substantially comply with the requirements that they act "(1) intentionally, (2) with understanding, and (3) without controlling influences that determine the action."[10] "Nonmaleficence" is the principle that "one ought not inflict evil or harm," and "beneficence" requires "preventing evil or harm, removing evil or harm, and doing or promoting good."[11] Formally, justice means that "equals must be treated equally, and unequals must be treated unequally."[12]

There are many theories of justice that try to describe when persons are equal and the respects in which persons ought to be treated equally. Beauchamp and Childress identify distributive justice (to whom should scarce resources be given) as a central problem in health care. They argue that several general conceptions can illuminate issues of justice and medical practice. Utilitarian conceptions of justice contribute the insight that in devising a rational system of distribution "we must balance public and private benefit, predicted cost savings, the probability of failure, and the magnitude of risks." Libertarian theory adds the perspective that a system of distribution should attend to "free-market procedures of acquiring property, legitimately transferring that property, and rectification for those who had property illegitimately extracted or otherwise were illegitimately obstructed in the free-market." Egalitarian theory emphasizes the need for "fair equality of opportunity."[13]

Beauchamp and Childress argue that none of the four principles is sacrosanct. Each creates a prima facie obligation that must be honored unless sufficient justification to overcome the obligation is offered. When the principles clash, they must be balanced and reconciled.[14]

Veatch has developed a similar theory. He posits three social contracts.[15] The first, among members of society, establishes basic ethical principles and rules for society: "It is what contractors taking the moral point of view (the outlook that other people's welfare is considered on the same scale as one's own) would invent or discover or have revealed to them as the basic ethical principles for society."[16] Veatch posits a second contract between society and a profession that specifies, from the same ethical point of view, "the special role-specific duties regarding interactions between lay people and professionals."[17] The only limit of this second contract is that it must not contravene the more basic social contract. Finally, within the context of these two contracts, individual professionals and patients can articulate, in a third contract, further terms, ethical and otherwise, of their specific relationship.[18]

The basic principles that Veatch derives to guide physicians are beneficence, promise or contract keeping, autonomy, honesty, avoiding killing, and justice. Most of these terms resemble the principles derived by Beauchamp and Childress. Veatch lumps nonmaleficence and beneficence together, and he observes that they can be calculated from the individual or societal perspective. In either event, because they are calculated from consequences, he judges them to be subsidiary to the nonconsequentialist principles. When the nonconsequentialist principles clash, they must be balanced and reconciled in a reasoned, proportionate manner.[19] Veatch also argues that, in many instances, it will be helpful to address recurring situations, to analyze them according to the principles, and then to generate more specific rules that will govern similar situations.[20]

Some ethical theorists criticize their colleagues like Beauchamp, Childress, and Veatch for undue attention to principles and rules. They argue that the virtues of the decision maker—the possession of morally excellent character traits—are more important than abstract theories, principles, and rules, and that specific theories, principles, and rules represent "cookbook" ethics.[21] Two important virtues that such writers emphasize for physicians are the desire to do what is right and the conscientiousness to exert the effort necessary to carry out the desire. Veatch observes that good intentions can lead to abhorrent ethical judgments, and he is skeptical of an exclusive emphasis on virtues.[22] Beauchamp and Childress express the same concerns but recognize that virtues play a significant role.[23]

A final ethical concept that should prove useful to physicians is "reflective equilibrium,"[24] the ideal end point of a dialectical process whereby decision - makers strive to match their general ethical principles to their considered moral judgments about concrete cases. The goal (which may never be fully realized) is to arrive at a small set of mutually consistent general principles that not only are consistent with, but also support, the full range of concrete considered moral judgments. In this process, one may revise general principles formerly found attractive if they clash with more confident, considered judgments. Adjustment may proceed in the other direction as well: Awareness that a particular judgment is inconsistent with a general principle to which one is deeply committed (and which supports many other particular judgments about which one is very confident) may lead one to jettison the particular judgment while retaining the general principle. The basic principles that Beauchamp and Childress articulate can be supported by the method of reflective equilibrium, as well as by hypothetical contract reasoning.

To summarize to this point, conflicts of interest cannot be defined without ethical analysis; ethical analysis is possible; although no perfect ethical theory exists, metaethical criteria to judge the relative merits of ethical theories do exist; ethical theories must account for general moral sentiments and avoid partiality and bias that favor particular interests; and the contractarian theories constructed by Beauchamp and Childress and by Veatch can assist physicians in ethical decision-making. Relevant principles include respect for autonomy, nonmaleficence, beneficence, justice, promise or contract keeping, honesty, and avoiding killing. These principles should be honored unless they clash or unless strong justification is presented. When they clash, a reasoned accommodation must be undertaken. Ethical decision-making is not like solving a mathematical equation. There is often considerable dispute about which principles and rules should be adopted generally or applied in a specific case, and there is no easy method by which to weight conflicting values. Nevertheless, physicians must embrace the virtue of conscientiousness, that is, the willingness to undertake ethical reasoning and abide by its results. Furthermore, the method of reflective equilibrium can supplement or substitute for contractarian approaches to the articulation of systematic ethical views for physicians and others. These conclusions should be kept in mind as we continue the search for insight into the ethical requirements of the physician role and proper management of conflicts of interest by exploring literature regarding that role, as well as pertinent legal and ethical code principles that have been applied in various clinical settings.

Literature on the Physician–Patient Relationship

Drawing on the notion of a contract between society and physicians espoused by Veatch and others, this section will seek insights into the nature of that contract—particularly its provisions related to obligations to third parties and society generally—by examining various articulations of the physician–patient relationship. We draw on an article authored by Drs. Ezekiel and Linda Emanuel: "Four Models of the Physician–Patient Relationship."[25] Drawing from previous writing on the physician–patient relationship, the authors describe four models: *paternalistic, informative, interpretive*, and *deliberative*. The Emanuels explain:

> [T]he models are Weberian ideal types. They may not describe any particular physician–patient interactions but highlight, free from complicating details, different visions of the essential characteristics of the physician–patient interaction. Consequently, they do not embody minimum ethical or legal standards, but rather constitute regulative ideals that are "higher than the law" but not "above the law."[26]

We do not advance these models to prescribe physician behavior or to suggest that all cases or certain cases be treated as suggested by any one model. Rather, we explore these models to illuminate physicians' roles in specific cases. The goal is to distinguish situations or motives that involve conflicting interests, on the one hand, from conflicts of interest, on the other hand. The models can be explored by examining their treatment of several common issues: patient autonomy, patient values, the role of the physicians' values, the role of third-party and societal interests, physicians' overall role, and conformity with the ethical principles espoused by Beauchamp, Childress, and Veatch.

The paternalistic model gives little content or weight to the patient's autonomy or values. At most, the patient assents to the physician's recommendations. The physician determines what is best for the patient's well-being, and the model assumes that what is best for the patient is objective, common to patients generally (though perhaps different from the patient's short-term preferences), and knowable to the physician with little interaction with the patient. The physician's overall role is essentially one of guardian.[27] This model focuses exclusively on beneficence and nonmaleficence. In relegating patient autonomy to a secondary position, the model clashes with the theories of both Veatch and Beauchamp and Childress. The model also pays no attention to third-party or societal interests.

The informative model conceives of patient autonomy as "choice of, and control over, medical care." Patients' values are assumed to be fixed and salient to them as individuals. This model requires the physician to describe all potential management options so that the patient can choose among them based on his own preferences. There "is no role for the physician's values, the physician's understanding of the patient's values, or his or her judgment of the worth of the patients values."[28] The interests of third parties or society are given no attention unless the patient's preferences explicitly include such interests. The overall role of the physician is to be "a competent technical expert."[29] This model favors patient autonomy (albeit a crimped version) over beneficence and nonmaleficence.

The interpretive model resembles the informative model by providing the patient with information regarding the nature of his condition and the risks and benefits of possible interventions. The conception of patient autonomy, however, is not of "control" but rather of "self-understanding relevant to medical care." The caregiver "assists the patient in elucidating and articulating his values and in determining what medical interventions best realize the specified values."[30] Although the physician helps the patient understand his own values, he does not inject his own values into the process. His role is that of "counselor or adviser" rather than "friend or teacher." Consequently, the physician does not interject third- party or societal interests unless that is necessary to elucidate the patient's own values.[31] This model emphasizes the same principles as the informative model, but it embraces more sophisticated definitions of autonomy and truth telling.

The deliberative model—the Emanuels' preferred model—conceives patient autonomy as "moral self-development relevant to medical care." The patient must make the ultimate choices, but the physician, as "friend or teacher," is encouraged to draw on his own values in an attempt to influence the patient's choice and development of values. The Emanuels caution: "The physician discusses only health-related values, that is, values that affect or are affected by the patient's disease and treatments; he or she recognizes that many elements of morality are unrelated to the patient's disease or treatment and beyond the scope of their professional relationship."[32] The deliberative model thus *allows* interjection of third-party and societal interests that are not directly relevant within the other models.

The Emanuels give the example of a physician recommending a course of treatment for a 43-year-old premenopausal woman with a (lymph) node-negative breast cancer to illustrate the differences between the deliberative and interpretive models. She was recently divorced and has gone back to work. The physician has recommended lumpectomy and radiation treatment rather than more extensive surgery. Regarding chemotherapy, the deliberative physician might explain that participation in a study involving chemotherapy could ensure excellent medical care and altruistically contribute to developing knowledge that might benefit women with breast cancer.[33] On the other hand, the interpretive physician might discourage chemotherapy, explaining that it would prolong therapy for months without any certain benefits at a time when the patient is undergoing a great deal of other stress.[34]

Brief consideration of this case study illuminates the usefulness of the models articulated by the Emanuels to analysis of conflicts of interest. Assuming that "interpretation" did not discover altruistic sentiments, the interpretive physician would deviate from the ethical requirements of his role if he were to recommend consideration of a clinical trial involving chemotherapy for altruistic reasons. He would arguably be guilty of a conflict of interest by foisting his own sentiments on an already burdened patient. On the other hand, the deliberative physician would be expected to engage in such "altruistic" discussion. He would not be guilty of any conflict of interest by so doing. Indeed, if he declined to discuss altruism because of fear of offending and losing his patient, along with the fees involved, he would, in that event, arguably be guilty of a conflict of interest between his obligation to science and future patients and his own selfish interest in keeping his patient and her fees.[35]

The deliberative model also emphasizes generously defined principles of autonomy and truth telling over beneficence. However, it also gives weight to considerations of justice toward society, and it is willing to risk at least some maleficence or harm (or at least the absence of maximal benefit) to patients to achieve such justice. This is demonstrated by the hypothetical case that allows risking harm to the patient's feelings by suggesting that she give weight to altruistic concerns about future patients.

The Emanuels briefly mention and quickly reject a fifth, *instrumental* model in which "the patients' values are irrelevant; the physician aims for some goal independent of the patient, such as the good of society or furtherance of scientific knowledge."[36] He does not try to influence the patient's values to encompass broader interests, but directly acts to further those interests regardless of the patient's values. They cite the infamous Tuskegee syphilis study on unwitting black men as an example of the instrumental model in practice.[37] The Emanuels have too quickly glossed over this model because, in fact, there are aspects of the physician role that turn to third-party and societal interests. These aspects are not necessarily founded on improper use of the patient as a means to some higher goal. Instead, a thorough account of the physician role must recognize that both physicians and patients are parts of human communities.

We propose, therefore, a sixth, overarching model of the physician: the *good citizen* model. The physician always occupies this role, regardless of the model that characterizes his direct interaction with specific patients. As a *citizen*, the physician must act for the good of specific third parties or society when the patient poses a threat of disproportionate harm. What constitutes "disproportionate" harm is an ethical judgment concerning the principle of justice, which we will discuss further in the section, "Law Relevant to the Physician Role and Conflicts of Interest" (see below). We emphasize that the presumption is in favor of patient interests, and overcoming this presumption requires strong justification.

As a good citizen, the physician is not required to become directly involved in any political or service groups typically associated with social status. However, he is required to act in all of his affairs so as to benefit his patients and society. When he does speak to or become involved in public issues, he speaks for the good and right rather than for his self-interests or the special interests of the medical profession. We base these mandates on our assumption, using Veatch's general theory, that persons adopting the ethical position—that is, a position not based on self-interest—would make them provisions of the contract between society and the medical profession. As Buchanan points out in Chapter 5, society has a right to expect such public-spirited behavior as a quid pro quo for the special economic and regulatory privileges afforded to physicians.

Law Relevant to the Physician Role and Conflicts of Interest

While some law reflects nothing more than majority or special interest group preference, other law is rich with sound moral content. Legislative acts are the legal pronouncements most likely to be based on majority or special interests.[38] The legislative process is not designed to perform the dialectic analysis most helpful to discovery of the good and right. Thus, we will not explore legislative acts to gain insights into the ethical expectations of the physician role but will focus instead on court decisions. However, we mention several categories of laws that show that our society often *requires* physicians to consider third-party and societal interests: laws that (1) require physicians (or others) to ask relatives of brain-dead patients whether they are willing to donate the patients' tissues or organs ("required request"); (2) require reporting of infectious diseases, injuries (such as gunshot wounds) indicative of criminal conduct, and child and elder abuse; (3) provide for involuntary civil commitment; (4) allow breach of confidentiality to permit utilization and quality review; (5) require immunizations; and (6) specifically speak to physicians' financial conflicts of interest. As to the latter, Hall, Mitchell, Moore, Morreim, and Rodwin explain in Chapters 8, 9, 10, 11, and 13 that various federal and state laws prohibit certain physician conduct on the basis of conflicts of interest.

Although this chapter will not address legislation, it will explore two general areas of law—negligence and constitutional law—insofar as they affect certain clinical settings that are rife with conflicting interests. Negligence law and constitutional law are rich with moral content. They are substantially grounded in a search for what is fair for society *and* individuals.[39] They are generated, moreover, in a dialectic process that is compatible with discovery of the good and right. The formulation, litigation, and adjudication stages provide ample opportunity for articulation of competing perspectives, policies, concerns, and values. Moreover, deliberation by neutral judges and juries bound by broad standards based on individual rights and community values approximates the "moral perspective" hypothesized by Veatch. Therefore, negligence and constitutional law decisions can indicate which provisions of the social contracts—among persons, between society and professions, and between individual professionals and clients/patients—Veatch's "ideal" contractors might choose.

Yet, juries, trial judges, and appellate court justices often disagree. Therefore, one must carefully examine legal opinions for their underlying logic, sensitivity, and resonance with moral sentiments. Lines of opinions, concepts, and values can serve as ethical guideposts. Here we chart the outlines of various legal approaches to facilitate consideration of interests, values, and norms relevant to conflicts of interest in clinical practice and research.

Negligence is a civil law concept that basically provides that all persons have a duty to behave as a hypothetical "reasonable person" so as to avoid harming others. When a professional is involved, the hypothetical reasonable person steps into the shoes of the professional. Doctors, then, are expected to behave as the hypothetical "reasonable doctor."

Generally, one cannot be held liable for refusing to act unless one has a specific duty to do so. A duty positively to help as opposed simply to refrain from inflicting harm generally is created only when there is a special relationship between the injured party and the one alleged to have been negligent. Such an affirmative duty is generally placed on doctors only when a physician–patient relationship has been created.

Such a duty can be breached only if the physician acted unreasonably. Here the law has been especially deferential to the medical profession. It has generally held that the reasonable standard of care is to be determined by what physicians presumably commonly know or do. On the other hand, there is always a possibility that the entire community of physicians will be found to have been unreasonable in their lack of knowledge or adequate practice. Ultimately, the determination of "reasonableness" is an ethical determination about what is right in the given situation—precisely because it is always an open question whether an entire community of physicians has been negligent. The determination takes into account the interests of the plaintiff, the defendant, directly interested third parties, and society. It has been described as a "moral calculus of risk" that balances the benefits and costs of the defendant's conduct.[40] It is not, however, a simple utilitarian calculation. The determination of reasonableness is to be guided by underlying goals, including compensation or placement of losses on the party at "fault," deterrence of improper conduct, retribution for aggravated conduct (rarely), and protection of important rights.[41] The judge instructs the jury as to the law. The jury then finds the facts and applies its "community" moral sentiments and the law imparted to it. The law embodies ethical norms and moral judgments. The judge can set aside the jury's determination if it does not comport with the law or with any conceivable version of the facts. These determinations are then subject to review by appellate courts. The substantive determination of reasonableness—especially in recurring sets of circumstances—is, therefore, an ethical judgment generated in a dialectic process of discovery.

Constitutional law is uniquely tied to ethics because, among other points: (1) constitutions speak in particularly vague, but value-laden, phrases such as "due process of law" that invite judges to perform ethical analysis, and (2) the very idea of federal and state constitutions is to place certain rights beyond the reach of majoritarian political processes. The best judges draw on history, public policy, morality, and ethics to interpret the broad and ambiguous statements in constitutions. In theory, judges, especially judges with lifetime tenure, are in a position to approach the ideal of fully informed but disinterested decision-makers posited by some social contract theorists.

Consider, then, how negligence and constitutional law have spoken to selected clinical settings, chosen for the insight they might give into the physician role and conflicts of interest that arise in that role. We will attempt to address the neglected issue of physicians' obligations to third parties and society by examining particular contexts: (1) where physicians are hired by persons or entities to examine "patients" for the sole benefit of the hirer; (2) where physicians are hired to provide care to patients for the dual benefit of the hirer and the patients; (3) where the physician simultaneously treats two or more related patients; and (4) where the law might either *require* or *forbid* physicians to act to protect third-party or societal interests that might diverge from the interests of their patients.

The Primary Client Is Not the Patient

One situation where the patient's interests alone cannot control occurs when the physician is hired to examine patients for the benefit of the hirer—for example, a physician performing preemployment physicals. In some circumstances, the physician might consider it to be in the best interest of the prospective employee to withhold information the employer has explicitly contracted to receive. Nevertheless, if the contract is valid, the physician has a legal obligation to provide the information that he has promised to obtain and supply.

Here models of the physician–patient relationship seem generally beside the point. Indeed, some courts approach such situations by assuming that the physician's only duty is to refrain from affirmatively harming the prospective employee, in effect denying that a physician–patient relationship exists.[42] Other courts, however, hold that a physician has a duty at least to *disclose* critical information—such as a diagnosis of cancer—found within the scope of the examination ordered by the employer.[43] Some authority finds, more stringently, that the physician has a duty to act reasonably so as to *find* and disclose important information that a reasonable physician would discover within the scope of the examination ordered by the employer.[44]

None of the legal authorities envisions involvement of the physician beyond the modicum that might be required by the informative model of the physician–patient relationship. (The paternalistic model is also not applicable because it requires the physician to act as the patient's agent and to focus on the patient's interests alone.) A proper ethical position would place the physician's obligation where the most stringent legal approach places it: The physician must refrain from inflicting injury and must competently find and disclose pertinent information within the scope of the intended examination.[45]

It can be argued that an employer might legitimately wish to forbid an examining physician to give *any* information or advice to patients, reasoning that the physician and the employer could be exposed to lawsuits for giving incorrect information, but that not giving any information protects them. It can be further argued that the physician could fulfill any obligation to the patient by simply disclosing that (1) he will not disclose pertinent information to the patient and (2) he should not be held responsible for or relied on competently to perform the examination ordered by the employer. We reject these arguments because they do not comport with what persons acting from the moral position would find to be terms of the contract between the medical profession and society. Society must demand of and foster in physicians an unremitting desire and inclination to respect and communicate with patients. Telling patients they have no remedy for harm caused by incompetent examinations or intended nondisclosure of important information breeds contempt for physicians and undermines their self-respect. It would violate the principle of beneficence. Moreover, the principles of autonomy and truth telling mandate that patients be fully informed before the examination that pertinent categories of information will be disclosed to the employer, and that they be told after the examination whether further care by another physician is advisable.

Putting this in terms of conflicts of interest, examining physicians, in a descriptive sense, always have a conflict of interest or obligation.[46] The structure of their role is such that they have duties to both employers and employees/patients. Moreover, the interests of employers and employees often conflict. For example, an employer might wish to discover an infirmity that a prospective employee wishes to hide and perhaps does not even consider to be an infirmity. The potential for improper reconciliation of these conflicting interests merits characterization of the examining physician role as one of conflict of interest. Nevertheless, the examining physician role is socially necessary, and we accept the conflict of interest that it entails. We might label this, then, a "soft" conflict of interest—that is, a conflict of interest that is socially acceptable.

Within the ethically expected role we have described for examining physicians, there would be a "hard" conflict of interest (i.e., one that should not be tolerated) if, whether out of self-interest or undue solicitude toward the employer, an examining physician planned either (1) to not inform the patient of the scope of the proposed examination and expected disclosure to the employer or (2) to not competently find and report to the patient information reasonably available within the scope of the intended examination.[47] Conversely, the physician would be guilty of a hard conflict of interest if, in a misguided benevolent attempt to help a person get a job, he planned not to disclose information the employer had legitimately contracted to receive. In this instance, the physician would deviate from his socially expected role by ignoring his duties to the employer. This example highlights the dual nature of the physician's duties. It might be useful to capture such situations within another model of the physician–patient relationship—a dual agency model. In this model, the relationship between the physician and the examinee is a physician–patient relationship, with the special or fiduciary duties that entails. The relationship between the physician and his employer or hirer, on the other hand, is simply a contractual one.

Case Study 1. Consider an actual case in which a physician is hired to determine an employee's fitness to return to work. In *Anhert v. Wildman,*[48] a railroad fireman was hospitalized for depression. When he was discharged by his attending physician, the railroad's physician did not allow him to return to work for several additional months. His health insurance policies required certification of inability to return to work before payments would be made. The fireman's attending physician refused to fill out the forms, presumably because he felt that the patient could work. The company physician also refused to fill out the forms, for undisclosed reasons, but one can speculate that the employer had a policy against such involvement. One can further speculate that the employer did not want to assist any insurance claims that might worsen its employees' claims experience and lead to higher future premiums.

The fireman sued the company physician. The court held that although a treating or attending physician has a legal obligation to fill out insurance forms, an examining physician has no such duty. His relationship and duty generally run solely to the one who hired him.

We disagree, arguing that the company doctor had a conflict of interest and unethically refused to fill out the forms. Professionals must not only meet minimum legal requirements but also act morally. They must, to some extent, place patients' and society's interests above their own. This entails some sacrifice, but that is part of what it means to be a professional.[49] We argue that sacrifice is part of the quid pro quo physicians promise to society in return for the substantial autonomy and privileges granted to the medical profession. One can reasonably conclude that, in this case, it is not ethically permissible for the physician to place either the employer's weak and greedy interests, or even the physician's legitimate concern with possible retaliation by his employer,[50] above the fireman's strong claim to be given either his right to work or the insurance benefits promised to him when unable to work. We endorse the line of cases that hold that an examining physician owes a duty to competently examine, find, and convey information to patients. Any other view would demean physicians in the eyes of patients, fail to minimize harm to patients, breed shoddy habits, and undercut physicians' self-respect. Here the dual agency model comes into play. The physician has an ordinary contractual obligation to the employer. However, he has a higher obligation—a fiduciary duty—to the employee/patient. The ethical calculus of risk entailed in negligence law requires no less, and the best legal authorities have recognized this. Moreover, the principles of autonomy, beneficence, and truth telling all require proper diagnosis and disclosure. The same conclusion is dictated through determination of the requirements of the principle of justice by discovering what persons contracting from the ethical point of view would require of physicians in the contract with society, regardless of individual contracts between specific doctors and patients. The narrowest legal authorities, which only require refraining from inflicting harm, are most likely based solely on the utilitarian principle of nonmaleficence.

Case Study 2. Another case that can be analyzed within the dual agency model is *Urbanik v. Newton.*[51] Urbanik suffered a head injury with secondary neck and back strain while working as a machine operator. He sought worker's compensation benefits, alleging inability to work. He was examined by Dr. Newton, who was retained by the attorney for the employer's insurance company in litigation over the industrial claim. In the course of the neurological examination, Dr. Newton fastened reusable metal electrodes to Urbanik's body. When Urbanik was leaving the office, he told Dr. Newton's nurse that she should carefully sterilize the electrodes because he was HIV positive. He emphasized that his HIV status should not be revealed in any report. Dr. Newton prepared a report attributing Urbanik's symptoms to stress—perhaps related to his HIV status—rather than to his work injury.

The court reasoned, first, that there was no physician–patient relationship and, consequently, no duty of confidentiality growing out of such a relationship. It reasoned, second, however, that there was a claim for invasion of privacy under a California constitutional provision because Urbanik "revealed his HIV positive status at a time and for a purpose that had no connection with the medical examination for his workers' compensation case."[52]

Second, concerning the irrelevance of Urbanik's HIV status to the medical exam, it appears that HIV-positive status could *conceivably* cause stress and resulting neck and back pain. That Urbanik was courageous enough to disclose his HIV status does not make it irrelevant. On the other hand, Dr. Newton was all too quick to publicize this information. This is not surprising because it is common knowledge among attorneys that certain physicians embroil themselves in a conflict of interest by becoming "hired guns" for employers or employees (and other contending groups) in litigation. The conflict lies in the apparent desire to invite repeat business from satisfied customers. Whether Dr. Newton acted out of such motives is not clear, but, in any event, if the facts were as Urbanik alleged, Dr. Newton acted unethically. Even if it is assumed that his position regarding the cause of Urbanik's symptoms was correct, he should have reported only that there appeared to be alternative explanations —such as stressful life situations—for Urbanik's symptoms. In broadcasting Urbanik's HIV status, Dr. Newton clearly did not heed the American Occupational Medical Association Code of Ethical Conduct for Physicians Providing Occupational Medical Services, Principle 7 (1976), which admonishes physicians to disclose as little specific information as is necessary.[53] Dr. Newton was an agent for both Urbanik and the employer, but he erroneously acted as if his higher duty was to the employer rather than the patient.

Case Study 3. In *Wickline v. California,*[54] Medi-Cal authorized payment for an aorta-femoral graft and ten days of postoperative hospitalization for a woman with Leriche's syndrome. Surgery was uneventful, but several hours later the patient developed acute circulatory problems in the right leg. She was taken back to the operating room, and a fairly large clot was removed through an arteriotomy. Subsequently, the patient had constant pain in the right lower leg, experienced hallucinatory episodes, and showed marked vascular spasm of the leg, leading to a right lumbar sympathectomy five days after the initial surgery.

Following the latter surgery, the patient seemed to progress well, and her discharge from the hospital was planned for the last day of the authorized stay. However, the day before the scheduled discharge, the vascular surgeon, believing her to be at risk for infection or another thrombotic episode, submitted to

Medi-Cal a request for an eight-day extension of her hospital stay. Medi-Cal, which acted through a reviewing nurse and a nonspecialist physician, granted only a four-day extension. The surgeon did not petition Medi-Cal for reconsideration, and on the fourteenth postoperative day the patient was discharged. At that point, she was stable and her leg seemed to be progressing satisfactorily.

Two days later, she started to experience pain and a change in the appearance of the right leg. The patient assumed that these changes were normal and did not tell anyone about them. On the third day after discharge the pain became severe, and the leg turned grayish. The patient then asked her husband to contact the assistant surgeon, who reassured them and increased the dose of her analgesics.

Over the next few days the pain worsened, and the leg went from grayish to bluish in appearance. When the pain became excruciating and the analgesics no longer worked, the husband contacted the assistant surgeon again. This time he readmitted the patient to the hospital on an emergency basis which did not require pre-authorization from Medi-Cal.

On admission the physician found an infected wound at the site of the right femoral incision and a mottled, cold, and pulseless right leg. Conservative therapy consisting of anticoagulants, antibiotics, bed rest, analgesics, and whirlpool failed. Exactly one month after the initial surgery, the patient's right leg was amputated below the knee. Nine days later another amputation—this time above the knee—was performed.

The patient sued Medi-Cal only. At the trial, the vascular surgeon testified that he believed Medi-Cal had the State of California's, rather than the patient's, interests in mind in authorizing the patient's limited hospital stay. He also testified that he believed Medi-Cal had the authority to dictate to him, the treating physician, when a patient must be discharged. For these reasons, he failed to challenge Medi-Cal's decision, even though his medical judgment was that an eight-day extension was warranted. Both the vascular surgeon and the assistant surgeon agreed, however, that discharge seemed appropriate at the time, in light of the patient's apparently stable condition. However, as the vascular surgeon pointed out, had she remained hospitalized for eight more days, he could have observed the changes in her condition and intervened to save her leg. The court held that Medi-Cal had a duty to act reasonably in its coverage determinations, although this duty was not breached in the instant case. It noted that this duty was limited because Medi-Cal was a government entity, and it implied that non-government third-party payers might have greater obligations. It also observed that treating physicians have an independent duty to advocate for their patients and to act reasonably, regardless of the third-party payer's actions.

At this point, we will only consider the roles of the physicians who participated in promulgation and application of the Medi-Cal guidelines. The former were not addressed at all in the *Wickline* opinion, and the latter were mentioned only in passing. Certain clinical guidelines are developed at a general legislative or executive level, and these are generally immune from legal attack. For example, if, at the highest levels, a state explicitly decides not to cover liver transplants for adults—an exclusion adopted by many public programs—there is no question of liability.[55] The same is true regarding private health plans and *explicit*, properly communicated exclusions from coverage. However, after basic coverage categories are identified and when questions arise about authorized hospital stays, medications, and treatments for disorders not specifically mentioned in the general plan or agreement under a general mandate or agreement to provide "medically necessary care," physicians become at least ethically, and in certain instances probably legally, responsible for the promulgation and application of guidelines.

A December 1992 Report and recommendation[56] to the AMA House of Delegates by the AMA's Council on Ethical and Judicial Affairs (subsequently adopted by the Delegates) speaks to the obligations of physicians in what it calls "administrative roles":

> Physicians in administrative and other nonclinical roles must put the needs of patients first. At least since the time of Hippocrates, physicians have cultivated the trust of their patients by placing patient welfare before all other concerns. The ethical obligations of physicians are not suspended when a physician assumes a position that does not directly involve patient care."

Questions arise as to which "patients" the "administrative physicians" have obligations to. Administrative physicians who promulgate guidelines directly affect groups of patients rather than individuals. Other administrative physicians apply the guidelines to specific patients. Nevertheless, physicians who promulgate guidelines know that if they are too strict, they will inevitably harm individual patients, while physicians who administer the application of guidelines can foresee that if they are too lax, the system might go over budget and perhaps not be able to treat future patients. The question becomes: Where should administrative—and even treating—physicians draw the line between individual and group or societal needs?

Guidance can be found in authorities that examine the related question of society's ethical obligation, if any, to ensure access to a certain level of health care to all citizens. Taken together, these authorities suggest that there is a societal ethical obligation to provide care that is justified by appropriately weighing patients' needs, the care's likely benefits, and alternative uses for the resources consumed by the care—that is, providing "proportionate care." For example, Daniels supposes that parties to a social contract would allocate "fair shares" of basic social goods like health care over a lifetime.[57] Danis and Churchill have built on such reasoning to argue that, within a system that guarantees minimum access to all persons, patients and physicians have duties to society to demand and administer only proportionate care.[58] The President's Commission for the Study of Ethical Problems in Medicine and Biomedical and Behavioral Research has espoused a similar view.[59] Likewise, administrative physicians should only be required to make decisions in favor of proportionate care.

Of course, this leaves unanswered the question of precisely where one draws the line. "Proportionate" is a vague, value-laden term like "due process of law" or "negligence." We can only conceptualize the line here; it must be drawn over time in individual cases, which together will become patterns to guide future conduct. In this process, negligence law will play an important part because it will attach liability to physician line drawing that is determined to be "unreasonable" ("unreasonable" being the legal term of art analogous to the moral term "disproportionate").

Many bioethicists argue, however, that physicians should have no part in making such "rationing" decisions.[60] However, we agree with Hall, who argues in Chapter 10 that such decisions, if properly contained, are inevitable and beneficial. We need not go that far, however, to justify administrative physicians in making such judgments because their role is precisely to prevent disproportionate use of resources. Consider examples of rationing decisions we think appropriate even when made by treating physicians. It would be disproportionate to attempt heart transplants for all persons in cardiac failure for whom no other treatment is available and who have some possibility of benefitting from them. On the other hand, there is a consensus that it would be unreasonable to deny to pregnant women trained medical personnel to attend their labor and delivery despite the rarity of complications.[61]

We essentially endorse, then, the obligations set forth in *Wickline* and the notion of proportionate care espoused by various authorities. All physicians are expected to place individual patients' interests first. This does not mean that they are obliged to be blind to the disproportionate use of resources. On the other hand, administrative physicians cannot, as some have done,[62] argue that their only duty is to the concerns of their corporation or group.

As to treating doctors, they must advocate for their patients whenever the bureaucracy is being intransigent. In close cases, they should resolve doubts in favor of the patient. Under *Wickline*, liability will attach to them whenever they unreasonably capitulate to external pressures. What is reasonable will be determined by reference to what the hypothetical reasonable physician would have done and through application of the moral calculus of risk entailed in negligence law. Author Spece proposes, however, a more stringent standard. As will be explained below, although all physicians are held to the (theoretically) *objective* standard of what is expected from a reasonable physician, physicians with superior knowledge or skills are required to exercise their best judgment. Similarly,

Spece proposes that although all physicians must act reasonably when interfacing with payers, physicians should also be required to act on their *subjective* judgments about payers' proposed limitations of care. In other words, for example, even if a reasonable physician might have acquiesced to the refusal of the requested eight-day extension of hospitalization in *Wickline* (after all, the treating physician opined at trial that the denial was not negligent), the treating physician initially felt the denial was inappropriate and based on illegitimate pecuniary concerns. In such cases, where physicians *subjectively* determine that payers' refusal to authorize care is not right, Spece proposes that physicians be held liable for not appealing and advocating as far as possible within the existing system, even if the hypothetical reasonable physician would have acquiesced. Just as a physician must exercise his best medical judgment if it is superior to that of the hypothetical reasonable physician, he must act on his ethical determinations even if it is inconvenient to do so.[63]

Author Shimm dissents from Spece's position because the obligation Spece would recognize can serve as a disincentive for physicians to ask tough ethical questions. If they ask such questions, they will be held liable if they do not act accordingly. If they persist and protest, however, they will be subject to bureaucratic sanctions with only the notoriously weak protections accorded to whistle blowers.

To summarize the foregoing in conflict of interest terms, an administrative physician is guilty of a conflict of interest if his actions favor the selfish concerns of his organization, while a treating physician is guilty if he either overzealously advocates disproportionate treatment for a patient or lazily fails to advocate for the patient before what he perceives to be a misguided and intransigent bureaucracy.

When a Third Party Hires a Physician to Provide Care to Patients

Another context in which physicians must consider interests other than those of patients is when a third party hires a physician to examine or treat patients for the dual benefit of the hirer and the patients. One example is a sports team hiring a physician to examine and care for its players. This setting is unique. Often physicians actually *pay* professional teams for the privilege of serving as the team doctor. The compensation is the prestige, camaraderie, and visibility the doctor receives with the position. Sometimes the interests of the team and its players are one. For example, the player-patient and the team both generally benefit when the team doctor makes an early and correct diagnosis that results in appropriate treatment and quick recovery. Moreover, the player and the team could both successfully sue if the physician negligently diagnosed or treated the player and this resulted in protracted inability to perform.

However, player and team interests can also be diametrically opposed. The team might feel, for example, that a player is concealing the severity of an injury in order to negotiate a more favorable contract. On the other hand, the player might feel that the team or coach is ready to sacrifice his long-term health interests to obtain immediate success. It is naive to suggest that in such cases the physician can reconcile any conflict by simply doing an excellent technical examination and disclosing the results to both the player and the team.

Consider the applicability of models of the physician–patient relationship to this context. The paternalistic model, which requires the physician to act solely in the best interests of his patient as the physician sees those interests, would not be appropriate because it would totally disregard the interests of the team in truthful disclosure. This would institutionalize a conflict of interest consisting of undue attention to the patient's interests alone.

The informative model might suffice here because presumably the information given to the patient under this model would be the same accurate information the team would be entitled to. Even here, however, the patient might be hesitant to share all facts with the physician so that the physician could adduce the correct information to disclose to both the player and team. Indeed, it appears that players should mistrust their physicians. One commentator has reported that in all sixty-seven National Football League arbitration hearings involving injuries, the team physician testified against the athlete on behalf of the team. Yet players won thirty-nine of these proceedings.[64] Although the AMA Code of Ethics does not directly address team physicians, it does clearly state that the primary duty of an employed physician who provides treatment is to his patient, not his employer: "A physician–patient relationship does exist when a physician renders treatment to an employee, even though the physician is paid by the employer."[65]

If team physicians would take the appropriate perspective, the interpretive and deliberative models would be most promising. These models' focus on values beyond the patient's naked preferences would arguably enable the physician to encourage the athlete to be truthful and respect his duties to the team. Arguably the interpretive model would allow focus on obligations to the team only insofar as such consideration would spring from the patient's own values. The deliberative model would empower the physician to attempt to persuade the patient to embrace new values of cooperation and respect. The physician should not, however, go any further than trying to persuade the patient "to do the right thing." For example, the team doctor should not testify for the team as an expert witness. The same result would follow under the dual agency model we have suggested. Although the physician has a contractual duty to the team, his higher duty is to the patient. Since an examining physician's role is to adduce certain information that might be useful to the employer and possibly detrimental to the employee, and since he must warn the patient of his limited and potentially adversary role, his duty to the employer requires testifying against the patient if litigation ensues. The team physician, however, is in a different position. He has a continuing relationship with the patient, and his role is to provide diagnosis and treatment. Taking an adversary role in litigation is wholly inimical to this relationship.

One might argue that the contract with the team and the role of good citizen should require more physician fealty to the team whenever there is any hint that the player-patient is not giving 100 percent. However, testifying against the patient as an expert witness would harm the physician–patient relationship and engender mistrust of physicians by athletes and patients generally. An equally important consideration is that putting the team first demeans the physician's self-respect, could breed the habit of always putting others before one's specific patients, and could be taken to symbolize physicians' untrustworthiness and identification with institutions over individuals. The pecuniary or emotional damage to the team is not a sufficiently serious interest to invoke the good citizen model and its focus on interests beyond those of the patient. The physician should, of course, give truthful factual testimony if subpoenaed and ordered to testify, but he should not give expert opinions against the player. Those can be obtained from independent physicians.[66]

When the Physician Is an Employee of a Total Institution

Another context where the physician has at least certain obligations to persons other than the patient is when the physician is employed by an institution that has control over the care of the patient—for example, the prison physician. To simplify, the prison physician has two types of duties: (1) duties peculiar to the prison setting and (2) routine medical care like that provided outside the prison. A physician working in a jail or prison in the United States might be asked to act entirely as an agent of the correctional authority and only circumstantially, if at all, on the prisoner's behalf. This could include searching for drugs or weapons; obtaining blood or urine specimens for drug testing; medically clearing patients for the punishment block; and preparing medical or psychiatric reports for the court, parole board, or prison authority.[67]

While these activities may be necessary for the proper functioning of the jail or prison and may require medical expertise, to ask a physician responsible for the care of a prisoner to perform these duties violates the physician's obligation to honor the confidentiality of the prisoner's medical record and to act to the benefit of the patient. Furthermore, if a prisoner is concerned that information provided to a prison physician might be used against him—for example, in a parole hearing—he would be reluctant to avail himself of the physician's services. Nonetheless, because this conflict of interest is so readily identified, it is relatively easy to propose a solution. When a physician is needed for any of the functions listed above, it should be one other than the individual identified as the physician responsible for prisoners' routine care.

It is very important that the prisoners be aware that the physicians performing these nontherapeutic medical functions for the prison authority should not be considered "their" doctors. Further, especially when the outside physician is a psychiatrist preparing a report for the court, parole board, or prison authorities, this individual should clearly inform the prisoner that their interview does not establish a physician–patient relationship and that anything the patient says might be used against him. In addition, since psychiatrists are professionally trained to be empathetic in order to draw out their patients' often hidden sentiments, it is incumbent on them to avoid the appearance of empathy in such evaluations in order to minimize the likelihood that the prisoner would unwillingly disclose information against his interests.[68]

In other instances where prison physicians perform conventional medical activities like those performed in routine practice, the peculiar requirements of the prison setting introduce elements of conflict of interest. Unlike the conflicts outlined above, these are less stark and therefore more problematical to deal with. These situations include dealing with prison security requirements, managing prisoners suspected of malingering, and handling special requests. The manacles and leg irons that may be required for maximum-security prisoners can interfere with proper physical examination, and close surveillance by correctional officers can threaten the confidentiality of the examination. On the other hand, to eliminate these measures might jeopardize not only the physician's safety but also the safety of other prisoners and correctional personnel. They simply present unavoidable conflicting interests.

In dealing with a potential malingerer, a conscientious physician must consider the potential organic causes for the patient's complaints, labeling the prisoner as a malinger only as a diagnosis of exclusion. On the other hand, many prisoners are skilled manipulators, and for the physician to accede too readily to requests for drugs with high abuse potential, for lighter work assignments, or for confinement in the hospital would contribute to prison corruption and undermine discipline. Non-religious requests for special diets often require approval of the prison physician; while the prison physician might prefer that dietary preferences be respected, to allow individual diets for the entire prison population would unduly burden the administration.

Unlike the conflicts of interest described earlier, where the physician is being asked to perform duties for the benefit of the prison authorities and where conflicts of interest are readily identified, these conflicting interests arise in the course of ministering to the prisoners' needs and are inseparable from the business of patient care. One absolutist point of view—that one should do *all* one can for one's patients—leads to the indiscriminate prescription of narcotics and other abusable drugs, and generally undermines the authorities' ability to run a disciplined prison, while the other absolutist point of view requires a degree of callousness that few physicians would willingly adopt. Both would transform conflicting interests into conflicts of interest. Perhaps a reasonable compromise, which honors the physician's responsibility to his patients while respecting the legitimate role of the prison system, is for the physician to assume a degree of paternalism that, while not acceptable in medical practice outside prison, can be justified in a correctional institution. While hard and fast guidelines are not possible, as Thorburn states,[69] the patient's interests should be foremost, provided that the physician does not invariably equate the patient's best interests with the patient's expressed wants.

A delicate balance of the prison's and prisoner's interests could be achieved via either the paternalistic model or the deliberative model. The interpretive model does not seem too promising because it would require elucidation of the prisoner's values. Although prisoners do not forfeit all their rights, nor are they necessarily totally evil, it appears much more feasible either to impose standard values on them through the paternalistic model or to seek to shape their values through the deliberative model. For example, a patient's sincere desire for a stay on the prison medical ward might not comport with his long-term interest in *avoiding* momentary retreats from reality. Confrontation rather than retreat might be necessary for rehabilitation, and the physician might paternalistically confront the prisoner. At the same time, the deliberative model has much to offer; it entails moral education and encouragement consistent with the goal of rehabilitation. We cannot dogmatically state that one model is definitely superior to the other in the prison setting. However, the physician must address the problem and adopt an approach that allows conscientious consideration of the interests of individual patients, the institution, and its residents as a group. It is not necessary that only one model be used. The paternalistic model might be appropriate for relatively minor decisions, such as whether the prisoner should visit the infirmary for a professed minor ailment. On the other hand, a model more respectful of the prisoner's autonomy should be adopted for vital decisions, such as whether a competent prisoner should take antipsychotic medication. Here too the dual agency model might illuminate analysis. The physician has contractual duties to the institution, but his higher obligation is to the prisoner/patients.

Case Study 4. Deciding whether a prisoner/patient should be forced to take a psychotropic medication that he competently refuses is a particularly challenging situation considered by the U.S. Supreme Court in *Washington v. Harper.*[70] A convicted felon, Harper was housed in a prison designed for persons with serious mental disorders. He was diagnosed as manic-depressive. After about eleven months, Harper refused to continue taking the psychotropic medication prescribed by the prison physicians. The prison policy allowed treating doctors to recommend forced medication. A hearing was then to be held before a committee consisting of a psychologist, a psychiatrist, and an associate superintendent of the prison to determine whether the patient should be forcibly medicated because he suffered from mental illness and was, as a result, dangerous to himself or others. Forcible medication could continue beyond seven days only after approval by an identically constituted committee. Treating doctors were not allowed to sit on the initial committee, but they could serve on the committee authorized to permit extended medication. The patient could appeal, finally, to the prison superintendent.

Harper argued that the state could not medicate him against his will unless he was incompetent *and* it were found that, if competent, he would have consented to the treatment ("substituted judgment"). He also argued that the process for determining whether he could be medicated violated the "procedural" due process of law guaranteed by the Fourteenth Amendment to the U.S. Constitution, in part because it was tainted by conflicts of interest.

The majority of the Court reasoned that, in the challenged system, treatment could be forcibly administered because of danger to self and others only after a treating psychiatrist found voluntary administration of medication to be in the patient's best interest. The Court assumed that the patient might competently refuse even what was in his best interest. It erroneously reasoned, moreover, that the physician would necessarily act in the patient's, as opposed to the institution's, best interest because of being bound by ethical norms, including the Hippocratic Oath. Thus, the Court, by implication, accepted the paternalistic model of the physician–patient relationship, in which the physician determines what is best for the patient. Indeed, it implied that the paternalistic model was required by applicable ethical codes. In essence, the Court found neither conflicting interests nor conflicts of interest. There is no support for the Court's assumptions. The Court's uninformed application of the Hippocratic Oath is particularly troublesome. As noted earlier, the Hippocratic Oath is itself the product of ancient professional self-interest, and it is admittedly outdated and ignored by many groups of physicians. Even those who take the Oath could not confidently describe its guidance, if any, in the *Harper* case.

Dissenting, three members of the Court emphasized the conflicts of interest among the goals of the institution, institutional residents generally, and the specific patient. The dissenters made several important points.[71] First, the substantive criteria for forcing treatment do not necessarily entail a pristine determination that the treatment is in the patient's best interest, even from the paternalistic perspective. Institutional convenience and expense are clearly general conflicting interests. Second, the reviewers have specific conflicts of interest in (1) vindicating their own decisions in the specific case and (2) avoiding offending colleagues who might review their decisions in the future. Third, an effect on the decision in each specific case need not be demonstrated to condemn a conflict of interest as violative of due process.

The standards of the National Commission On Correctional Care support the dissent's view. Those standards provide that if a specific treatment is necessary, a nonmedical person may not countermand an order for it, regardless of the security risk or cost of the proposed treatment.[72] Yet the scheme attacked in *Harper* allowed the superintendent to countermand the treating physician and subsequent committees. It would appear, therefore, to allow administrative decisions prohibited by the Commission's accreditation standards.

We submit that the good citizen model should lead prison physicians to refuse to become involved in any substantive or procedural regimes that allow (1) substantive medical decisions to become tainted with administrative convenience, (2) nonmedical personnel to decide treatment options, and (3) prison medical personnel to sit on appeals committees within their own prison system. As to the last, the conflicts of interest mentioned by the *Harper* dissent are too compromising. Prison physicians should insist on a mechanism by which the prisoner can appeal to a physician or medical committee independent of the institution. The provision of an independent medical review should not preclude judicial review. The court system must make the ultimate ethical/constitutional determinations entailed in coercive treatment.[73]

Prison physicians should not allow political officials to foist on them a role incompatible with the term of the contract between society and the medical profession that requires physicians to act solely in the interests of patients unless there is strong justification otherwise. The bureaucratic inconvenience and expense associated with stricter protections (e.g., independent reviews) do not constitute strong justification.

In this situation, moreover, the standards of the National Commission on Correctional Care indicate how ethical codes or practice standards can advance ethical practices. They allow physicians to speak against an unfair practice as a united group, thus relieving individual physicians of the need to carry the burden alone.

Situations Involving Multiple Patients: Marriage and Genetic Counseling

Marriage counseling and clinical genetics represent settings where physicians have multiple patients with conflicting interests. Suppose, for example, that a couple seeks genetic testing to determine the risk of their future children having a genetic disorder. The testing inadvertently discloses that the man could not have been the biological father of the couple's only child. The doctor shares this information with the mother, and she does not want it disclosed. We are not aware of a published opinion on this point. We can find guidance in the similar context of marriage counseling because there, too, the physician or other provider has two patients with apparently mutual goals but possible conflicting interests.

Horak v. Biris[74] is an instructive case. Mr. and Mrs. Horak sought marriage counseling from Dean Biris, a certified social worker. Mr. Horak sued Biris, alleging that he was negligent by becoming sexually involved with Mrs. Horak, failing to guard against the transference phenomenon, failing to inform Mr. Horak about the sexual liaison and the resulting conflict of interest, and failing to terminate the relationship with Mrs. Horak as soon as the conflict of interest arose.

Biris cynically alleged as a defense that his only wrong, if any, was directed at Mrs. Horak, and that, in any event, there was no clear standard of care for social workers that he breached. The court answered that Biris had a relationship with both Mr. and Mrs. Horak and that standards for the profession were embodied, in part, in a code of ethics adopted by the National Association of Social Workers. The latter was not binding, but it was sufficient, along with statutes providing for certification of social workers, to indicate that a jury should be allowed to determine whether Biris acted below determinable minimum standards of social worker practices.

This is an easy case. It presents not only conflicting interests but a hard conflict of interest as well, and it would be decided the same under any model of the provider–patient relationship. It illustrates, moreover, that a physician or other provider should be particularly wary when he simultaneously represents two parties. Whenever possible, he should withdraw from the relationship and make an appropriate referral if a direct and serious conflict between the interests of the two patients arises. At a minimum, he should withdraw from the representation of one of the patients. It is better, except in extraordinary cases, to withdraw altogether so as to avoid an appearance of favoritism or improper use of the confidences of one patient to favor the other patient. Obviously, moreover, the physician should avoid creating conflicts of interest by becoming sexually involved with patients. The only close question, which we will not resolve here, is whether withdrawal without express disclosure of the nature of the conflict of interest is permissible. Autonomy would seem to require both telling the truth to the husband and maintaining the confidentiality of the wife. Even if one determined, on balance, that disclosure would be warranted under the principles of autonomy and truth telling, it might seriously damage the interests of one or both patients, thus violating the principle of nonmaleficence. For example, disclosure by Biris, or another therapist in a similar position, might destroy an otherwise salvageable marriage that the therapist has helped make precarious.

Do the *Biris* case and the models and ethical principles discussed above give us any insight to a proper resolution for the clinical geneticist who is asked to keep a husband from knowing that another man conceived his wife's child? The geneticist's case is distinguishable because he did not create the conflict of interest. Moreover, withdrawal could be problematic because many areas do not offer patients convenient or competent alternative genetics providers. The cases are similar, however, in that truth telling and autonomy (information is needed to exercise choice) seem to indicate disclosure, while beneficence or nonmaleficence seems to counsel silence. Since, in Veatch's system, beneficence and nonmaleficence are consequentialist and subordinate to the nonconsequentialist principles of autonomy and truth telling, the latter principles would seem, under Veatch's theory, to require disclosure. On the other hand, perhaps the husband would prefer not to know the truth. Foisting the information on him might rob him of the choice for ignorance and his autonomy.

One might turn to models of the physician–patient relationship to resolve this apparent clash of principles. The paternalistic model might enable the physician to reason that it would be best for the mother, father, child, and/or the family either to know or not to know. The interpretive model would seem to require that the physician explore, if at all feasible, whether the father (and the child, if mature enough to understand) would want to know and whether the wife really wants to tell. The deliberative model would perhaps indicate that the physician should convince the wife that she should disclose. The good citizen model does not seem to provide additional insight here because we are dealing directly with duties to patients, not to third parties or society. Similarly, the dual agency theory does not help because both principals are patients to whom a fiduciary duty is owed.

The physician could not avoid the conflict by withdrawing because this would really be deciding for nondisclosure (or indirect disclosure) by pretending not to decide. The problems in actually resolving this case indicate that there is no cookbook approach for resolving conflicting interests. Indeed, in this situation, we submit that there is no single right answer. The physician must have the virtue and strength to work through such dilemmas with every practical and ethical resource at his disposal. If he intends to and in fact does so, there are conflicting interests but neither a conflict of interest nor a breach of obligation.

However, with additional facts, a clear answer might emerge. For example, were it necessary for medical reasons—such as a search for a compatible donor of bone marrow or an organ to treat a fatal illness—to reveal the nonpaternity to the child and/or the father, then the value in saving a life would, we submit, require disclosure even if the mother refused the same after appropriate counseling. Nondisclosure would then constitute a breach of obligation. Similarly, if the father spontaneously voiced doubts about his paternity and explicitly asked the physician whether the genetic tests provided any pertinent information, the principle of truth telling would require disclosure.

*Forced or Permissible Consideration of Third Parties' Interests Even When a
Single Patient Has Retained the Physician*

Perhaps the most obvious requirements that physicians assume obligations possibly inconsistent with their patients' interests are those that obligate physicians
to breach confidentiality to protect potential victims of violent patients. The most
serious required action is coercive commitment—which often entails some form
of coercive treatment—when the patient is a danger to others because of a mental disorder. Even if the patient is not committable, the physician is expected to
warn potential victims. In this instance, the law creates specific incentives to
encourage physicians to consider victims' interests above patients' interests.
Most authorities hold that a physician can be held civilly liable if he fails to take
steps to protect a *specific* potential victim.[75] A few authorities require warning
even if the danger is only to society generally.[76] Liability is sometimes premised
on mere negligent failure to diagnose dangerousness, while in other jurisdictions
liability can only be found if the physician actually determines that the patient
poses a *bona fide* threat and then fails to take reasonable steps to protect the victim.[77] In addition to requiring certain disclosures, the law invariably provides
physicians who are involved in the commitment process or who warn potential
victims with either total immunity or limited immunity that allows liability only
for aggravated misconduct.[78]

The paternalistic model might justify commitment or warning under the reasoning that it might prevent greater harm that might befall the patient were he
to act on his violent propensities. The informative model would seem to allow
no more than warning the patient about the severe consequences *for the patient*
that might accompany a violent assault. The interpretive model would allow the
physician to elucidate any patient values inconsistent with assault, while the
deliberative model would allow the physician to attempt to persuade the patient
to alter his values and embrace nonviolence. Obviously, none of these approaches is definitive. However, the good citizen model is clearly applicable here.
Regardless of the patient's preferences or objective best interests, a citizen simply cannot tolerate preventable violent action toward another member of the
community.

The good citizen model is not necessarily based on a simple utilitarian calculation. In fact, it might be the case that the practice of requiring warnings will, in
the long run, lead to violent patients eschewing therapy and actually committing
more assaults. If so, at issue would be the immediate interests of specific persons
or the community where the dangerous patient presently operates versus the interests of the class of future potential victims generally. The principle of avoiding
killing espoused by Veatch or the principle of nonmaleficence adopted by both
Veatch and Beauchamp and Childress might come into play. This is not clear
because these principles are primarily explained by these bioethicists insofar as

they relate to the physician not killing and doing good to his specific patients. Much more work needs to be done regarding the application of these (and additional) principles to the protection of third parties and society.

Veatch's specific thoughts on the dangerous patient problem offer some guidance. He argues that the social contract between physicians and society includes a provision requiring breach of confidentiality to protect potential victims at some given level of danger. This is based on the equal regard due all persons or the disproportionate harm possibly posed to members of society. Veatch does not determine the exact boundary, but he argues that the medical profession must not be allowed unilaterally to determine the degree of danger necessary to justify warning. Rather, the line that separates conflicting interests from conflicts of interest must be drawn as a result of negotiation between the profession and society.[79]

The *Tarasoff*[80] case, which first recognized the duty to warn, contains additional insights regarding conflicting duties to patients and third parties. First, recognition of the duty to warn was based, in part, on the Principles of Medical Ethics of the AMA (1957), Section 9: "A physician may not reveal confidences entrusted to him in the course of medical attendance . . . unless he is required to do so by law or unless it becomes necessary in order to protect the welfare of the individual or of the community." This shows how ethical codes can be used as evidence of a legal duty to undertake some action and of moral sentiments held by members of the profession itself.[81]

Second, the American Psychiatric Association filed an amicus brief and, in so doing, took a position that seemed to be based on the profession's self-interest rather than a studied conclusion regarding what would be right. The APA argued that no duty to warn should be imposed because psychiatrists are not capable of predicting dangerousness.[82] A psychiatrist cannot be found liable, however, unless the jury is convinced, based at least in part on expert testimony, that she *unreasonably* failed to diagnose dangerousness. It is obvious that at least certain levels of behavior, albeit perhaps rare, indicate sufficient danger to reasonably require warning. As good citizens, physicians should speak for the *public* interest. It does not appear that APA physicians did so in *Tarasoff*.

Clinical genetics also raises the issue of obligations to third parties. Information obtained by the geneticist might well have implications for family members outside the nuclear unit. The frequency and severity of dilemmas faced by clinical geneticists are apt to increase as a result of advanced technological capacities likely to be engendered by the Human Genome Project. This multi-billion-dollar long-term government commitment to finance research aimed at mapping and sequencing the human genome will likely enable us to identify, economically test for, and perhaps treat many more genetic disorders (though it is easy to overestimate the degree of predictability we are likely to get). The number and type of conflicting interests among nuclear and extended families, spouses, parents, and children will be increased by these developments. For example, if it becomes economical to test for susceptibility to deadly cancers that are heavily influenced by diet, clinical geneticists might have to consider disclosing such possible susceptibility to patients' relatives. A similar problem already exists concerning relatives' increased risk of conceiving children with genetic disorders. Moreover, there is some ability to predict relatives' increased susceptibility to certain forms of cancer through family histories or expensive experimental procedures. The present consensus is, however, that there is no legal obligation to inform relatives of such risks, especially over patients' objections.[83] Indeed, an ethical guideline of the National Society of Genetics Counselors provides that patients' genetic information must remain confidential in the absence of patients' waiver.[84] This inflexible guideline implies that considering disclosure constitutes a conflict of interest.

Wertz, Fletcher, and Mulvihill[85] have surveyed clinical geneticists from several countries. A majority stated that they would disclose relatives' increased risk of bearing defective offspring even if their patients refused to share that information. Their moral sentiments seem to contradict the formal ethical statement of the National Society of Genetic Counselors. It could well be that the code statement is based on provider self-interest. Given the present state of the law, it is highly unlikely that a court would find a provider liable for not disclosing information to relatives. Furthermore, such disclosure of information is a good way to lose patients. At the same time, it is possible that providers would be found liable for breaching genetic confidences. There are, in short, political and liability reasons for clinical geneticists to disfavor disclosure. Is the National Society of Genetics Counselors' statement another example of providers, as a group, acting out of self-interest rather than as good citizens? Have they erroneously found a conflict of interest (telling relatives) because of a conflict of interest (fear that telling will create personal problems)?

The models of the physician (or other provider)–patient relationship described by the Emanuels do not do much to help resolve the problem of patients' versus relatives' interests. As in the team physician context, the paternalistic and informative models would seem to make relatives' interests irrelevant. The interpretive model would allow elucidation of any patient values favoring broad family well-being, but only the deliberative model would permit direct attempts to convince patients to change their values and inform relatives.

Some authority has hinted at redefining the "patient" as the extended family.[86] The argument is that increased genetic information enabling us to predict dangers more precisely, not only to offspring but also to relatives themselves, expands the class of persons to whom the physician's ministrations are relevant. This perspective seems to greatly extend the paternalistic model. It does not define the obligations of an existing relationship to be paternalistic in nature. Rather, this perspective assumes that a relationship is formed with the class of persons who can be helped by the physician. Carried to its greatest lengths, this perspective could hold that all of society is the patient of each physician under a eugenic paternalism. Of course, this perspective emphasizes beneficence toward relatives over autonomy of immediate patients.

It is true that determining when and with whom a physician–patient relationship is formed, as well as the nature of the relationship, is essential to identification of conflicts of interest. If the relationship is only with the individual or couple directly tested and counseled, and if one assumes a paternalistic model in which only the immediate patients' interests are relevant, it would constitute a conflict of interest for the physician to make disclosures to relatives. On the other hand, if the patient were assumed to be the extended family, disclosure would seem to be required.

It appears that, given the dearth of attention to the physician role outside the physician–patient relationship, commentators are attempting to solve the problem of obligations to third-party family members by recasting it as a problem of defining the patient. This deals with a possible conflict-of-interest problem by defining it away and, in so doing, glosses over the principles and values at stake for physicians, patients, and society. What probably underlies the impulse to solve the problem by definition is a sense that present legal and ethical approaches will not accommodate the interests of relatives.

We propose the following approach. As we noted earlier, the presumption is in favor of honoring the patients' wishes. Their wishes can be overcome only by strong justification. Legally and ethically, the risk of serious illness or bodily harm has been clearly recognized as essential to justification. However, there are often additional requirements: that the harm be highly probable, imminent, and sometimes directed to a specific person. As Dr. Donald Francis has pointed out concerning AIDS, however, our very survival as a species might be tied to our ability to confront adequately crises that unfold over decades.[87] We cannot act only when harm is imminent. Ethical and public policy calculations must consider the nature and magnitude of the harm as well as its probability and imminence. Some harms can only be averted by measures undertaken in their incipient stages. Moreover, physicians are often in a position to identify potential harms at their beginning.

Applying these requirements to clinical genetics requires further guidance. Here we turn to guidelines for whistle blowing adduced by Gene James.[88] Whistle blowing is similar to physician disclosure because agency law provides that an employee has a prima facie duty to maintain confidentiality of any data that is either proprietary or, on the other hand, detrimental to his employer. James argues that professionals have a greater obligation to risk their self-interest on the public's behalf than do non-professionals. He then advises: "Make sure the situation involves illegal actions, harm to others, or violation of people's rights, and is not one in which you would be disclosing personal matters, trade secrets, customer lists, or similar material. If disclosure of the wrongdoing would involve the latter, make sure that the harm to be avoided is great enough to offset the harm from the latter."[89]

Of course, physician disclosure does involve "personal matters." The pertinent point, however, is that the physician must balance the expected benefits and harms of disclosure. Once again, in doing this, he should consider the nature and magnitude of the harm as well as its imminence and probability. Applying these criteria to clinical genetics, the harm involved can be the birth of a severely disabled child a couple would not have conceived or carried to term; harm to disabled offspring; harm to existing children within the family; and even great bodily harm to a relative who could have altered his lifestyle over many years so as to minimize the risk of a serious disease such as cancer. Although these harms often unfold over many years, they strike at vital reproductive and health interests of the sort that could justify overcoming the presumption in favor of patient confidentiality.

The question remains whether a clinical geneticist is either ethically *free* to sacrifice patient confidentiality or *required to do so* when vital reproductive or health interests of relatives are at stake. Given the present formal ethical guideline of genetics counselors' advising *against* disclosure, it would appear Draconian to consider disclosure *obligatory*. We submit that the question should be left to a careful case-by-case analysis. A jury might decide, based on a given set of facts, that a physician was unreasonable (i.e., negligent) in not disclosing information. For example, the patient might have announced that the reasons for nondisclosure are spite and ill will rather than legitimate privacy concerns. Moreover, we recommend that physicians be allowed to disclose data to relatives without imposition of liability as long as they are not grossly negligent or in bad faith (i.e., in making the diagnosis or projecting inheritance, and in the accuracy and manner of presentation). This departure from the usual rule of liability for mere negligence might seem odd in light of our usual presumption in favor of patients' interests. It is informed, however, by our perception that the physician role has been defined as one that too readily ignores the interests of third parties, especially grievous harms that can unfold over a significant time period. We believe that the approaches we suggest are consistent with terms of the social contract that would be agreed to by persons acting from the ethical point of view.

Whenever disclosure is ventured, the physician must first sensitively attempt to convince the patient to carry it out or agree to it. If the patient refuses, he should be informed that it will take place. It should be carried out in a manner that accommodates any legitimate concerns of the patient that can be assimilated into the process, and it should be as narrow as possible to achieve the desired warning effectively. It should be undertaken, moreover, only if there is a significant possibility that the information will be used in an appropriate way.[90] Further, any information disclosed should be conveyed solely to the directly interested relatives.

Circumstances in Which the Physician Is Not Allowed to Consider Third-Party or Societal Interests

Part IV of this book focuses on clinical research. Some contend that the very notion of research involves "using" patient/subjects to further the good of science or society.[91] Therapeutic research is designed to benefit patients directly while also advancing knowledge. In nontherapeutic research there is no claim of direct benefits to the subjects; they might even be healthy but at risk from participation. The law requires, however, that physicians act to further the interests of their patients, without regard to the benefits to science, unless the patient freely and informedly agrees to certain acceptable sacrifices. Consider two cases.

First, in *Burton v. Brooklyn Doctor's Hospital*,[92] a pediatric resident caring for a premature infant ordered the baby's inspired oxygen concentration reduced to minimize the risk of retrolental fibroplasia. Two days later, a member of the hospital staff who was an instructor in pediatrics at the hospital's affiliate, the Cornell University Medical College, on instructions from the chairman of the Department of Pediatrics, ordered that the baby's inspired oxygen concentration be increased in accordance with an ongoing clinical study. The department head and the instructor entered the order without examining the baby or consulting with either the resident or the parents. The national standard of care allowed the greater oxygen concentration because the trade-off between the risk of death or retardation, on the one hand, and blindness, on the other hand, was not known. Although the national standard of practice for such infants was to use a high oxygen concentration (with a consequently higher risk of blindness), the concentration necessary to maximize the chances of survival without either mental retardation or blindness in premature infants had been established through earlier, albeit not widely known, studies nationally and at the very hospital in question. The infant was blinded.

Although a physician usually is not liable if he comports with the customary knowledge and practices of physicians, a refinement of this rule is that a physician must exercise his *best judgment* whenever his skill or expertise surpasses the standard of care customarily exercised by or expected of the reasonably prudent physician. The rule is rarely invoked, and the plaintiff must prove that the doctor did not use his best judgment. The best judgment rule most commonly comes into play in large, highly specialized teaching institutions. The department head was aware that the infant had progressed well under the diminished oxygen therapy. Although most physicians at the time believed that a high dose of oxygen was essential to the survival of premature infants, the studies at the institution in question showed that high levels of oxygen were unnecessary and potentially dangerous. This was particularly important in this case, since the resident had already successfully treated the infant with a reduced oxygen concentration. The department head did not use his superior knowledge. He had in mind a possible future benefit to other infants but risked the welfare of his specific patient. The jury found that the physician failed to do that which he himself considered proper and necessary. He had ignored his own best judgment.

The department head did not act as a good citizen. At best, he acted under what the Emanuels describe as the instrumental model, in which the patient is used as a means to an end (such as the advancement of science). Whether he acted for the good of future patients or out of selfish motives, the Department Head's conduct evidenced a hard conflict of interest. His overriding concern here should have been the interests of his patient.

An equally cynical position was taken by the physicians in *Moore v. Regents of the University of California*.[93] John Moore had his spleen removed at UCLA Hospital for the treatment of leukemic reticuloendotheliosis. Without obtaining his informed consent, Moore's physicians used his tissue from the operation to develop a cell line capable of producing pharmaceutical products. Moreover, under the pretense of needed medical follow-up, his physicians induced him to make trips back to California from his home in Seattle at his own expense. During these trips, the physicians collected additional tissue samples. When Moore learned the truth, he sued the physicians for conversion of his property and other torts. The intermediate appellate court recognized a conversion theory (essentially, civil "theft" of property), but the California Supreme Court held that he should only be given the opportunity to convince a jury that the physicians either breached their fiduciary duty to him or failed to obtain informed consent.

Although the court found the facts alleged to be unprecedented, it indicated that some legal theory must be recognized to prevent physicians from engaging in such conflicts of interest between their own (selfish or altruistic) interests and those of their patients. Ironically, the majority of the court refused to recognize the conversion theory under the rationale that it would retard the development of science by encouraging patients to file huge claims for profits that might be engendered through the use of human tissues. In other words, the court found that patients' autonomy and bodily privacy needed to be honored somewhat, but this right had to be balanced against the utilitarian goal of advancing science and commerce. Arguably, the court, by not allowing the greater recovery entailed in a conversion theory, did to Mr. Moore for the benefit of society and advancement of science what it held the physicians should not have done to further their own interests, pecuniary or otherwise, in the advancement of science.

This case would be decided the same way under any legitimate model of the physician–patient relationship or ethical theory. The paternalistic physician would act here to benefit solely the patient, which was not done. The informative physician would have disclosed the truth. The interpretive physician might have elucidated any of the patient's values that would favor scientific advancement. The deliberative physician might have encouraged altruistic donation, but he would have been open with the patient. The good citizen would not have jeopardized either his own relationship with the patient or professionals' relationship with society by engaging in such unethical tactics. Only the instrumental physician would have behaved as the defendants in *Moore* did. In doing so, they ignored the principles of truth telling, autonomy, nonmaleficence, and justice. Their motivations evidenced a hard conflict of interest.

Conclusion

Conflicts of interest can be identified and properly dealt with only by determining the physician's ethically expected role in specific situations. We have examined various sources of insight concerning the physician role: ethical theory, literature regarding the physician–patient relationship, ethical codes or guidelines, and legal materials (particularly negligence and constitutional law principles). Concerning ethical theory, we have identified metaethical criteria to judge the relative merits of ethical theories, two related contractarian theories that yield similar broad principles (autonomy, honesty, promise or contract keeping, justice, beneficence, nonmaleficence, and avoiding killing) to guide decision-making, and the importance of the virtue of conscientiousness (diligently applying logic, moral sentiments and intuitions, ethical principles, feelings, and accurate factual determinations to reach a state of "reflective equilibrium" in which one is satisfied that he has reached the best decision).

We have explored various shortcomings of ethical codes as a source of data concerning physicians' ethically expected roles, but we have nevertheless examined the application of various ethical code or practice guidelines to specific cases. We have observed that although ethical codes or practice guidelines can serve as tools of physician self-interest, they can also allow physicians to justify ethical behavior that might not please parties to whom they owe certain obligations. For example, administrative physicians who devise treatment protocols can diffuse criticism from corporate superiors who believe the protocols to be unnecessarily cautious and expensive by pointing out that their fealty to patients as a class is mandated by a specific medical ethical code provision.

We have also described models of the physician–patient relationship that facilitate examination or discovery of the ethically expected course in given situations: the paternalistic, informative, interpretive, deliberative, instrumental, citizen/leader, and dual agency models. Similarly, we have described negligence and constitutional law principles that speak to physicians' ethically expected behavior concerning conflicting interests and conflicts of interest. In an effort to distinguish conflicting interests and reasonable accommodations of them from conflicts of interest and breaches of obligation, we have applied the various models of the physician–patient relationship, values that underlie these models, and negligence and constitutional law principles to categories of cases: where the primary client is not the patient, where a third-party hires physicians to treat patients, where the physician simultaneously cares for multiple patients, where physicians are permitted or forced to consider third-party and societal interests even when they have been retained by a single patient, and where they are forbidden to consider third party or societal interests.

Although negligence and constitutional law are rich with ethical content, actual cases often differ on what is expected in given situations. We suggest that although the law is a source of ethical guidance, it should generally only be considered a source of minimally expected conduct. Moreover, when different legal authorities disagree as to the correct approach, physicians generally should follow the course that is most generous to patients. Professionalism requires going beyond minimally required conduct. On the other hand, although physicians' first obligation is to patients, and although this obligation can only be overcome by strong justification, physicians must consider the nature and magnitude, as well as the probability and imminence, of harm to third parties and society when determining the ethically proper course. Legal and ethical authorities have neglected physicians' obligations to third parties and society. Much work needs to be done in this area. One of the important issues it raises is the proper approach to harms—for example, the AIDS epidemic and the effects of environmental toxins—that insidiously unfold over many years. The law should encourage and accommodate physician consideration of third party and societal interests by holding physicians liable if they do not *reasonably* consider such interests, and by holding them liable when they do consider such interests *only* if they are grossly negligent or act in bad faith. The determinations of reasonableness, gross negligence, and good faith are ultimately ethical judgments our law invites us to discover and implement.

Notes

1. Writings on "professions" and "professionalism" generally are also useful background sources. *See, e.g., Ethical Issues in Professional Life* (Joan Callahan, ed., 1988); T*he Sociology of the Professions* (Robert Dingwall and Philip Lewis, eds., 1983); *Professional Ethics* (Michael Bayles, ed., 1981); and Alan Goldman, *The Moral Foundations of Professional Ethics* (1980).

2. *See, e.g.*, Ezekiel and Linda Emanuel, Four Models of the Physician–Patient Relationship, 267 *N. Engl. J. Med.* 2221 (1992); Robert Veatch, Models for Ethical Medicine in a Revolutionary Age, 2 *Hasting Cent. Rep.* 3 (1975); Thomas Szasz and M. H. Hollander, The Basic Models of the Doctor–Patient Relationship, 97 *Arch. Intern. Med.* 585 (1956); and M. Siegler, The Progression of Medicine from Physician Paternalism to Patient Autonomy to Bureaucratic Parsimony, 145 *Arch. Intern. Med.* 713 (1985).

3. For example, although Veatch *and* Beauchamp and Childress—whose general theories are discussed in the text at notes 7 to 21—specifically consider certain obligations to society, the discussions of their major principles are almost solely devoted to the physician's obligations to his patients. *See also, e.g.*, Edmund Pellegrino and David Thomasma, *A Philosophical Basis of Medical Practice* (1981); and H. Tristram Engelhardt, *The Foundations of Bioethics* (1986). The exception to focus on individual patients' concerns in all these works is consideration of general problems of allocation and distribution of resources ("distributive justice"), particularly health care resources.

4. Robert Veatch, *Medical Ethics* 7–9 (1989); Robert Veatch, *A Theory of Medical Ethics* 19–24 (1981).

5. Telephone interview with Jill Hirt of the AMA, September 27, 1993.

6. Readers with formal ethical training may wish to skip ahead to the section, "Literature on the Physician-Patient Relationship".

7. John Rawls, *A Theory of Justice* 136 (1971).

8. Tom Beauchamp and James Childress, *Principles of Biomedical Ethics* 45–47 (4th ed., 1994).

9. We have included a brief bibliography of additional readings in ethical theory following note 90 for those who wish to explore additional theories and their conformance with metaethical principles. Ethical theories that fare as well under these metaethical criteria as any theories promulgated with medical practice in mind are those of Beauchamp and Childress and Veatch discussed in the text. See the bibliography.

10. Beauchamp and Childress, *supra* note 7, at 1230.

11. *Id.* at 190–192.

12. *Id.* at 192.

13. Tom Beauchamp and James Childress, *Principles of Biomedical Ethics* 265–275 (3d ed., 1989).

14. *Id.* at 101–106.

15. Robert Veatch, *A Theory of Medical Ethics* 120–138 (1981).

16. *Id.* at 137.

17. *Id.* at 138.

18. *Id.*

19. *Id.* at 296–305.

20. *Id.* at 306–315.

21. *See, e.g.*, A. MacIntyre, *After Virtue* (1981); D. G. Smith and L. Newton, Physician and Patient Respect for Mutuality, 5 *Theor. Med.* 43 (1984); *Virtue and Medicine* (E. C. Shelp, ed., 1985).

22. Robert Veatch, *A Theory of Medical Ethics* 9 (1981).

23. Tom Beauchamp and James Childress, *Principles of Biomedical Ethics* 386 (4th ed. 1994).

24. See John Rawls, *A Theory of Justice* 20, 48–55 (1971).

25. Ezekiel Emanuel and Linda Emanuel, Four Models of the Physician-Patient Relationship, 267 *JAMA* 2221 (1993).

26. *Id.*

27. *Id.* at 2221, 2224.

28. *Id.* at 2221.

29. *Id.* at 2221, 2224–2225.

30. *Id.* at 2221–2222, 2225.

31. *Id.*

32. *Id.*

33. *Id.* at 2223.

34. *Id.*

35. It is implicit in the Emanuels' analysis that the deliberative physician does not have a duty to encourage altruism independent of the patient's values.

36. *Id.* at 2221, 2222.

37. *Id.*

38. Indeed, some political theorists argue that the legislative process is and should be one of pork barreling among representatives of various special interest groups. Hans Linde, Due Process of Lawmaking, 55 *Neb. L. Rev.* 197, 222–235 (1976). Others argue that legislators, although representing constituents, must ultimately look after the common good, as well as minority and individual rights. Scott Bice, A Rationality Analysis in Constitutional Law, 65 *Minn. L. Rev.* 17 (1980).

39. However, some theorists pursue negligence law (and tort law analysis generally) from a "pure" efficiency standard. Special Committee on the Tort Liability System, *Toward a Jurisprudence of Injury: The Continuing Creation of a System of Substantive Justice in American Tort Law* 2-16 to 2-17 (1984).

40. *Id.* at 4-13 to 4-21.

41. *See id.* generally regarding purposes of tort law. As to "fault," see 4-146 to 4-150.

42. J. P. Ludington, Annotation, Physician's Duties and Liabilities to Person Examined Pursuant to Physician's Contract with Such Person's Prospective or Actual Employer or Insurer, 10 A.L.R.3d 1071, 1076–77 (1966).

43. *Id.* at Sect. 4, p. 1071 (supp.).

44. *Id.* at Sect. 5, p. 1074 (supp.).

45. Conversely, it would appear unethical (under the principle of justice) to expect a prospective employer or the physician to pay for the physician's time and involvement contemplated by the interpretive and deliberative models.

46. We do not distinguish between conflicts of interest and conflicts of obligation or loyalty.

47. We will not attempt to characterize the situation were the physician *negligently* to fail to find or disclose. See the discussion at note 45.

48. 376 N.E.2d 1182 (Ind. App. 1978).

49. *See, e.g.*, William May, Contract or Covenant, in *Ethical Issues in Professional Life* 92, 93 (Joan C. Callahan, ed., 1988). But see Chapter 10 by Hall in this volume (professional sacrifice is an erroneous and boundless concept). *See also* Buchanan's discussion of limited altruism in Chapter 5.

50. Physicians should be somewhat comforted that although the law previously allowed employers to terminate physicians and other employees without any reason, many legal principles now provide some protection against employer retaliation. Many jurisdictions provide that an

employee cannot be fired for reasons that either breach an implied obligation of good faith toward the employee or violate "public policy." One or both of these doctrines are likely to protect from retaliation physicians who conscientiously act to accommodate the interests of employers and examined patients.

51. 226 Cal. App. 3d 1128 (1991).
52. *Id.* at 1135.
53. American Occupational Medical Association, *Code of Ethical Conduct for Physicians Providing Occupational Medical Services*, Principle 7 (1976).
54. 192 Cal. App. 3d 1630 (1986).
55. *See, e.g.*, Dexter v. Kirschner, 984 F.2d 979 (9th Cir. 1992) (a state Medicaid program director was within his authority in refusing to fund a chronic myelogenous leukemia patient's bone marrow transplant even though the state legislature had decided to fund autologous bone marrow transplants for which state facilities were available).
56. Report of the Council on Ethical and Judicial Affairs, *Ethical Guidelines for Medical Consultants*, Report: B (I-92), adopted by the AMA House of Delegates, December 8, 1992. See *AMA Policy Compendium* 117 (1994).
57. Norman Daniels, *Just Health Care* 12, 54, 103, 105 (1985).
58. Marion Davis and Larry Churchill, Autonomy and the Common Weal, 21 *Hastings Cent.* Rep. 25 (1991).
59. *See* the Commission's Volume 1: *Report, Securing Access to Health Care*, particularly the Introduction at 4, 6 ("Society has an ethical obligation to ensure equitable access to health care for all. *** Equitable access to health care requires that all citizens be able to secure an adequate level of care without excessive burdens." The report also observes that disproportionate use by those with the ability to pay undermines the goal of access for all); and Chapter 1, "An Ethical Framework for Access to Health Care" 39–40 (professional judgment is one way to define adequate care and limit utilization, but professionals are likely to allow too much care).
60. *See, e.g.*, Robert Veatch, DRGs and the Ethical Reallocation of Resources, 16 *Hastings Cent.* Rep. 32, 38 (June 1986); and Edmund Pellegrino and David Thomasma, *For the Patient's Good: The Restoration of Beneficence in Health Care* 172, 173, 187 (1988).
61. President's Commission Report, note 58 at 38 (there is a consensus regarding access to trained professional attendance during delivery).
62. *See, e.g.*, Michael L. Millenson, Health Care Debate Rages: Cost-Paring: Good Business or Bad Medicine?, *Chicago Tribune* 1, 3–5 (June 14, 1987) (quoting Dr. J. Kristin Olson-Garewal, former medical director of University Family Care, an HMO in Tucson, Arizona, in answering a question about possible conflicts of interest in convincing doctors to use less expensive medications: "When I became the medical director, I represented the payment entity").
63. *See* text at note 90 regarding discussion of the "best judgment" rule.
64. Charles v. Russell, Legal and Ethical Conflicts Arising from the Team Physician's Dual Obligations to the Athlete and Management, 10 *Seton Hall Legis.* J. 299, 316 (1987).
65. American Medical Association, *Principles of Medical Ethics*, Sect. 5.09 (1989).
66. The authorities agree that a treating physician has a duty to cooperate with the patient by, for example, filling out insurance forms or making reports required in adversarial proceedings. *See, e.g.*, Anhert v. Wildman, 376 N.E.2d 1182 (Ind. App. 1978). This does not mean that the treating physician must review *additional* materials or formulate *new* opinions in a patient's malpractice suit against another physician. Moreover, both plaintiffs' attorneys and their clients' treating physicians must be sensitive to interference with the physician–patient relationship that might ensue in *certain* situations if the physician testifies *for* his patient. For

example, if a treating oncologist testifies that a plaintiff in a case of failure to diagnose cancer has a dim prognosis, this might help the patient's case by making the damages greater. However, it might also destroy his hope in any ongoing therapeutic relationship.

67. Professional groups have increasingly opposed physician "participation" (very broadly defined) in executions. *See, e.g.*, Lee Ann Lodder, Who Will Aid The Executioner?, *American Medical News* 2 (March 1, 1993). We will not explore this controversy.

68. Daniel Shuman, The Use of Empathy in Forensic Examinations, in *Ethics and Behavior* (B. Sales, ed., 1992).

69. Kim Thorburn, Croakers' Dilemma—Should Prison Physicians Serve Prisons or Prisoners?, 134 *West. J. Med.* 457 (1981).

70. 494 U.S. 210 (1991).

71. Id. at 251–154.

72. National Commission on Correctional Health Care, *Correct Care* 3 (January-February 1993) ("Questions and Answers" discussing the Commission's Standard P-02, J-02, on medical autonomy).

73. We reject any notion that punishment entails attenuation of the physician–patient relationship.

74. 474 N.E.2d 13 (Ill. App. 1985).

75. Fay Anne Freedman, The Psychiatrist's Dilemma: Protect the Public or Safeguard Individual Liberty?, 11 *U. Puget Sound L. Rev.* 255 (1988). The landmark case is Tarasoff v. Regents of The Univ. of Cal., 551 P.2d 344 (1976).

76. Petersen v. State, 100 Wash. 2d 421, 671 P.2d 230 (1983), limited by subsequent legislation, Wash. Rev. Code § 71.05 120(2) (1987), as reported in *supra* note 73.

77. *Id.* at 262–263.

78. See Joseph H. King, Jr., *The Law of Medical Malpractice in a Nutshell* 190-192 (2d ed., 1986).

79. Robert Veatch, *A Theory of Medical Ethics* 184–189 (1981).

80. Tarasoff v. Regents of the Univ. of Cal., 551 P.2d 334 (1976).

81. But some courts do not allow introduction because they fear this will create incentives for ethical codes to be too restrained and legalistic. *See, e.g.*, Criton Constantinides, Professional Ethical Codes in Court: Redefining the Second Contract Between the Public and Professionals, 25 *Georgia L. Rev.* 1327 (1991); Horne v. Patton, 287 So.2d 824, 829 (Ala. 1973) (AMA's *Principles of Medical Ethics* used to help establish the duty of confidentiality); and Bryson v. Tillinghast, 749 P.2d 110, 114 (Okla. 1988) (medical ethics "aspirational in nature and not enforceable by law," so a report of information leading to the patient's conviction for past rape was not actionable).

82. 551 P.2d at 344.

83. *See, e.g.*, Lori Andrews, Torts and the Double Helix: Malpractice Liability for Failure to Warn of Genetic Risks, 29 *Houston L. Rev.* 149, 174–182 (1992).

84. National Society of Genetic Counselors, Inc., Position Statement re Confidentiality of Test Results (adopted 1991).

85. D. C. Wertz, J. C. Fletcher, and J. J. Mulvihill, Medical Geneticists Confront Ethical Dilemmas: Cross-Cultural Comparisons Among 18 Nations, 45 *Am. J. Hum. Genet.* 1200 (1990).

86. D. C. Wertz, The 19-Nation Survey; Genetics and Ethics Around the World, in *Ethics and Human Genetics—A Cross Cultural Perspective* 1, 16 (D. C. Wertz and J. C. Fletcher, eds., 1989); and Robert Wachbroit, Making the Grade: Testing for Human Genetic Disorders, 16 *Hofstra L. Rev.* 583 (1988) (not speaking of patients' interests in test results but rather of various individuals' interests in the information).

87. Donald Francis, Toward a Comprehensive HIV Prevention Program for the CDC and the Nation, 268 *JAMA* 1444, 1447 (1992).
88. Gene James, In Defense of Whistle Blowing, in *Ethical Issues in Professional Life* (Joan Callahan ed. 1988).
89. *Id.* at 319.
90. One might argue that disclosure of an increased risk of having a child with a genetically caused disease should take place only if there is a significant possibility that the information would alter the receiving party's reproductive decision-making. On the other hand, there might be significant benefit in simply being briefed or forewarned. *Cf.* Sandi Wiggins et al., The Psychological Consequences of Predictive testing for Hereditary Disease, 327 *N. Engl. J. Med.* 1401 (1992).
91. *See, e.g.*, Samuel Hellman and Deborah Hellman, Of Mice But Not Men: Problems of the Randomized Clinical Trial, 324 *N. Engl. J. Med.* 1585 (1991).
92. 452 N.Y.S. 2d 875 (1982).
93. 793 P.2d 479 (Cal. 1990).

The following are selected readings on ethical theory (generally and as applied to medical practice and research) that we suggest for health care practitioners who wish to delve further into the area:

John Rawls, *A Theory of Justice* (1971).

William Frankena, *Ethics* (2d ed., 1973).

Bernard Williams, *Morality: An Introduction to Ethics* (1973).

Alan Donagan, *The Theory of Morality* (1977).

Ronald Dworkin, *Taking Rights Seriously* (1977).

Encyclopedia of Bioethics (Warren T. Reich, ed., 1978).

Richard Brandt, *A Theory of the Good and the Right* (1979).

Edmund Pellegrino and David Thomasma, *A Philosophical Basis of Medical Practice: Toward a Philosophy and Ethic of the Healing Professions* (1981).

H. Brody, *Ethical Decisions in Medicine* (1981).

Alasdair MacIntyre, *After Virtue* (1981).

James Childress, *Who Should Decide? Paternalism in Health Care* (1982).

Charles Culver and Bernard Gert, *Philosophy in Medicine: Conceptual and Ethical Issues in Medicine and Psychiatry* (1982).

Samuel Gorovitz, *Doctor's Dilemmas: Moral Conflict and Medical Care* (1982).

Michael Sandel, *Liberalism and the Limits of Justice* (1982).

Tom Beauchamp and Laurence McCullough, *Medical Ethics: The Moral Responsibilities of Physicians* (1984).

H. Tristram Engelhardt, *The Foundations of Bioethics* (1986).

Ruth Macklin, *Mortal Choices: Bioethics in Today's World* (1987).

Health Care Ethics: An Introduction (Donald VanDeVeer and Tom Regan, eds., 1987)

Consequentialism and Its Critics (Samuel Scheffler, ed., 1988).

Edmund Pellegrino and David Thomasma, *For the Patient's Good: The Restoration of Beneficence in Health Care* (1988).

Ethical Issues in Modern Medicine (John Arras and Nancy Rhoden, eds., 1989).

John Bruhn and George Henderson, *Values in Health Care: Choices and Conflicts* (1991).

David Rothman, *Strangers at the Bedside: A History of How Law and Bioethics Transformed Medical Decision Making* (1991).

4

Conflict of Interest in the Classic Professions

Geoffrey C. Hazard, Jr.

Conflict of interest is the central ethical problem of a profession, and indeed the problem that gives a profession its defining characteristic. By definition the function of a professional is to serve interests beyond the professional's own self-interest. The concept of "conflict of interest" is a reflexive definition of this fundamental characteristic, for it implicitly identifies those other interests that the professional must recognize. Accordingly, to analyze the problems of a profession's conflicts of interest is to probe the essence of the profession itself.

My analysis of conflict of interest is presented in terms of the professions of medicine and law, the classic professions along with the priesthood. The antecedents of medicine and law in antiquity were, respectively, the healer and the judge; the cognates of medicine in modern society include the healing professions generally, such as nursing, clinical psychology, and physical therapy; the modern cognates of law include such callings as accounting, public relations, and personnel management. In their modern forms these professions all encounter conflict-of- interest problems that have the multi–dimensional structure described in this chapter.[1] Accordingly, the discussion of doctors and lawyers that follows may well have more general significance.

The Structure of Conflicts of Interest

Economics of Professional Services

As a preliminary matter, it is useful to call attention to the economics underlying the relationships between doctor and patient and lawyer and client in modern practice settings. In modern industrialized societies, the cost of most medical treatment is borne by a third-party payer, such as an employer, an insurer, or a government funding program. Accordingly, in the case of medicine, the risk of financial exploitation, considered below, is felt primarily by the funding source rather than by the patient himself. The cost of some legal services to individuals is also borne by third-party payers, notably through legal aid (particularly in criminal cases) and liability insurance (particularly in automobile accident cases). In these situations, the third-party payer is at risk of financial exploitation similar to that in medical-care insurance. On the other hand, most legal services (measured by lawyer remuneration or any other quantifiable standard) are provided to organizations, including businesses and governmental departments. In most instances it is these organizations themselves that pay for the services, so that they are vulnerable to financial exploitation. At the same time, however, organizational clients are especially vulnerable to another kind of conflict of interest—that between the interests of the organization itself and the interests of the organization's employees and other operatives.

These important differences in the economics of modern medical and legal services significantly limit the direct comparisons that can be made between professional ethics in medicine and those in law. After all, economic incentive is one of the strongest interests that conflicts of interest norms are designed to address and counterbalance. That said, problems of financial exploitation arise in both medicine and law, but in both settings they are only one aspect of conflicts of interest.

The Dimensions of Conflict

A member of a profession faces conflicts of interest along three general dimensions. One dimension is that of conflict between the professional and the patient/client. Here the essential problem is exploitation of the patient/client by the professional. The second dimension is that of conflict between the patient/client and the interests of specific third parties, that is, parties who have a special relationship with either the professional or the patient/client. The typical specific third person in the case of a doctor is a member of the patient's family who is somehow involved in the treatment situation, such as the parent of a sick child. The typical specific third person in the case of a lawyer is another client whom the lawyer also represents, for example a copartner in a business partnership. In this second dimension of conflict, the essential problem for the profession is balancing the interests of the patient/client and the concerned third party. A third dimension of conflict of interest concerns the interest of the public or society. Here the essential problem is exploitation of the public interest for the benefit of the patient/client, with the assistance or acquiescence of the professional.

These various types of conflict of interest can occur in isolation or in combination. Depending on the situation, one dimension or the other of conflict may be given emphasis, sometimes to the exclusion of the other. However, more sober consideration suggests that all three dimensions are ever-present in a professional's work. In this light, it can be seen that the professional's role requires exercise of control along three different lines. The first is self-control to prevent the professional's exploitation of the client; the second is mediation of tripartite relationships including the professional, the patient/client, and a third party; and the third is the professional's imposition of restraint on the patient/client for protection of the public interest. In shorthand, these professional responsibilities for dealing with conflict of interest can be referred to as "self-control," "mediation," and "civic responsibility."

The multidimensional structure of these obligations means that the professional must think, speak, and act in orientation to at least three different goals. It is therefore illusory to suppose that the professional's sole obligation is to the patient/client, although the patient/client's interest is always the salient concern. Rather, the fact must be confronted that the professional cannot have an unequivocal commitment to the welfare of the patient/client. Hence, there is an unavoidable indeterminacy in the professional's ethical responsibility, a corresponding tension in the professional's orientation to his work, and complexity in the concept of professional integrity. Given the heavy burden of personal accountability entailed in a professional's work, it is very difficult for the professional to recognize and accept these ethical ambiguities in his calling. This circumstance may help explain why the concept of professional ethics generally held within a profession is at variance with the concept that the outside world demands. The profession's ethical definition of itself presupposes self-discipline, indeed self-denial, and focuses on service to the client. It obscures the necessity for making ethical choices that could subordinate interests of the patient/client. From an outside perspective, the duty to make such choices seems an essential element of professionalism.[2]

Forms of Conflicts Controls

Professional Codes, Statutes, and Regulations

In the modern context, the controls on conflicts of interest are expressed primarily in codes of ethics, augmented by statutes, regulations and interpretive decisions. These forms of normative direction coexist with older forms of control, including the conscience of individual professionals, shared lore and tradition within the professions, and the example of practice provided to apprentices by established practitioners. Not surprisingly, the codes governing the legal profession, and the corresponding body of interpretive decisions, are highly developed: When lawyers contemplate the control of behavior, they tend to think in terms of rules.[3] The parallel codes and interpretive decisions in medicine are much less fully developed.[4] However, codes of rules have come to assume a central place in the increasingly impersonal and bureaucratized settings in which medicine is now practiced. Many of the rules now governing medical practice originate from government regulation that is a concomitant of government payment for medical services. The professional codes of ethics do not cover professional ethics fully or with complete accuracy. The codes do not express their own presuppositions—for example, that doctors have a high social status that affects their relationships with patients, or that lawyers' social status has always been morally ambiguous ("first thing, let's kill all the lawyers"), which in a different way affects their relationships with clients. Nor do the codes take account of the discrepancies between the "book rules" and normative standards actually exhibited in practice. Nor do the codes face the most difficult ethical problems with complete candor. It is difficult, for example, for either doctors or lawyers as a group to speak openly about psychological exploitation of patients and clients.

Nevertheless, the professional codes do respond—even if sometimes obliquely—to the basic conflict–of–interest problems that have been identified here as self-control, mediation, and civic responsibility. The professional codes, particularly when read with sensitivity to nuance, are a useful template for analyzing conflict–of–interest problems.

Regulatory Techniques

In addressing these conflict–of–interest problems, the ethical codes reflect four control techniques: prophylactic rules; disclosure or "informed consent" requirements; reference to recognized professional standards; and intraprofessional consultation, or "second opinion."

Prophylactic rules categorically prohibit certain forms of conduct by a professional on the ground that the possibilities for exploitation in such conduct outweigh any efficiencies or other gains that might be achieved. For example, rules governing doctors generally prohibit them from having ownership interest in a pharmacy, although they may dispense from their offices, and rules governing lawyers in many jurisdictions prohibit a lawyer from representing both the buyer and seller in a real estate transaction. "Informed consent" rules, as the term implies, require that, with respect to certain procedures, the consent of the patient/client be obtained on the basis of an adequate explanation of the risks involved. For example, the legal ethics rules require that a client have an opportunity to obtain an independent consultation when entering into a business transaction with his lawyer. Reference to standards of practice requires that a professional use a generally accepted procedure in dealing with a situation or be prepared to justify a deviation to his peers or perhaps to civil authority. Intraprofessional consultation requires that a colleague's concurrence be obtained before undertaking a proposed procedure or that there be a review consultation promptly afterward. The "tumor board" in medical practice functions in this fashion post hoc; many law firms now require that written opinions have the concurrence of two partners.

Limitations of Regulatory Technique

All techniques for controlling conflicts of interest have inherent limitations, as will be more fully suggested in the following discussion. The net effect is that the professional rules of ethics do not—and, in my view, cannot—resolve fundamental aspects of conflict of interest. In particular, they cannot fully address the problem of uncertainty. As a practical matter, prophylactic rules cannot be used to impose categorical prohibition on practices that usually have beneficial effects, even though they also entail the risk of exploitation. Prohibition of such practices would throw out the baby with the bath water. For example, requiring that one standard fee be charged for all services of a specified kind would inhibit service in cases of unusual complexity.

There are counterpart limitations on what can be accomplished through informed consent or disclosure rules. As a practical matter, disclosure rules at best require communication only of that which can be made intelligible to the patient/client. This leaves open situations that are not fully intelligible to the professional himself, that is, situations of uncertainty. Rules governing informed consent or disclosure require the professional to acknowledge uncertainty and risk, and these days, prudent regard for malpractice liability is a strong inducement for compliance. The effectiveness of these rules is attenuated by the uncertainty in trying to communicate about uncertainty and by the anxiety that the professional himself experiences about the uncertainty.[5] Ethical rules that incorporate professional standards also incorporate these elements of uncertainty and hence are question-begging. The same is true, to a lesser degree, of the requirement of intraprofessional consultation.

Thus, there remain features of professional practice that are unfathomable from an external perspective. *Professional practices that cannot intelligibly be described cannot be rendered into fully intelligible ethical standards.* At the point beyond which effective communication is impossible, trust has to be placed in the professional, inasmuch as there is no practical alternative. For this very reason, there also remains an irreducible need for self-consciousness and personal discipline on the part of the professional. An ingredient in meeting this need is serious analysis of the ethical dilemmas in professional practice, as well as various procedures for fully opening our minds to these dilemmas.

Exploitation of the Patient/Client

Exploitation of the patient/client for the benefit of the professional takes several basic forms, with infinite variations in practice. The crudest and most obvious form is financial exploitation. Less direct is exploitation by the professional for the purposes of improperly dominating the relationship with the patient/client. Least direct and more subtle is exploitation for the purpose of controlling the problem of uncertainty in the professional's mind. All three forms of exploitation ultimately derive from the fact that a professional's services involve both special knowledge and elements of judgment that respond to unresolvable uncertainty and unavoidable risk.

Financial Exploitation

Financial exploitation consists of charging more for the services provided than ought to be charged. Excessive charges can take various forms. These include using a fee basis higher than that used in other similar situations; providing and charging for unnecessary services; charging for services not performed; giving services actually performed a higher classification for which higher charges can be made; charging for phantom support services and expenses; when auxiliary services are required (such as prescription drugs ordered by a doctor or a land title report ordered by a lawyer), referring the patient/client to a captive or affiliated supplier in which the professional has a profit interest; when services of a coprofessional are required, receiving a kickback for making the referral. These abuses are all too familiar.

Another form of financial exploitation occurs where a professional undertakes a case, and the opportunity to garner fee income from it, when professional competence indicates that the case should be referred elsewhere. The medical profession has reduced this incentive through its elaborate system of specialist accreditation, an institution of both self–advancement and self-denial that the legal profession has declined to impose on itself. Lawyers are now permitted to advertise fields of specialization, but doing so does not necessarily require limitations of practice.[6] However, the development of multimember practices—the clinic in medicine and the firm in law—has greatly reduced this source of conflict. In such arrangements, the individual professional has little incentive to perform services that should be undertaken by a different kind of specialist, for such specialists are part of the individual professional's own professional enterprise. Of course, problems may remain where an unusually difficult case should be referred to a superspecialist outside the clinic or firm. It seems fair to say, however, that the clinic and the firm are important controls against exploitation through incompetent performance.

Moreover, the rising risk of malpractice liability, itself a form of legal regulation, is a deterrent against undertaking services that the professional is not qualified to perform. Many forms of service entailing the risk of financial exploitation are prohibited altogether or are inhibited by disclosure requirements. For example, doctors are generally prohibited from owning interests in pharmacies, and similar controls have been imposed by legislation on clinical laboratories in which the referring doctor has an interest. Similarly, lawyers who use the services of captive title insurance companies in real estate transactions are generally required to disclose the relationship and to charge separately for the legal services and title insurance. However, some arrangements readily susceptible of financial exploitation remain permissible despite persistent criticism from inside and outside the professions. Thus, doctors have been permitted to own interests in clinical laboratories to which they refer patients, and lawyers in all states are permitted to accept what amount to referral fees where personal injury cases are forwarded from a general practitioner to a personal injury specialist.

This is not the place to consider whether there should be tighter controls against financial exploitation or to lament once again the professional venality that makes them necessary. It seems sufficient to make three observations. First, no system of direct regulation can be fully effective. Such a system seeks to regulate the prices not of standard commodities such as bread or beer but relatively amorphous services. For this reason, direct regulation of professional exploitation is necessarily indefinite in its terms.

Second, control is stronger where someone involved in the patient/client's interest is in a position to inhibit exploitation by monitoring the professional's performance. Thus, patients are better off complaining to their company's health plan about poor treatment at the hands of a plan doctor than trying to complain to the doctor directly, which involves unpleasant confrontation. The same point holds for legal services. However, the professions resist such arrangements on the ground that they interfere with the sanctity of the professional relationship—which is, of course, what the arrangements are intended to do. Finally, another source of control is effective competition among professionals coupled with the opportunity for patient/clients to compare services over time. This kind of control appears to have expanded in recent decades, particularly through greater availability of price and service information. It would be impossible to prove the matter one way or the other, but it would appear that financial exploitation by doctors and lawyers of their patients/clients is a less serious problem today than it was one or two generations ago. The problem of financial exploitation of health insurance is, of course, another matter and is referred to below.

These observations apply as well to the other forms of exploitation considered below.

Psychological Exploitation

Much more difficult to deal with is the professional's psychological exploitation of his information advantage. Psychological exploitation is easy to define in words but often difficult to delineate in practice. As a matter of definition, it is the professional's use of superior position and knowledge to induce the patient/client into inappropriate acceptance of the professional's definition of their relationship, their respective spheres of authority, and the course of services to be provided. As a matter of practice, however, it is difficult to specify normatively what is inappropriate in a given relationship between professional and patient/client and even more difficult to specify objectively the relationship's actual characteristics. For example, what seems to the professional to be a careful explanation may be perceived by the patient/client as condescension; what seems to the patient/client to be maddening delay may to the professional be careful reconnoitering of the situation; and so on. Who is to arbitrate the elusive evidence as to what the relationship really is?

Superior Knowledge. Nevertheless, psychological exploitation is widespread. To a large extent, psychological exploitation is simply another form of the possibility of financial exploitation. The practice of medicine and the practice of law involve special science and art that are beyond the average patient/client's knowledge and experience. This knowledge differential is the very reason why people to go to a doctor when their health malady goes beyond a common cold or contusion and to a lawyer when their legal malady goes beyond the common conflicts of everyday life. That is to say, most people simply endure most of their bodily and legal injuries, and wisely so. It is when people do not understand how to deal with a problem of health or with a transaction in finance or with the government that they feel it useful to seek professional help. Hence, the patient/client's deficiency in information is not merely an incident of a professional consultation but rather its very inducement.

The patient/client's information deficiency can be moderated by explanations given by the professional. In the practice of medicine, this process is called "informed consent" on the part of the patient; in the practice law of it is called "adequate consultation" with the client. The professions today have rightly given increasing attention to this vital professional responsibility. Adequate communication with the patient/client is recognized as important as a matter both of substance and of style. However, the patient/client's information deficiency cannot be fully overcome.

In the first place, the nuances of many technical problems in law and medicine are very difficult to explain, as everyone who has taught in medical or law school knows. In the second place, many recipients of professional services have modest or little education and correspondingly limited capacity to understand even rudimentary concepts and terminology. It may not be popular to note this fact, but it is fatuous to ignore it. In the third place, patients and clients are usually in a more or less anxious frame of mind when they come to see the doctor or the lawyer. This frame of mind is not conducive to learning.

Finally, and most fundamentally, beyond a limited threshold it is often frustrating for both parties to the transaction for the professional to give an elaborate explanation of the professional's diagnosis and proposed course of action. I say this with recognition that questioning the efficacy of informed consent goes against the trend of both professional ethics and legal requirements. The fact of the matter is, however, that the best a doctor or lawyer can do is to sketch the objective and the procedure, and possible alternatives, along with the corresponding costs and risks, and convey care and concern in doing so. This is not to disparage the need for adequate communication, informed consent, and sympathetic engagement with the patient/client. It is notorious that many professionals are very poor in meeting these needs, so that no reiteration of their importance is redundant. Nevertheless, the notion of full and equal partnership in the service relationship between the professional and the patient/client is an illusion. The patient cannot know all that the professional perceives, any more than the professional can know all that the patient or client feels and fears. When it comes to knowing what is going on and how to deal with it, there is an unavoidable element of dependency on the part of the patient/client, and therefore an unavoidable element of fiduciary responsibility on the part of the professional. That is, the professional must act as a trustee for the patient/client's interests.

This dependency results in a parental (or "paternal") relationship, no matter what might be demanded by egalitarian philosophy. Formerly it was held that the professional always knew best and that a patient/client simply had to trust the professional. That philosophical regime of simplistic paternalism no longer holds sway. But neither has a day dawned of participatory democracy in the relationship between professional and patient or client. The relationship between professional and patient/client entails an inherent and unavoidable risk of psychological exploitation.

The task for ethical control against psychological exploitation therefore could be viewed not as seeking to abolish paternalism in the relationship but to redefine the character of paternalism. Modern mothers and fathers realize that they must talk with, work with, and think of their children in a more interactive way than in the past. They must recognize that children, albeit inexperienced and dependent in matters of life, have minds and wills of their own and a capacity to communicate and to accept risks. Yet responsible modern mothers and fathers also realize that in most crisis situations the judgment calls are theirs to make, if they have any rapport at all with their children. Even in this era of informed consent, the professional has similar power and therefore similar responsibility.

Uncertainty. The problem of psychological exploitation has a root still deeper than that of the professional's superior knowledge. The most fundamental characteristic of a professional's service is that the professional deals with uncertainty in what is to be done in nonroutine cases. Indeed, it is not incorrect to say that dealing with uncertainty is a professional's essential function. In that task, the professional is necessarily isolated from the patient/client. If the doctor or lawyer cannot foresee the course of events in the undertaking, the patient or client certainly cannot. Moreover, in dealing with uncertainty, the professional is often isolated from the effective scrutiny of peers. Even a requirement of concurrence by a professional peer usually involves an element of communication and, in any event, involves allocation of responsibility for finally making a judgment call.

The problem of uncertainty takes infinite forms. In medicine the essential problem is whether the curative gain that is possible with a given procedure is offset by the risk of loss in well-being that is a concomitant of the procedure. Is the surgery worth it? Will the therapeutic regimen yield results commensurate with its inconvenience and discomfort? Is it worth the financial cost? In concrete terms, will surgery arrest the cancer?

The explosive development of modern health technology continually relocates the boundaries of uncertainty but does not eradicate them. To be sure, procedures that formerly were problematic become routine and thereupon are relegated to the provinces of paraprofessionals. However, by the same token, new knowledge poses dilemmas not previously perceived. Indeed, among the most profound dilemmas today are those posed by techniques that will succeed, but only temporarily and at great financial and existential cost.

The practice of law presents corresponding problems, although ones that usually involve jeopardy to property and liberty rather than to life itself. The most painful dilemma in litigation is whether to settle a case, and on what terms, when the client honestly and justifiably believes his cause is just. However fervent and well grounded the client's conviction may be, the fact is that the court and the jury may see the case differently. If that happens, not only is the case lost, and often large sums of money with it, but the client's whole structure of belief and self–confidence is put under severe strain. Yet forecasting the outcome of close cases is necessarily a matter of informed guesswork on the part of the client's lawyer.

Similar uncertainty attends the other primary legal service: negotiation by a lawyer concerning an important client interest. This service is performed in all sorts of business counseling: the formation of business enterprises such as corporations, major contracts such as franchise deals, finance agreements and securities issues, real estate transactions, and the like. These transactions involve uncertainty as to whether a deal will be consummated on any terms, uncertainty as to price, and uncertainty as to the risks that should be addressed in the terms of the transaction. The client, especially an experienced business client, of course, knows as much about most of these uncertainties as the lawyer. However, the lawyer has to calibrate these uncertainties to the resulting legal consequences and eventual legal remedies if the transaction encounters misfortune. That process involves professional judgments no less impalpable than those made by the medical practitioner.

The ethical problem is how the professional presents this uncertainty to the patient/client and how he deals with it in his own mind. The classic approach in medicine and law relied heavily on the authority implicit in the professional's superior knowledge. Accordingly, the professional presented himself as having special insight into the facts of a situation and special access to the wiles of fortune. The professional's conversance with the occult was manifested in special costumes for professional performances (doctors and lawyers both wore robes), the use of obscure terminology (especially Latin), and the solemnity of professional theatrics.

The apparatus of modern professions for dealing with uncertainty is less obvious. In modern medical practice, the mystique of science has supplanted, or perhaps simply reinforced, the use of special ceremony and terminology. In modern American legal practice, the lawyer's apparatus is primarily his conversance with the uncertainty of the legal process itself. It is popular knowledge and a commonly held fear that courts, juries, and regulatory agencies are prone to perversity. The lawyer can exploit this fear to cover the limitations on his own ability to deal with the situation.

Systematic efforts can be made to reduce the professional's reliance on irrational ways of dealing with the uncertainties inherent in practice. Simpler language can be used to give more candid explanations of the professional's science and art. The ceremony in professional service can be reduced, if not eliminated. The patient or client can be encouraged to confront the uncertainty along with the professional. Greater care can be taken to probe the patient/client's sensitivity to risk.

However, as my colleague Dr. Jay Katz has so well explained,[7] the professional's greatest difficulty in dealing with uncertainty is how the professional himself deals with it. Dr. Katz believes that many doctors fear the uncertainties they confront, leading them to perceive the uncertainties in an unrealistic way (either exaggerating or ignoring them) and to function in unrealistic ways in response. The elaborate and often superfluous tests used by many doctors may be a manifestation of such fearfulness. So may be the loudly voiced fear of malpractice liability.

The same analysis can be made of legal practice. For example, fear of the unknowable unknown helps explain the elaborate and often superfluous pretrial discovery used by many trial lawyers. A similar explanation may underlie the elaborate and often superfluous documentation that many office lawyers employ in transactions that can bear the cost of such procedures.

The basic problem here is not simply financial exploitation or purposive exploitation of patients and clients. The basic problem is that of self-deception. This could be considered a conflict of interest between the professional's mind and his soul—perhaps, as the poets recognize, the ultimate problem of self-control.

Mediation

Many professional tasks involve not only the professional and the patient/client but an intimately concerned third party to whom the professional owes some kind of responsibility as well. In many situations, it is impossible to fulfill both responsibilities completely. At a minimum, there are limits to the professional's time and attention. Beyond this, measures that serve the patient/client's interest may conflict with the interests of the concerned third party, and vice versa. In such circumstances the professional has to mediate the conflict; in some situations, the professional may be obliged to withdraw, entirely or partially. The latter course of action itself requires mediation to the extent of justifying the choice to withdraw and of ameliorating its consequences.

Three-Party Relationships

In medicine the third party is typically a member of the patient's family—the patient's parent, child, spouse, sibling, or relevant other. In modern medical practice, a relationship that is becoming increasingly common is that between aging parent and adult child, where the latter, in addition to the family relationship as such, has responsibilities of care, custody, and financial assistance. In situations where treatment resources are in radically short supply, medical professionals may have the additional responsibility of rationing their services by some sort of triage procedure; in administering such a system, they engage in mediation of an especially grim form.

Ethical problems arising from immediate third–party interests are ubiquitous in law practice. The third party may be another client, as where a lawyer represents both husband and wife in estate planning or all the partners in a business partnership or several codefendants in litigation. The third party may be a person to whom the lawyer's client owes a fiduciary responsibility—for example, where the client is a trustee or an executor charged with managing a trust fund or an estate. A lawyer representing a corporation owes primary allegiance to the corporation as a legal entity, but he necessarily has confidential working relations with members of corporate management and, in the case of a closely held corporation, with the stockholders. In these corporate relationships, there is an ever-present risk that the interests of the corporate "constituents"—management, employees, stockholders—will conflict with the collective interest of the corporation as such.

In such situations, the governing ethical rules specially define or limit the professional's scope of action. In law practice, the conflict–of–interest rules preclude a lawyer from representing more than one client in certain types of transactions or impose special constraints on the professional initiatives that may be undertaken. For example, a lawyer ordinarily may not bring suit against a person whom he represents in another transaction, even if the transactions are unrelated; the theory is that the hostility incident to litigation is incompatible with the open and trusting relationship that should be maintained between lawyer and client. When joint representation is permitted in law practice, it must be predicated on especially careful informed consent.

The interests to be protected are those of loyalty and confidentiality. The biblical injunction that "no man can serve two masters" implies that no risk of compromising loyalty or confidentiality should be permitted. However, such an injunction would prove too much, for taken literally, it would preclude any professional undertaking that involves duties to multiple interests. As we have seen, orientation to multiple interests is inherent in a professional calling.

Nevertheless, serious compromise of the professional's loyalty must be avoided. In law practice the ethical formula is that the division of loyalty should not create "significant risk" of a "material adverse effect" on the lawyer's responsibilities to the client. Application of this standard is highly fact specific and accommodates a range of thresholds of sensitivity. In practice, the matter reduces to this: If actual conflict is present or foreseeable, a lawyer who proceeds takes the risk that unmanageable conflict may eventuate, and he must be prepared to deal with it or take the consequences.

The same considerations apply to maintaining confidentiality. If the situation requires confidences to be shared among the participants, this must be done in a way that minimizes the risk of embarrassment to the client and the relevant other.

In medicine, the same problem has long been recognized in psychiatric practice and is governed by similar principles. The problem also arises in any situation where the patient's condition may be a source of embarrassment or conflict in regard to the third person. Pregnancy of an underage girl, venereal disease, AIDS, Alzheimer's syndrome, and other conditions are familiar illustrations. The poignant question of whether to continue heroic lifesaving measures—as in the

Karen Quinlan case—is addressed in hospitals every day, whether openly or otherwise. Beyond this, a serious medical condition of any kind can pose the question of how much personal responsibility the relevant other is to take in caring for the patient and paying the cost of treatment. For example, if a young child or aged parent is to recuperate at home rather than in the hospital, the burden on the family is correspondingly increased. Often, though not always, recuperation at home is not only less expensive to the funding source but faster and less stressful for the patient.

How are the interests to be weighed in such situations, how articulate will be the choice, and whose judgment will be determinative? A formula calling on the doctor to pursue the "best interests of the patient" with "due regard" for the family's interest seems about as indeterminate as the counterpart formula governing a lawyer's mediation of conflicting interests. A substantial element of professional judgment is necessarily involved.

The Mediating Task

There are several common threads in the mediation required in these situations. In the first place, all the possibilities for exploitation of the patient/client discussed earlier are also present in a three-party situation. That is, the professional has an incentive to exploit the situation, has superior knowledge through which to accomplish exploitation, and confronts uncertainties that conduce to interpreting the situation in accordance with the professional's own wishful thinking. An additional variable has been introduced, that of the third party's interest, but this only complicates the situation. Indeed, real or ostensible concern for the third party's interest can mask exploitation of the patient/client.

By the same token, the indeterminacy of the ethical controls is greater. What was a two-party relationship between professional and patient/client now requires an equation taking account of the interests of an interested third party. For example, when informed consent is required, not only is an additional respondent involved but delicate questions arise as to how far confidences received from one can be used in informing the other. Indeed, in a three-party situation there can be diametric opposition between the professional's duty to protect the confidences of one respondent and the duty to make full disclosure to the other. So, application of prophylactic rules becomes correspondingly problematic. Should a doctor never be allowed to minister to members of the same family? Should a lawyer never be allowed to counsel members of the same family?

These complications are compounded when, as is often the case in modern practice, two or more professionals provide services in the case. Their relationship involves questions of scope of responsibility, communication, possibly divergent professional judgment, cost and risk considerations, and uncertainty in their relationship. Especially risky procedures are shadowed by the potential for later recrimination if things go wrong.

In the second place, when a situation involves two clients, or both a patient and a relevant third party, choices have to be made that entail the risk of being detrimental to one of them. In medical practice it may appear, for example, that the patient will actually be better off in a skilled nursing care facility rather than recuperating in the family member's home. But that choice, by whomever made and on whatever ostensible grounds, could turn out to be wrong. In law practice it may appear that the managers and directors of a corporation can all be advised effectively by one legal counsel, but that choice too could turn out to be wrong. The aware professional knows that the choices carry this risk, and that he may suffer recrimination and other consequences if things go badly.

In the third place, it is inevitable not only that the professional will influence the choice but also that the outcome will affect his interests, at least his interests of self-esteem and reputation. Yet the rules concerning conflict of interest pretend to preclude a choice that could be detrimental to a patient/client. The rules require that if a procedure involves significant conflict of interest, then the interests of the patient/client are to prevail; if it is impossible to make those interests prevail, then the professional should not proceed. But even here the controls are predicated on a difference between significant risk and insignificant risk; mediating that distinction is the professional's responsibility.

On analysis, therefore, a professional is inevitably called on to mediate conflicts between the interests of a patient/client and those of someone else. That duty, in turn, inevitably results in some outcomes that may be adverse to the patient/client.

Civic Responsibility

The problem of civic responsibility is much more conspicuous and has been experienced longer in the practice of law than in the practice of medicine. Hence, it is convenient to begin with the ethical problems it presents for the lawyer.

Whereas compliance with law is a basic civic responsibility, law practice by nature involves pressures to overstep the law. Litigation, the activity of trial lawyers, involves direct and aggressive assertion of the client's interests, subject to constraints of fairness imposed by procedural law and professional ethics. Thus, for example, a lawyer is not permitted to use testimony he knows to be false or evidence he knows to be fabricated. However, being constrained by such rules makes it more difficult to win—and sometimes impossible. The incentives to break the rules, or at least to bend them, are correspondingly strong. The opposing party, of course, is a watchful monitor of the lawyer's compliance with his duties under procedural law. However, many unethical maneuvers can go undetected or at least unprovable. The lawyer himself therefore is the principal safeguard against exploitation of the situation for the benefit of his client.

The same point holds for the office lawyer. Negotiation and other office practices always proceed in contemplation of potentially adverse interests of third parties. A contract, by definition, involves the legal rights of another party; a business enterprise, those of partners or stockholders; a lending agreement, those of a creditor and a debtor. Most such transactions involve positive–sum gains in the sense that all parties stand to gain if things go well. However, zero-sum elements are also involved, particularly division of net gain and allocation of losses. Resolution of these issues pits the lawyer against the third party on behalf of the client.

Under governing legal and ethical rules, the lawyer in negotiation is prohibited from making false representations and may not assist a client in doing so. On the other hand, the rules generally do not require the lawyer to be forthcoming to the opposing party. The lawyer is not required, indeed ordinarily is not permitted, to disclose background facts that might affect the opposing party's calculations in the transaction, or to reveal contingencies that the opposing party may not have considered. Here again, there is often an incentive to bend the rules. The difference between a prohibited misrepresentation and a permissible nondisclosure is often one merely of nuance; the lawyer is trained to be a master of nuances.

There is a public interest in ensuring that litigation and negotiation are conducted according to the rules of the game. The rules governing litigation are technically complex; so are those governing certain kinds of contracts—for example, securities and real estate transactions. However, in general, when statements are made they must be truthful. Only in this way can the parties peacefully resolve matters requiring exchange of information, a process that, in turn, is integral to an orderly and productive society. The lawyer, as professional facilitator of that process, shares a civic responsibility to maintain the integrity of litigation and negotiation and thereby their continuing public value.

Another target of potential exploitation on behalf of the client is the government. Government has manifold interactions with individuals and businesses, including taxation, regulation, recordkeeping requirements, contract relationships, and various types of grants and subsidies. These transactions involve submission of information to the government and sometimes direct negotiation or other presentations, activities in which lawyers may be involved. Opportunities for misrepresentation and illegal manipulation are ubiquitous. In general, the lawyer is constrained by the same governing legal principles that apply to everyone else. The basic dividing line is drawn between misrepresentation, which is prohibited, and presentations nuanced in favor of the private client, which are permitted.

Unfortunately, in practice, the governing ethical principles are often disregarded. Sometimes this is conscious, for there are dishonest and rapacious lawyers. More often, however, violation of the legal interests of others proceeds from self–persuasion, rationalization, and self-delusion. The lawyer's ministrations on behalf of the client are protected by confidentiality, and many clients are happy to cheat the government through the instrumentality of their lawyers. Even under close regulation, lawyers are often able to persuade themselves of the virtue of unvirtuous practice, as the current wave of financial scandals attests. The legal profession is widely and properly criticized for the complicity of many of its members in such exploitations. Less often there is similar criticism of the clients, who ordinarily understand what is being done for them.

Similar opportunities have become salient ethical problems for doctors. Now that third parties pay most of the cost of medical care, doctors face ubiquitous opportunities for exploiting third-party payers for the benefit of their patients. In earlier days, the cost of care was a matter between the doctor and the patient or the patient's family. The potential for fraud was limited to providing unnecessarily elaborate care to rich patients, which was not unheard of, or concealing malpractice, which was also not unheard of. Today, however, most of the income of most doctors comes from third–party payers, including the government.

It is distressing, but surely not surprising, to find that doctors are exposed to the same incentives for misrepresentation and manipulation that lawyers have always confronted. It is also not surprising, even though it is distressing, that many doctors have a substantial capacity for self-persuasion, rationalization, and self-delusion in these matters. After all, what can be more humane than helping into a nursing home a patient whose family would be severely stressed, psychologically as well as financially, if the placement is not arranged?

In medicine, as in law, the professional has an irreducible obligation to safeguard the public interest against the interest of the patient/client. It is often in the immediate interest of a lawyer's client, but not in the public interest, for the client to evade taxes, disregard government regulations, exploit the unwary in business transactions, and encroach on or misappropriate other people's property. It is often in the immediate interest of a patient to get treatment that the patient would not request, and that the doctor would not prescribe, except for the fact that the cost is being covered by an insurer or government funding. The professional has special knowledge of the facts of the transaction, which are shared only with the patient/client and which is covered by rules of confidentiality. The professional has special expertise in the technical standards—medical or legal, as the case may be—that determine whether a proposed procedure is legitimate. Against these circumstances, the professional has a legal and an ethical obligation at least not to employ his services in the aid of criminal or fraudulent purpose on the part or on behalf of a patient/client.

A problem now concerning the practice of medicine, but not soberly confronted, is rationing medical care, particularly care based on clinical considerations alone. The blunt fact is that the "need" for medical services—want of clinically legitimate procedures that the patient cannot afford—not only is greater than what patients will pay for but is becoming more than the community at large will pay for. There is a paradox in the public's wish for wider availability of health care (reflecting a personal standard of demand) and antipathy to higher taxes and premiums to pay for such care (reflecting an economic standard of supply). The difficulty is in determining what clinically justifiable services will be denied to whom, on the basis of what criteria applied by which decision-makers.[8] The question here is not one of fraud or exploitation but of withholding justified treatment because of cost. Under the old fee–for–service regime, withholding was accomplished by the market—patients who couldn't pay were left out—and by limits on the willingness and ability of doctors and hospitals to take charity cases. That decision process was diffuse, low in visibility, and unaccountable in terms of legal or professional ethics. There was a recognized moral duty to serve the poor, and professional and public honor in doing so, but no enforceable obligation.

The same situation prevailed regarding legal services, and to a large extent still does. Under the fee-for-service regime, people who need legal assistance—criminal defendants, for example, or people having legal troubles with a landlord or an automobile dealer—often cannot afford what it takes to vindicate their legal rights. They are therefore dependent on the generosity of friends, public charity or publicly subsidized services. Legal assistance, however, was and is in grievously short supply compared with the clinically justifiable need. Moreover, poor criminal defendants and those otherwise entangled with the law are not attractive in public sentiment in the same way that the sick and disabled are. Hence, justice—that is, legal assistance necessary to obtain justice—has to be rationed. As in the case of medical services, rationing was done in a diffuse, low–visibility process in which no one was specifically accountable.

However, once medical care and legal assistance become entitlements, the rationing process changes and with it the civic responsibility of the involved professionals. Under an entitlement system, defined categories of citizens are entitled to defined types of benefits. For example, all persons with incomes below a certain level could be entitled to nursing home care, among other coverage; similarly, all persons charged with felonies or facing driver's license revocation could be entitled to legal representation. Whatever the system, the relevant professionals will be involved at two basic levels: shaping the definition of covered persons and covered benefits, and administering the definitions in practice. Making the policy choices is remote from individual cases, but making clinical decisions in terms of program eligibility is not. In the latter context, the legal aid lawyer's civic responsibility inevitably requires withholding service from a potential client who meets professional standards of need and is morally deserving. The medical profession must make similar choices, either personally or by delegation to paramedical staff. In both contexts, civic responsibility in the rationing process conflicts with the ethics of professional dedication.

In rare situations, the public may have to be protected against sinister purposes of the patient/client—a physical or homicidal attack. Often the target can be anticipated, but sometimes not. The problem is endemic in psychiatric practice, an incident of which led to the notorious *Tarasoff* case.[9] The psychiatrist's patient disclosed an intention to kill the object of his deranged infatuation, and then acted upon the intention. The psychiatrist in fact took preventive steps, which unfortunately failed. The courts held that the professional had a legal duty to use reasonable efforts to head off the patient. On a similar basis, legal ethics permit, and in some states require, breach of a client's confidence if necessary to prevent the client from committing homicide or serious bodily harm.[10]

In all such circumstances, whether the imminent act threatens life or merely property, the professional has an ethical obligation to counsel the client to refrain. Failure to carry out that obligation may subject the professional to legal liability. These inducements are intended to counterbalance the professional's primary commitment to the patient/client, thus posing a delicate and often excruciating conflict of interest. Uncertainty and ambiguity permeate the facts of the matter being confronted, the intentions and perceptions of the participants, and the possible outcomes. On the one hand lies the prospect of irreparable harm to an innocent victim—harm with which the professional will be associated morally, if not legally. On the other hand lies the prospect of betrayal of the patient/client's confidences and trust.

This combination of circumstances puts the professional in the position of a gatekeeper responsible for safeguarding a public interest where the potential predator is the patient/client. The professional accordingly must monitor and judge the patient/client and, when necessary, interdict the patient/client's purposes. In an extreme case, the professional has to go to the public law enforcement authorities. Fulfilling these responsibilities poses the sharpest of all professional conflicts of interest.

Conclusion

Conflicts are endemic between the professional and the patient/client, between the interests of the patient/client and those of specific third persons, and between the interests of the immediate parties and those of the general public. The interest of the patient/client generally has priority, but not in all circumstances. At a minimum, the professional cannot assist the patient/client in wrongfully harming other interests and may be obliged to take positive action to prevent such harm. More prosaically, the professional in ordinary practice must continually make choices among competing interests, including choices that are adverse to the patient/client. Professional lore obscures this obligation, as though practice would not be ethically governed if any interest were allowed to compete with that of the patient/client.

Nevertheless, the ethical codes, the law, and comparison of professional ethics make it clear that professional have obligation to accommodate conflicting interests and to make ethical choices accordingly. Direct acknowledgment of those obligations is necessary for fulfilling them intelligently and humanely.

Notes

1. *See* R. Gorlin, ed., *BNA Codes of Professional Ethics* (2d ed., 1990) (compilation of codes of professions for law, health care, and business professions, with a bibliography).
2. Compare S. Koniak, Between the Bar and the State, 70 *North Carolina L. Rev.* 1389 (1992) (comparison between the legal profession's view of its ethical duties and that of the courts).
3. The American Bar Association Model Rules of Professional Conduct, adopted in 1983 and since amended, are promulgated by the legal profession's national voluntary organization. The Model Rules have no legal force but have been adopted by most states and most local federal courts. For analysis and commentary, see Geoffrey Hazard, Jr. & L. Hodes, *The Law of Lawyering: A Handbook on the Model Rules of Professional Conduct* (2d ed., 1990). For annotations to judicial decisions and ethics committee opinions, see American Bar Association/Bureau of National Affairs, *Lawyers' Manual on Professional Conduct* (1992).
4. *See* American Medical Association, *Principles of Medical Ethics* (1980). For commentary, see, e.g., Thomas O'Rourke and Dennis Brodeur, *Medical Ethics: Common Ground for Understanding* (1987) (Catholic orientation).
5. *See* J. Katz, *The Silent World of Doctor and Patient, passim* and chap. VII (1984).
6. Lawyers are permitted to designate themselves as specialists, as a form of advertising, and some states have formal certification procedures and requirement. *See* ABA Model Rule 7.4 ("A lawyer may communicate the fact that the lawyer does or does not practice in particular fields of law"). The principal fields so far thus developed include trial advocacy, particularly plaintiffs' personal injury matters, and domestic relations. However, specialist qualification has not yet come to be recognized as the primary basis for referral.
7. *See* Katz, op. cit. supra note 5.
8. *See* Guido Calabresi and Phillip Bobbitt, Tragic Choices (1978).
9. Tarasoff v. Regents of the University of California, 17 Cal.3d 425, 131 Cal.Rptr. 14, 551 P.2d 334 (1976).
10. See *ABA Model Rules of Professional Conduct*, Rule 1.6(b).

5

Is There a Medical Profession in the House?

Allen E. Buchanan

Concern Over Conflict of Interest

There is a growing awareness that the new conditions under which medicine is practiced in this country are creating or at least exacerbating conflicts of interest in the physician–patient relationship. On the one hand, private insurers and government agencies are exerting pressure on physicians to cut costs by reducing utilization of services. The result is that physicians increasingly practice under incentives for *underutilization of services*—that is, for utilizing fewer services or lesser quantities of given services than would be optimal from the standpoint of the patient's best interest.[1] On the other hand, hospital administrators and entrepreneurial physicians themselves are creating incentive structures designed to increase revenues even at the price of *overutilization of services*—that is, providing services that exceed what is optimal from the standpoint of the patient's best interest.[2] Whenever the incentive structure under which physicians practice either rewards or penalizes them for utilizing services that are not in the patient's best interest or for not utilizing services that are in the patient's best interest, a conflict of interest exists.

To the extent that private or government cost containment measures employ incentives that serve to reduce *unnecessary* services—those that cannot reasonably be expected to produce any net benefit for the patient—they are morally

105

uncontroversial and involve no conflict of interest. However, some of the cost-containment measures now employed by private insurers and government agencies provide incentives for physicians to reduce not just unnecessary (i.e., nonbeneficial) services, but also services that can reasonably be expected to provide a net benefit—sometimes a very significant benefit—to the patient.[3] Current cost-containment strategies give physicians an incentive to *ration* services, not simply to eliminate waste.

Underutilization (relative to the patient's best interest) can result in inadequate treatments that fail to relieve pain or to restore or preserve normal functioning, or failure to detect conditions that may later become untreatable or very difficult and costly to treat, and can shift costs to the patient or the patient's family (as when patients are discharged early from the hospital and must recuperate at home). Overutilization (again, relative to the patient's best interest) can lead to iatrogenic injuries, unnecessary discomfort, inconvenience and waste of the patient's time, increased out-of-pocket expenses (copayments, deductibles), increased private insurance premiums, and more taxes to support government-reimbursed coverage such as Medicare and Medicaid.

A recurrent theme in the literature and in public discussions concerning conflict of interest in contemporary medical practice is the declaration that pressures for cost containment and entrepreneurial behavior are eroding patient trust and undermining medicine as a profession.[4] Entrepreneurial behavior is especially troubling to some. They worry that when physicians are themselves motivated by the thirst for profit or are the virtual employees of those whose dominant concern is the bottom line, medicine becomes a mere business rather than a profession. It is this worry upon which I wish to focus in this chapter.

Unexamined Assumptions About the Nature, Existence, and Desirability of a Medical Profession

Instead of adding to what I believe to be rather inconclusive and speculative predictions about how entrepreneurial arrangements will or will not erode patient trust and extinguish professionalism, my objective is to uncover and critically examine certain highly problematic but rarely articulated assumptions that frame the debate about conflict of interest. The most fundamental assumptions are these: (1) the reduction of patients' trust in physicians as professionals is bad; (2) unless physicians are regarded as professionals, trust in them and the benefits it brings for patients will not exist; and (3) there currently is in this country a medical profession according to a conception of what a medical profession is that makes it desirable that there be such a profession. Together, these assumptions constitute what I shall call the "myth of professionalism."

To explicate and criticize these three fundamental framing assumptions, it is first necessary to clarify what is meant in this context by a profession and then to explain the *justification* or *rationale* for according a particular occupational group the status of a profession. In addition, it is necessary to distinguish clearly between the existence of a profession and belief in its existence, but in such a way as to take into account the fact that for this type of social entity, belief is partly constitutive of the entity itself. Finally, it is important to clarify the relationship between professionalism and trust. In particular, we must examine critically the assumption that the extinction of professionalism means the end of trust.[5] A secondary aim of this chapter is to show just how constraining the three major framing assumptions are. I shall argue that these assumptions seriously restrict the range of policy options for dealing with problems of conflict of interest in the context of increasing pressures for rationing and growing entrepreneurial activity. In brief, acceptance of the myth of medical professionalism tends to prevent us from dealing with—and indeed, even from adequately understanding—the problem of conflict of interest.

The Concept of a Profession and the Justification of Social Inequalities

The extensive literature on professions yields two distinct but overlapping conceptions of a profession. The first may be called the "ideal" conception. It includes the following elements.[6]

1. Special knowledge of a practical sort (whose application is the distinctive activity of the profession.)[7]
2. A commitment to preserving and enhancing the special knowledge.
3. A commitment by the members of the profession to achieving excellence in the practice of the profession (in other words, practice of the profession is *not* motivated only by the desire to earn a living.)
4. An intrinsic and dominant commitment to serving others on whose behalf the special knowledge is applied. (To say that the commitment is intrinsic is to say that it is not exclusively instrumental, that is, derived from other motives, such as the desire for personal gain. The commitment is dominant in the sense that, at least in many cases, it overrides other desires or commitments with which it may come into conflict.) This element may be referred to as the "*service commitment*."
5. Effective collective self-regulation by the professional group, including the articulation of standards of competence for the profession, measures for inculcating in individual members the commitment to these standards, *and* sanctions (including expulsion from the professional group) for ensuring compliance with them.[8]

It is worth noting that at least in the case of the medical profession, and perhaps in all of the so-called caring professions (e.g., nursing and social work), elements 4 and 5 may not be clearly distinguishable. If serving the needs and interests of others is essential to the characteristic activity of the profession, then an intrinsic commitment to performing the characteristic activity well (element 4) already includes an effective disposition to put the patient's (or client's) interest first. If the professional allowed her own interests to interfere with providing appropriate care for the patient (or client), this would be a departure from excellent performance. In other words, excellent performance requires that the activity be directed toward some goals and not others. Accordingly, a commitment to excellence in performing the activity—at least this kind of activity—includes a commitment to putting the patient's interest first. In that sense, the commitment to excellence and the service commitment, according to the ideal conception of a medical profession, are not distinct.[9]

Some have equated what I have referred to as the service commitment with *altruism*.[10] In this context, however, the term "altruism" is misleading unless it is qualified with the adjective "limited" (or "particularized"). Sometimes altruism is understood as a rather *general* disposition to act so as to serve the interests of others (other people generally), and to do so even when this means *sacrificing* one's own interests. The service commitment differs from altruism so understood in two ways. First, it does not imply a general disposition, that is, a disposition to serve the interests of all persons or even of all persons in need of medical care, but rather only a disposition to put the interests *of one's patients* first. Second, the service commitment need not (usually) involve sacrificing one's own interests, and we need not think of the professional as one who, by virtue of superior moral will, ruthlessly suppresses his own most basic interests (at least as far as his most important interests are concerned, as the notion of sacrifice suggests). Instead, the service commitment is better understood as *limited* (as opposed to generalized) *altruism* that is substantial, though not necessarily literally self-sacrificing. To put it in a slightly different way, the service commitment focuses attention on the interests of certain others, not all others. The professional, by striving to perform the characteristic activity with excellence, focuses on the interests of the patient, since the characteristic activity is the application of his special knowledge for the purpose of serving *those* interests, not his own. What (generalized) altruism and the service commitment, or limited altruism of the professional, have in common is that both involve *not* being guided primarily by the goal of maximizing self-interest.

This first conception of what a profession is may be called the ideal conception because it is normative, not purely descriptive. Even if it could be shown that most physicians do not exhibit some or all of the characteristics listed in elements 1–5, it would not follow that the concept of a medical profession is vacuous or nonsensical. Instead, one might conclude that there are few "true" medical professionals. Similarly, the concept of a virtuous person or of a good carpenter is an ideal rather than a purely descriptive concept: It expresses a norm, a prescription, about how things should be, not simply about how they are. In other words, the ideal conception functions as a standard for evaluating the behavior of physicians: Those who conform to it are said to be professionals (or "true" or "genuine" professionals); those who do not are condemned for unprofessional conduct or for not being ("true") professionals.

The second conception of a profession I wish to distinguish is what may be called the "sociological" conception—the conception that is most prevalent in sociological analyses of the professions. It incorporates all the elements of the ideal conception, but in a way that wavers between pure description of the actual characteristics of those whom we call professionals and a report of the social perception of the occupational group in question, at least under conditions in which the "professionalism" of the group is not widely called into question. For example, according to the sociological conception of a profession, members of the group in question avow a commitment to service and are generally thought of as actually having such a commitment, at least when there is not a "legitimation crisis" with respect to the public's attitude toward the profession.

The sociological conception also includes another element, which is purely descriptive:

6. Special status for members of the group (public acknowledgment of worth, marks of prestige, etc.) and special privileges, including financial advantages (such as public subsidies for training and education and insulation from economic competition) and a significant sphere of autonomy, that is, substantial freedom from external regulation of the characteristic activity.[11]

It is crucial to point out that at least some components of this sixth element are quite separable, at least in principle, from the preceding five. In particular, there is no obvious connection between elements 1–5, on the one hand, and the favored economic position of medical professionals, on the other.

Professions are *social constructs*, not facts of nature. As such, they are appropriate subjects for critical appraisal. It makes sense to evaluate them and, indeed, to ask whether it is a good thing that they exist. Indeed, professions, at least as far as they exhibit the features listed in item 6, are *socially constructed inequalities*. And with respect to any socially constructed inequality, it is appropriate to ask: What is the justification for this unequal treatment? Why should some occupational groups (such as physicians) and not others (such as automobile mechanics or butchers) receive special status, reap exceptional financial rewards, and be accorded an exceptional degree of freedom from external regulation in their activities?[12]

Two different putative justifications may be distinguished: (1) *the simple appeal to expertise* and (2) *the social cost/benefit justification*. The former is at best capable of justifying only one aspect of that socially constructed inequality we call the medical profession: the relative freedom from external regulation. The idea is simply (indeed, as we shall see, simplistically) that only those who possess special expertise are qualified to exercise control over how the expertise is employed.

It is, of course, true that physicians possess special expertise.[13] But this is true of every specialized—that is, skilled—occupational group. Yet we do not generally assume that possession of a special skill exempts an occupational group from external regulation. Nor does the fact that the special skill of physicians is highly technical seem to be a good reason for allowing them to be free from external regulation in its exercise. A number of other occupational groups, including accountants, air traffic controllers, ships' captains, and mining and petroleum engineers, possess technical skills, yet they are not exempt from external regulation. Nor does the fact that a technically skilled occupational group works directly with people, in the service of their needs, seem to be a good reason for excluding external regulation: Financial advisors do just that, yet they are subject to external regulations in the form of legal obligations under the law of agency and fiduciary law.

Generally speaking, the question of regulating a group's characteristic activity arises only where the activity has the potential for seriously affecting the interests of others who are not in a position to protect themselves adequately. The physician/patient relationship—which, like other principal/agent relationships, is characterized by an asymmetry of knowledge and capabilities—creates just such a situation. The patient seeks a physician because the physician has knowledge and capabilities that the patient lacks.[14] But, as is also the case in other principal/agent relationships, the very asymmetry of knowledge or capabilities which makes it attractive for one person to engage another as his agent also creates the potential for a divergence between the agent's and the principal's interests and hence introduces "agency risk"—the risk that the agent will use his superior knowledge and ability to pursue his own interests (or the interests of others) at the expense of the principal's.

In attempting to justify its relative freedom from external regulation, the medical profession implicitly claims that patients in general are *not* able to provide adequate protection for themselves and that some other party must do so. But once it is assumed that some sort of regulation by another party is necessary, the question arises: Who should the regulator be? Surely the agent is not the most obvious candidate. Simply put, the agent—that is, the one who is placed so as to exploit the asymmetry of knowledge and capability that characterizes the principal/agent relationship—is the *least* obvious candidate for the regulator, assuming that some form of regulation is necessary. But if the physician as agent—the source of the risk that makes regulation desirable—is not the most obvious choice for the regulator, why should the collectivity of agents, the medical profession, be allowed to perform this function?

Self-regulation, whether individual or collective, generally is not the most plausible option for regulation. Indeed, a presumption against self-regulation is expressed in a wide range of our social institutions and practices, from the use of *civilian* review boards for complaints against the police, to government regulation of certain industries, to the system of checks and balances of constitutional government itself. In short, the mere fact that a group possesses special technical knowledge does not by itself defeat this presumption in the case of many other groups. So there must be something more than a simple appeal to (technical) expertise if the medical profession's relative freedom from external regulation is to be justified. The simple argument from expertise does not do the job.

What the simple argument from expertise overlooks is that effective regulation is to a large extent procedural or structural rather than content specific, or substantive. It is no doubt true that in formulating substantive standards of performance for a certain activity, external regulators must rely to a greater or lesser extent on advice from those who possess the special technical expertise. But once this crucial substantive input is available, an external authority can impose reasonable structural and procedural regulations. For example, effective regulation of railroad engineers or airplane pilots requires input from engineers and pilots regarding the types and levels of particular skills that are desirable and the training programs needed for them. But an external authority can then use this information to formulate, publicize, and enforce licensing and relicensing requirements designed to ensure that those who work as pilots and engineers initially possess and continue to maintain the skills in question.

Furthermore, even if reliance on those who possess the technical skills is necessary for formulating substantive standards, this is only one aspect of effective regulation. Another crucial point that the simple argument from expertise overlooks is that some central aspects of effective regulation have nothing whatsoever to do with technical skills or with standards for their maintenance. Much regulation has to do, instead, with eliminating or reducing situations and relationships that involve potentially dangerous conflicts of interest.

All regulation prohibiting or controlling self-dealing and self-referral practices is of this nature. In many cases, the situations and relationships in which conflicts of interests occur can be identified, and a measure to prevent or control them can be intelligently devised, without relying in any substantial way on the special expertise of those who are to be regulated. An example from the case at hand—the activity of medical professionals—will make this simple but significant point clearer.

One does not have to be an internist to understand that a situation in which internists refer their patients to their own diagnostic laboratories involves a conflict of interest. The conflict is between the service commitment of the physician to doing solely what is in the best interest of the patient and his own financial interest in securing additional revenue from referring the patient to a facility that the physician owns. The danger inherent in this conflict of interest is that the physician's referral will not be based solely on his judgment of what is best for the patient. A number of studies indicate that this danger is not merely speculative: Physicians who are owners of facilities to which they refer patients order the procedures in question much more frequently than nonowner physicians, and these higher rates of referral are *not* explained by higher incidences of the conditions in question in the populations that the owner-physicians treat.[15] The most stark example of such a conflict is an arrangement whereby the diagnostic facility pays the physician a fee for each patient he refers. Such arrangements have now been legally prohibited. But it is worth noting that self-regulation by the profession did not prevent them from flourishing before they were outlawed.[16]

The special expertise of physicians is not needed either to understand that such practices involve a conflict of interest or to appreciate the evidence that the physician's financial interest corrupts her clinical judgment. (In the latter case, all that is required is a basic grasp of the relevant data concerning rates of referral and rates of normal versus abnormal results from diagnostic procedures.) Further, the special expertise of physicians is not essential for determining whether the best strategy for coping with such a conflict of interest is to prohibit such self-referral arrangements. Whether prohibition is advisable depends on what the facts are—in particular, on whether prohibition would adversely affect the availability of such facilities by removing the incentive for physicians to invest in them. A sound prediction of whether the needed capital would come from sources other than the referring physicians themselves may require some technical expertise, but the expertise is economic, not medical.

To summarize the argument thus far: The attempt to justify the medical profession's special exemption from external regulation by a simple appeal to the special expertise of physicians fails. Two important aspects of effective regulation are less directly tied to special expertise than the simple argument from expertise assumes. First, much important regulation designed to ensure that technical standards are initially met and maintained is procedural or structural rather than substantive or content-specific. Second, some important regulation is a response to conflicts of interest and neither the identification of situations involving conflicts of interest, nor the development of policies to minimize these conflicts need involve the special expertise of physicians to such an extent that external regulation is not feasible.

It is worth emphasizing that even if the simple appeal to expertise succeeded in justifying the profession's relative freedom from external regulation, this would not suffice to show that the full range of inequalities involved in the existence of the profession is justified. In particular, it is not at all obvious that proper recognition of the special expertise of physicians requires that they be accorded such a favorable and secure economic niche.

A second, more promising justification for the medical profession as a socially constructed inequality is *the cost/benefit justification*. Again, the basic idea is simple. The special status, exceptionally advantageous economic position, and relative freedom from regulation enjoyed by the profession are *costs* to society, but they are worth bearing because they are more than compensated for by the *benefits* that these arrangements secure for society. These benefits include the preservation, advancement, and transmission of valuable practical knowledge, effective collective self-regulation by the profession, and the profession's inculcation of the service commitment in its members. The inequalities are justified because the benefits to society associated with them outweigh the costs.

As we shall see, the success of the cost/benefit argument depends on two problematic assumptions: (1) that the benefits to society in question are adequately provided (*e.g.*, is collective self-regulation by the profession adequate? Is the service commitment sufficiently pervasive and effective?) and (2) that there is no less costly (and morally acceptable) arrangement that does not involve these inequalities and that would provide the same benefits.

A variation on the cost/benefit justification is suggested by sociological discussions of the medical profession. It may be called the "social bargain model." The fundamental idea is that society grants special status, financial advantage, and exceptional freedom from external regulation to an occupational group *in exchange* for some significant expected benefits for society, benefits that either cannot be attained in any other way or that can be achieved most cheaply and effectively by this exchange. As with the cost/benefit justification, the benefits in question are indicated in the other five characteristics of a profession. In exchange for elevated social status, financial advantage, and substantial autonomy, the members of a profession are expected to preserve and enhance the special knowledge applied in their distinctive activity, to cultivate an intrinsic attachment to excellence in the performance of the activity, to be motivated predominantly by the desire to further the interests of those on whose behalf they act, and, perhaps most important, to exercise collective self-regulation. Presumably the rationale for allowing the group a substantial degree of autonomy in exchange for collective self-regulation is the assumption that self-regulation will be more cost-effective than external regulation.

To some, the social bargain model may be more attractive than the cost/benefit justification. It carries with it resonances of a long, distinguished tradition in social and political thought concerning the existence and justification of inequalities: that of the social contract. The social bargain model also has the advantage of making especially vivid the idea that the profession is a social creation, not an unalterable fact of nature, for one implication of the bargain metaphor is that the bargain may periodically be reevaluated and renegotiated or even not renewed.

The dangers of the social exchange model are, however, considerable. If taken too literally, it presents a falsely democratic picture of the way social institutions come about (by "society deciding to do such-and-such"). A literal construal of the model also mistakenly suggests that the social inequalities in question were created by someone's deliberate choice, rather than emerging from complex interactions of agents and groups pursuing much more concrete and limited purposes.[17] The cost/benefit justification has the advantage of avoiding these dangers. Nonetheless, partly because it makes the question of the medical profession's legitimacy more vivid and because it so clearly conveys the idea that the profession is a socially constructed inequality, I will, in the remainder of the chapter, frequently use the metaphor of a social bargain. However, all of what I say concerning the social bargain model will apply to the less rhetorically potent cost/benefit justification.

The social bargain model has explanatory import: It helps explain the distinctive features of professions by seeing them as elements in an exchange between an occupational group and society. But it also has *normative* significance: The social bargain model articulates the conditions under which the special status and exceptional autonomy of some occupational groups are *justified* according to a public standard of justification that appeals to the common good. Our focus will be on the justificatory function of the social bargain model.

It is worth emphasizing *why* it is appropriate to ask for a justification of the elevated status, favored financial position, and relative autonomy of the medical profession. The answer, in brief, is that a profession is a *social construct*, not an unalterable fact of nature. It is a particular kind of institution or social arrangement, one alternative among others. More important, it is a *socially constructed inequality*, an arrangement involving benefits for one group that are not generally available to other members of society. As such, it is appropriate to ask for a justification for it. In other words, those who endorse the continuation of a socially constructed inequality bear the a burden of justification. Even if inequalities per se do not require a justification, socially produced—that is, institutional—inequalities do. The social bargain model is one attempt to justify the socially constructed inequalities inherent in a profession.

Many analysts have emphasized one aspect of item 6, the favored financial position of professionals, that is in special need of justification. More specifically, they focus on the fact that professional organizations characteristically attempt to carve out a *sheltered economic niche*—to limit competition and keep income levels high.

The social bargain or exchange model explains, at least in principle, why such behavior might be tolerated, in spite of the fact that it is costly to society. According to the social bargain model, the only justification for allowing professionals to carve out a sheltered niche for themselves is the assumption that by doing so they *insulate* themselves from the more severe economic pressures that might undermine the commitment to excellence and to serving their clients' or patients' interests.[18] The idea is that if physicians are more or less guaranteed a comfortable and stable financial position, most will not succumb to venal impulses. (Interestingly enough, even one of the most acerbic critics of the medical profession, George Bernard Shaw, apparently accepted this assumption uncritically. He attributed venal behavior on the part of many of the physicians of his day to their poverty.)[19]

As we shall see later, there are actually two assumptions here that require more critical attention than they usually receive. The first is that a privileged economic position is an effective obstacle to corruption. The second is that the actual level of economic well-being currently available to medical professionals in this country is necessary to achieve whatever insulation against incentives for venality can be secured by according physicians a privileged and secure economic position. Even if (as seems highly unlikely) the first assumption is true as a broad generalization, it is an altogether different question as to whether the actual favored economic position of physicians in this country is optimal, from the standpoint of providing insulation against temptation, or whether it includes what we may call "surplus inequalities." There is the danger that if the economic rewards of being a physician are too high, the profession may attract the wrong sort of people—those whose primary interest is in money. Thus, if there are surplus inequalities, the assurance of a favored economic position would erode rather than encourage the service commitment. In other words, it is one thing to say that the physician lives comfortably enough so that the howling of the wolf at his door does not distract him from serving his patients' interests; it is quite another to say that physicians should be able to expect an income that is four times the average income of their fellow citizens.[20]

The Costs of the Bargain

In what follows, I offer what I hope is a comprehensive classification of the most serious costs of granting professional status to practitioners of medicine in our society under present conditions. Whether these costs are *excessive*—that is, whether, in the aggregate the cost of the social bargain exceed the benefits—is very difficult to determine. My aim in this chapter is only to show that the wisdom of the social bargain today is seriously in doubt. I offer no rigorous calculation purporting to *prove* that the bargain is a bad one from the social point of view.

Nevertheless, it is worth emphasizing where the burden of argument should lie in this matter. Given that the recognition of a particular occupational group as a profession ipso facto involves the granting of special status, privileges, and autonomy to that group, a convincing case must be made that such preferential treatment is justified. My contention is that a convincing case has not been made, and that for that reason the wisdom of the social bargain, and hence the legitimacy of the special status, privileges, and relative freedom from external regulation of practitioners of medicine, are in doubt.

The major costs of having a medical profession under current conditions can be classified under three main headings: (1) the costs of granting the authority for self-regulation (and of the correlative freedom from external regulation), (2) the costs of allowing or enabling the profession to construct for its members a sheltered economic niche, and (3) the costs of the public's trust in professionals qua professionals. I take up each of these classes of costs in turn.

The first class of costs is well known to economic analysts of the medical profession and to historians of organized medicine. A number of scholars have described the ways in which the medical profession has used its authority to maintain standards of excellence in order to stifle competition and keep the incomes of practitioners of orthodox medicine high.[21]

The profession's control over licensure is perhaps the most obvious example: Historically, organized medicine has steadfastly refused to require periodic demonstrations of competence to practice (unlike, say, airplane pilot licensing regulations). Instead, it has tended to erect barriers to licensure excluding alternative forms of medicine, some of which were not shown to be less efficacious than orthodox medicine, and to allow those who clear the initial hurdle to continue practicing even though it is known that some will lose their competence at some point after entering the profession. Other things being equal, a system of licensure with a high entry barrier and no comparable periodic re-licensing requirements clearly functions better to protect from competition those who succeed in entering than to protect the public by ensuring that standards of excellence are maintained.[22]

Moreover, continuing medical education requirements are almost universally recognized as both inadequate and subject to serious abuses. Physicians can receive credit for simply attending any of a wide range of conferences (of greatly varying quality) and merely sitting in the audience. Indeed, in some cases, physicians simply sign the attendance sheet the first day of the conference and then attend either sporadically or not at all, while receiving full credit for the entire conference. No examinations to demonstrate mastery of the material supposedly acquired in continuing medical education are required.

It will not do to reply, in defense of this system, that the continued competence of licensed physicians is adequately ensured by malpractice litigation and monitoring by state medical licensure boards. For one thing, most cases of malpractice are not even detected by patients, much less litigated or settled out of court.[23] For another, state medical licensure boards, which are physician dominated, have received a great deal of criticism for repeated failures to revoke licenses even from extremely incompetent and even dangerous physicians. Moreover, even if a state board of medical licensure takes the highly unusual step of revoking the license of a physician who has exhibited a pattern of malpractice, the physician can sometimes continue to practice in another state. Finally, even if malpractice litigation and revocation of license were much more effective than they apparently are, it would still be difficult to understand why serious periodic relicensing requirements (as for airline pilots) would not also be advisable.

By the very nature of the case, it is difficult to form even rough estimates of the social costs resulting from orthodox medicine's monopoly on licensure and, until very recently, its near monopoly on certification for reimbursement by government and private insurers. It is hard to know what magnitudes of cost savings or gains in medical outcomes *might* have occurred had alternative types of services and forms of practice been allowed to develop. We *do* know that some types of services and some forms of practice that finally gained legitimacy despite dogged resistance and outright persecution by organized medicine, such as midwifery and prepaid group practice (HMOs), have provided significant benefits.[24] And hence we know that society was deprived of these benefits during the many years in which organized medicine succeeded in suppressing them.

Defenders of the medical profession would be quick to point out that the question is not whether the profession's control over licensure and reimbursement has resulted in the exclusion of some high-quality and/or lower-cost alternatives. The question, rather, is whether, on balance, the profession's self-regulation has adequately protected the public. If the price of preventing quacks from inflicting themselves on the unwary is the mistaken suppression of some unobjectionable (or even superior) types of services or forms of practice, then this is a necessary, though regrettable, cost.

This defense of the status quo is inadequate for two reasons. First, the question is not simply whether the profession's self-regulation has adequately protected the public, but rather whether self-regulation, with all the social costs it entails, has provided the *least costly* method of ensuring an adequate level of protection. Pointing out that this system, like any other, is imperfect and that we must expect some "false positives" in the workings of any system designed to suppress quackery does not answer that question.

If, as I have already suggested, the burden of argument lies with any group whose activities seriously affect the well-being of others under conditions of conflict of interest, but that nonetheless claims that it ought to receive special authority for self-regulation and special exemption from external regulation, then this means that the medical profession or its defenders must show not only that the profession's actual record on self-regulation has been adequate, but also that self-regulation is more efficient than external regulation alternatives. This burden of argument certainly has not been borne.

Second, and more important, the most obvious objection to the way the medical profession has performed the task of self-regulation, as noted above, is independent of the question of whether the profession has done an acceptable job, on balance, of developing appropriate standards for distinguishing good medicine from quackery. That objection is that *regardless of the content* of the standards (i.e., regardless of what is counted as good medicine and what as quackery), the public would be better served by a system of periodic relicensing than by one that imposes high (and very narrow) barriers to entry at the beginning of a career and then allows those who clear them to continued to practice for the rest of their lives without a serious attempt to ensure that they are even continuing to meet the original standards, much less whatever new standards become appropriate in the light of advances in medical technique and knowledge.

So far, I have simply noted what several generations of sociologists and historians of medicine have documented: that the authority for self-regulation granted to medicine as a profession has often been exercised, especially in establishing licensing requirements, in ways that serve better to further the interests of physicians than to protect patients. The chief function of licensing requirements, at least in principle, is to articulate and enforce technical standards of competence. But there is another important function of self-regulation whose performance has been even more defective, if anything: the articulation and enforcement of ethical standards, especially these regarding conflict of interest in the physician–patient relationship.

As a broad generalization it is fair to say that organized medicine in the United States from before the beginning of this century through the present has tended to abdicate its responsibility for *effective, collective self-regulation* regarding conflict of interest. With few exceptions, the profession has not articulated clear standards of conduct regarding conflict of interest and establishing effective institutional sanctions to ensure an acceptable level of compliance. Instead, it has usually relied on rather vague ethical norms (often only after public disapproval has become widespread and the threat of government regulation has become imminent) and on appeals to the conscience and judgment of individual physicians rather than to collective mechanisms for compliance.

One of the best treatments of this failure of collective ethical self-regulation is found in Marc A. Rodwin's major work on conflict of interest in medicine, *Medicine, Money, and Morals: Physicians' Conflicts of Interest.*[25] Rodwin skillfully traces the history of organized medicine's responses to one of the most

prominent conflicts of interest—physician self-referral in its various guises—
from the 1890s to 1992. Rodwin documents the fact that the two most prominent medical organizations, the American Medical Association and the
American College of Surgeons, have for long periods entirely evaded the problem of self-referral, and that when they have taken positions on the issue, they
have only announced vague and ambiguous exhortations while relying on individual physicians to interpret and apply them to their own conduct.

Rodwin aptly characterizes this approach as "subjective." Perhaps more
important, the dominant approach of organized medicine to these crucial ethical
problems may be characterized as *individualistic*, as opposed to *institutional* or
collective, and *voluntary*, as opposed to *sanctioned*. Organized medicine has not
only opposed *government* regulation of self-referral; it has also refused to
undertake serious efforts at collective *self*-regulation.

Rather than using its organizational resources to articulate collectively
endorsed, substantive standards and to provide institutional sanctions to ensure
that physicians comply with them, the profession has narrowed its role to that
of offering rather general principles for the purely voluntary consideration of
individual practitioners. Especially after the mid-1950s, the AMA backed away
from anything resembling clear prohibitions against self-referral, asserting that
a physician could dispense drugs and devices he prescribed so long as, in his
own judgment, this was "in the best interests of the patient."

Similarly, in 1961, the AMA held that physician ownership of pharmacies
was permissible "as long as there is no exploitation of the patient." Again, since
no provision was made for authoritative, substantive guidance on what counted
as exploitation and what did not, and since no measures were developed for collective sanctions to ensure compliance with the vague prohibition against
exploitation, the approach was voluntary, individualistic, and nearly vacuous.[26]
The same approach was followed in 1976 when the AMA chose not to develop
specific guidelines concerning conflicts of interest arising from physicians'
investment in diagnostic technology. Instead, it approved of physician ownership of such facilities, saying only that "physician ownership of equipment
should not involve abuse or exploitation of the physician–patient relationship."[27] Issuing the stamp of approval to practices that clearly involve conflicts
of interest, while merely announcing the rather uncontroversial proposition that
physicians ought not to exploit patients (or, presumably, to murder or rob them),
hardly counts as self-regulation in any sense that could satisfy the normatively
adequate conception of a profession.

At present, the AMA's Principles of Ethics include no reference whatsoever
to conflicts of interest arising from self-referral practices. To the extent that it
has made any official pronouncements on the issue, it has spoken equivocally.
In 1989 the AMA's Council on Ethical and Judicial Affairs stated a presumption

against self-referral (but noted that there were cases in which self-referral was ethical). However, once again, no mechanism for enforcement was mentioned, and forty-three state medical associations failed to recommend that their members comply with the AMA's presumption against self-referral (Indeed, it is hard to know exactly what it means to comply with a presumption whose exceptions are left so vague).

Even this rather anemic response to the public outcry about self-referral was thought to be too restrictive by many physicians. The reaction against it culminated in June 1992, when the AMA's House of Delegates passed a resolution that contradicted the Judicial Council's position. The resolution stated that self-referral was ethical so long as physicians disclosed their ownership of facilities to which they referred. Again, enforcement mechanisms were not even suggested, and the problem of developing adequate procedures for disclosure was not addressed. Given mounting public pressure, the House of Delegates reversed itself several months later and condemned self-referral except to meet a special medical need or if the only way a center could be established were by the involvement of referring doctors.[28]

To the extent that the profession has relied chiefly on an individualistic, subjective, and voluntary approach to problems of conflict of interest, it has failed to discharge one of the chief functions of self-regulation: The development of ethical policies specific enough to provide substantive practical guidance, with collective sanctions to ensure a reasonable level of compliance. Yet, as we have seen, this self-regulatory function is essential to the social bargain that elevates an occupational group to the status of a profession.[29]

The second major class of costs of the professionalism consists of the costs of providing a sheltered economic niche for members of the profession. It is important to note that the much higher than average incomes of physicians cannot be explained simply as the result of average rates of return on the individual physician's investment in his or her own education and training, comparable to average rates of return on other investments in our society. Since physician education and training is heavily subsidized by public funding, physicians' incomes cannot be explained simply as returns on their own investment.[30]

It was observed earlier that, according to the social bargain model, the chief justification for the privileged economic position of physicians is that it supposedly reduces the temptation to behave venally. Another way to put this is to say that according to physicians, a privileged economic position is supposed to lower the physician's costs of focusing on the interests of his patients. If a physician is assured a high income, then he "need not weigh economic benefits to himself when considering treatment recommendations for his individual patients."[31] In the simplest economic terms, society buys the service commitment, the commitment of the physician to put the patient's interests first, by allowing physicians a favored economic position.

One result, of course, is that higher incomes for physicians mean higher health care costs overall—higher costs than would exist if physicians' incomes were determined solely by the operation of the market and normal rates of return on investment. This is the first and most obvious cost of providing medical professionals with a sheltered economic niche.

Until quite recently, physicians' income from professional activity was generated almost exclusively by third-party, fee-for-service payments. This system's incentives ensured a high degree of convergence between the financial interests of the physician and the patient's interests as a consumer of health care. (It is crucial to remember here that by the "patient" we mean only those individuals who are in need of health care *and who are insured.*) At least where copayments or deductibles are low, the physician can assure himself that in ordering all services that can be expected to produce any net benefit for the patient, he is serving the patient's best interest and his own financial interest as well. Under such a system of payment, the angelic voice of the conscience of the physician as fiduciary and the insistent whine of self-interest become one.

Moreover, since the level of fees was not determined by competition but according to the so-called reasonable and customary standard, which was largely determined by the providers themselves, regardless of their actual costs, the fee-for-service system turned out to be a very expensive way to ensure a privileged economic position for physicians. It became increasingly clear over the past decade that the price of ensuring this congruence of the patient's best interest and the physician's self-interest—the social cost of making the service commitment cheap for physicians—is unacceptably expensive health care. Indeed, the whole gamut of recent restrictions on straightforward fee-for-service payment, from diagnosis related groups to the myriad constraints on utilization imposed by various managed-care practice plans, can be seen as a renegotiation of the fee-for-service system "bargain" for ensuring high incomes for physicians.

The demise of unconstrained fee-for-service reimbursement has not, however, resulted in a decline in average physician income.[32] Physicians have found other ways of keeping their incomes much higher than average, including, most conspicuously, investment in health care facilities—laboratories; dialysis, radiation and imaging centers; outpatient surgical centers; and ancillary services of various sorts. And there can be no doubt that physicians are exceptionally well placed to reap high profits from such investment opportunities, in part because the higher economic position they have traditionally been assured, including the public subsidization of their education and training, has equipped them with more resources for investment than the average individual investor and greater knowledge about where to invest.

The question of whether the favorable economic position of physicians is a good bargain for society is correspondingly transformed. The issue now is whether the enhancement of physician altruism that physicians' higher economic status is supposed to produce is worth the cost to society associated with these new entrepreneurial sources of physician income. Those who argue that the new entrepreneurism exacerbates conflicts of interest in the physician–patient relationship—for example, when physicians refer patients to facilities that they own—doubt that it is a good bargain.

So far, I have only raised questions about whether the costs of ensuring physicians' high incomes in order to encourage the service commitment (limited altruism) to patients exceed the benefits. A more radical challenge to this element of the social bargain model is to cast doubt on the assumption that high incomes do in fact produce an exceptional level of the service commitment in physicians—that is, a service commitment that is deeper and more pervasive than that found in the population at large or in the population of those in occupations providing services to others.

There is, in fact, considerable evidence that, contrary to the myth of medical professionalism, physicians are not significantly more altruistic toward those they serve than many others whose altruism is not encouraged by exceptional incomes.[33] One need not adduce evidence that at least *some* physicians are more self-seeking than the average person—the all too familiar instances of Medicaid fraud, sexual molestation of patients, and so on. The relevant questions, rather, are these: (1) What evidence is there that physicians, as a class, are more likely to forego the pursuit of self-interest and cleave steadfastly to the interests of those they serve; if such evidence exists? (2) What additional evidence is there that this extraordinary (limited) altruism results (at least in part) from their being assured a favored economic niche? and (3) Is the additional level of service commitment thus secured worth the cost?

If, as I have already noted, the burden of argument is on those who would try to justify the favored economic position of physicians as the price we must pay for physicians' (alleged) exceptional (limited) altruism, then the first step is to marshall convincing evidence regarding statement (1) (the claim that physicians as a class really do possess the service commitment to an exceptional extent). Until this is done, the second and third questions cannot be answered. And unless the first question is answered affirmatively, they are irrelevant anyway.

To my knowledge, no empirical evidence that physicians as a class possess the service commitment to an exceptional extent (as compared with other service providers, including auto mechanics, roof repairers, etc.) has been presented. It is, of course, the business of a profession to encourage the belief that its members are especially altruistic to those they serve, and I suspect that the indignation that the mere request for such evidence brings in some quarters is a good indication that, in achieving this objective, the medical profession has been quite successful. But it is important to distinguish between the inadequately supported beliefs that compose the myth of professionalism and genuine evidence that professionals are especially altruistic.

There is considerable evidence that many, indeed perhaps most, physicians are not exceptionally altruistic individuals. This evidence surfaces once we reflect on some major patterns that emerge from the choices that physicians make *as individuals* (apart from the activities of organized medicine). First, individual physicians have a great deal of freedom to choose where they will practice. The resulting pattern of geographical distribution—or rather maldistribution—is hardly what one would predict if physicians as a class were imbued with an extra dose of altruism. On the contrary, there is persistent maldistribution of physicians. As Uwe Rheinhardt points out:

> Careful empirical research has established scientifically what was known to any cab driver all along: physicians, like everyone else, like to locate in pleasant areas where money is to be had. Thus our favorite areas have been vastly over-doctored, while other areas, notably the inner cities, have been sorely under-served.[34]

A second indication that physicians are not exceptionally altruistic is the maldistribution of physicians across specialties. A number of recent studies contradict any assumption that patient need is a good predictor of the choices medical students in the United States make regarding specialties when applying for residencies; and some recent studies indicate that expected financial gain is an important, even dominant consideration in such choices.[35] If physicians were exceptionally altruistic human beings, or even individuals who placed the health interests of others whom they could serve above the maximization of their own interests, we would expect a different distribution of physicians among specialties.

It is worth emphasizing that these are only two of many forms of evidence drawn from the behavior of individual physicians, that physicians are not exceptionally altruistic. If we concentrate on the behavior of organized medicine, there is perhaps even less reason to attribute exceptional altruism. Indeed, it is difficult to imagine how any impartial person familiar with the history of organized medicine in this country could sincerely conclude that it exhibits the triumph of altruism over self-interest.

A third bit of evidence that at least casts doubt on the assumption that physicians as a class are exceptionally altruistic is the fact that many physicians refuse to accept Medicaid patients because Medicaid reimbursement rates are lower than private insurance reimbursement rates. This phenomenon is in some ways more directly pertinent to evaluating the extent of the service commitment, since it indicates that significant numbers of physicians are willing to put their own financial interests ahead of the medical interests of patients in a very concrete way. Such physicians sometimes refuse to care for individuals who arrive at the physician's place of practice needing care. This is a more dramatic and direct example of not putting the patient's interests first than a situation in which a physician simply chooses not to go into a specialty in which practitioners are desperately needed or chooses not to locate in an underserved area.

Fourth, the studies cited earlier concerning the much higher rates of referral by doctors who own diagnostic facilities provides compelling evidence that the service commitment in these practitioners is far from robust. In the absence of any data to show that they are referring more because more referrals are medically indicated in their patient populations, the only reasonable explanation of their higher referral rates is that these physicians are pursuing their own financial interests rather than the best interests of their patients.

Of the evidence cited thus far, the self-referral studies bear most directly on the question of the extent of the service commitment. However, the cumulative import of all four areas of evidence (not to mention well-documented cases of Medicaid and Medicare fraud and other, more egregious abuses of the fiduciary relationship) is to cast serious doubt on the assumption that the service commitment in physicians is so deep and pervasive as to justify the exceptionally favored economic positions they occupy. And again, it is important to note that even if it could be shown that some degree of special economic reward did something to facilitate the service commitment, it would not follow that the extremely high level of reward that now exists is required to secure this benefit for society. For it is one thing to say that physicians will be better able to honor the service commitment if they are not poor or are financially comfortable and quite another to say that they must be rich.

So far, I have raised questions about whether the benefit of the service commitment is worth the economic costs of the favored economic position of physicians. Two other costs of providing medical practitioners with a secure and elevated financial position must be noted. The first is the creation of organized medicine as a powerful political force. The second, an effect of the way in which this political force has been deployed, is the barrier that the medical profession in this country has erected in response to repeated efforts to extend access to care to those who are unserved or underserved.

A prominent and dramatic theme in the history of organized medicine in the United States is the profession's largely successful efforts to block national health insurance, which many believe to be the only workable reform that would have a chance of making a truly significant impact on the access problem.[36] Organized medicine has traditionally seen national health insurance, as well as more radical proposals for extending access, as a threat both to physicians' income and status and to the profession's relative freedom from external regulation.

Despite strong initial opposition from organized medicine, Medicare and Medicaid were established in the mid-1960s. However, the price of securing the profession's cooperation in implementing these programs was a concession that became another major barrier to universal access: reimbursement rates for Medicare were set at such generous levels that the extension of publicly funded access to other populations became politically unfeasible.[37]

Here we see another significant—and perhaps largely unanticipated—cost of the social bargain: the creation of a highly concentrated, well-educated, and financially powerful political force, willing and able to place severe constraints on society's capacity to carry out major social reforms. The social "bargain" that allows practitioners of medicine to secure a sheltered economic niche also empowers the profession as a formidable political lobby—a class of individuals with exceptional resources and prestige, united by a common interest in maintaining and preserving these advantages. Moreover, if medical practitioners enjoy status trust and are thought to be exceptionally altruistic, this is likely to enhance the effectiveness of their lobbying efforts by fostering the perception that when they speak out on public issues, they have the common good, rather than their own good as an interest group, at heart.

According to some theories of social justice, the mere fact that any group, including the medical profession, enjoys such exceptional political power is itself a serious social cost—an infringement on the principle of political equality.[38] But even those who hold less egalitarian conceptions of justice must admit that the profession's tendency to use its resources to impede solutions to the access problem is a major cost of according physicians a favored economic position. It is also a cost that is *not* taken into account in the public understanding of the social bargain that is supposed to legitimate the existence of the profession. Once it is added to the reckoning, the desirability of the bargain, and hence the legitimacy of the medical profession, become all the more doubtful.

The third and final category of costs of professionalism consists of the costs of trust. Here it is important to distinguish clearly between two sorts of trust. According to what I shall call "status trust," the individual practitioner is deemed worthy of at least significant patient trust simply by virtue of being a member of the professional group—independent of evidence of his own conduct. The second sort of trust is what might be called "individually merited trust"—trust based on evidence about the actual conduct of the individual in question.

Some of the most prominent defenders of medical professionalism have explicitly held not only that the trust of patients in physicians is beneficial but also that what I have called status trust is a necessary concomitant of the social recognition of an occupational group as a profession.

> The sheer fact of having been socially "certified" as professionals means that clients [or patients] will typically take it for granted that professionals are [to be trusted].[39]

Defenders of the medical profession often stress the beneficial therapeutic effects of status trust. But before we can assume that anything that erodes status trust—including entrepreneurial or rationing behavior by physicians—is undesirable, we must first consider whether status trust provides a *net* benefit. And to do this, we must consider the costs of status trust, not just the benefits. We must attempt to compare whatever therapeutic benefits status trust provides with the costs associated with status trust, not in an ideal world in which status trust is justified by a profession that satisfies the normatively adequate conception of a profession, but in our real world.

If the argument thus far is correct, then it is far from clear that the actual medical profession in this country (as opposed to its idealized image, as portrayed in the myth of professionalism) possesses all the features it would have to have in order to be legitimated according to the social bargain model. In particular, there is at least serious doubt about its performance of the essential function of self-regulation. In addition, the burden of argument has not been borne to show that the elevated status and advantageous economic position of medical practitioners are both effective and necessary for securing the service commitment.

These same considerations cast serious doubt on the rationality of status trust. For status trust, if it can be rationally grounded at all, must be supportable by evidence that the profession is doing an adequate job of self-regulation, especially with regard to conflicts between the professional's and the patient's or client's interest, and that its members can be counted on to resist temptations that others would find irresistible.

The costs of status trust are many and significant. In some cases, patients wrongly assume that simply because an individual is a physician, his referrals or prescriptions for treatment are appropriate, or at least that they are motivated solely by concern for the patient's interest rather than by the desire for revenue. The results of such misplaced status trust range from death and disfigurement to merely unnecessary treatment and additional costs.

A more subtle but nevertheless significant cost of status trust is the inhibition that many patients apparently feel about questioning their physician. If the tacit assumption is that the physician is to be trusted as one whose motives are pure—simply because he is a physician, independently of having done anything to earn one's trust—then one may understandably be reluctant to ask certain pertinent questions.

For example, suppose one knows that one's physician is an owner of the laboratory to which he refers one for a test. How easy would it be for most of us to ask him if he is referring us there because it provides the best service for the money or because it is to his financial benefit to do so?

At least in some cases, such a query—and indeed any questioning of a physician's clinical recommendations—will be greeted with righteous indignation, if not hostility, from physicians who have been socialized to expect status trust.[40]

To the extent that status trust prevails, it is likely that many patients will find it difficult to raise questions that may challenge the physician's dedication to putting the patient's interest first. But if this is so, then status trust can seriously impede certain otherwise plausible strategies for dealing with conflict of interest. In particular, simply posting an announcement in the waiting room disclosing that the physician is the owner of the laboratory to which he refers patients will not be likely to empower patients to protect themselves.

As was noted at the beginning of this chapter, a number of prominent physicians bemoan the erosion of trust in medical professionals. What they fail to consider is the possibility that the erosion of misplaced status trust may be essential for developing realistic responses to the problem of conflict of interest. Instead of relying primarily on the service commitment of medical professionals and the supposed self-regulation of the profession, it is more reasonable to consider the entire range of possible arrangements for dealing with conflicts of interest.

Among the possibilities worth considering—but that we are not likely to take seriously if we cleave to the unsupported dogma that the medical profession is a self-regulating cadre of exceptional altruists—is the proposal that the law of agency, which applies to other principal–agent relationships, should be extended and adapted to provide protection against conflict of interest in medicine.[41] For example, federal or state legislatures could impose fiduciary standards on physicians in the same way they have already done for government officials, corporate directors and officers, lawyers, trustees, and certain financial specialists (often called "financial professionals"), including money managers and investment brokers. Self-referral, or certain forms of it, might be prohibited by such statutory fiduciary standards. Alternatively, or in addition, courts might award strict liability damages if patients are harmed when a physician engages in self-referral.[42]

Another possibility that emerges once the myth of professionalism is dissipated is that the resources of principal–agent theory should be utilized to protect patients from the adverse effects of conflicts of interest.[43] Contractual or other arrangements might be devised to ensure a closer congruence between the physician's and the patient's interest, for example, by financially rewarding exemplary physician decision-making. Alternatively, or in addition, arrangements external to the physician–patient relationship might also be employed to reduce agency risk to patients.

Indeed, three instances of the latter approach are already being employed with growing frequency. The first is the practice of seeking second opinions, with the implied threat of terminating the relationship. The second is the use of advance directives for medical care. As I have argued in some detail elsewhere, advance directives, as public documents rather than confidential instructions to one's physician, serve to avoid or cope with potential failures in the physician–patient relationship, understood as a principal–agent relationship.[44] This is clearest in the case of a proxy advance directive, a legal document that creates a *secondary* principal–agent relationship (between the patient and his proxy). Some patients may be led to create this secondary principal–agent relationship out of apprehension that the physician will not honor their wishes concerning termination of treatment. Similarly, if patients were thoroughly assured that their physicians would honor their wishes once they become incompetent, there would be little need for a witnessed, public document recording the patient's instructions, as opposed to a personal, confidential communication to the physician. The third method that is being employed with increasing frequency is the case manager approach. The use of a case manager, who tracks the patient throughout the complexity of a multi-specialty course of treatment, is an admission that the physician–patient relationship (or rather a series of such relationships) can put the patient at risk.

It is revealing to note that some physicians oppose all of these methods for reducing agency risk in the physician–patient relationship, contending that they signal a failure to trust the physician as professional. That is undoubtedly so. And that is precisely the point. To dismiss them and other related proposals that do not rely exclusively on physician altruism and existing collective self-regulation on the grounds that they are incompatible with professionalism is simply to beg the question of to what the alternatives are for protecting patients from conflicts of interest.

None of these approaches is exclusive of the others or exhaustive of the alternatives. The point is that one of the hidden costs of the recognition of medicine as a profession, at least so far as this carries with it widespread status trust, is the foreclosure of options for dealing with conflict of interest.

Some might protest that the imposition of legal fiduciary standards or the use of financial incentives to reduce conflict of interest would transform a profession into a mere business and *thereby* extinguish trust. This objection wrongly equates all trust with status trust and hence mistakenly assumes that if physicians are not regarded as professionals their patients will have no basis for trusting them. However, the erosion of status trust, even its total disappearance, need not mean the end of trust in the physician-patient relationship. Even if physicians came to be regarded not as professionals but as people in the business of providing health care (or rather certain forms of health care, since much health care is provided by nonphysicians), this would not mean that trust would not be an important element in the interaction between physicians and patients. It would merely mean that trust would have a different basis. Nor would the disappearance of medicine as a profession necessarily mean the end of the provision of medical care within a framework of moral norms.

In recent years, social scientists and legal theorists alike have increasingly emphasized the vital role of trust and of moral norms at the very heart of the market exchanges that purveyors of the myth of professionalism have portrayed as "mere business." Of particular importance is the recognition that the complex exchanges that characterize many contemporary business activities flourish only within a framework of trust built up by compliance over time with norms of reciprocity and fairness.[45]

Conclusions

The main conclusions of our investigation can be summarized briefly:

1. The most plausible justifications for according certain occupational groups (and not others) the status of a profession are (a) that the benefits to society of this socially constructed inequality exceed the costs (and that this way of securing the benefits is the least costly morally acceptable alternative) or (b) that such recognition can be viewed as the outcome of a social bargain.

2. According to the latter justification, in exchange for certain social benefits, including exceptionally altruistic behavior and cost-effective self-regulation by a group that applies special knowledge on behalf of those lacking this knowledge, society grants special status, a favored and secure economic position, and considerable freedom from external regulation.

3. A profession is a social construct and, more precisely, a socially-constructed inequality whose justification depends on whether the benefits of having the profession exceed the costs or upon whether the social bargain is fair and mutually advantageous.

4. Whether the costs do exceed the benefits, or whether the bargain is fair and mutually advantageous, depends on whether there is convincing evidence that the elevated status and favored economic position of physicians in fact promote an exceptional service commitment in the members of the profession, and on whether there is convincing evidence that the profession is exercising collective self-regulation that is not only adequate but superior to other forms of control.

5. At present, convincing evidence for an exceptional service commitment or for adequate collective self-regulation is lacking. Nor is it clear that there is good reason to think that the extremely high level of financial reward available to physicians in this country is necessary for securing whatever depth and extent of service commitment in fact exists. Those who wish to legitimate the socially constructed inequality known as the medical profession have not produced convincing evidence of a deep and pervasive service commitment. Moreover, neither the history of organized medicine nor the patterns of career choices of individual physicians support the hypothesis of exceptional physician altruism

toward patients. Furthermore, for the most part, the past century of organized medicine's history exhibits an abdication of the responsibility for effective collective self-regulation. On the one hand, the exercise of self-regulatory authority in medical licensure has been a qualified success at best, imposing strenuous initial barriers to entry that historically have kept physicians' incomes high while excluding some forms of practice and certain types of services that could have produced valuable benefits. At the same time, licensing regulation has failed to ensure the continued competence of licensed physicians.

6. While there is little hard evidence that the favored economic position of the medical profession has enhanced altruism toward patients by insulating them from crass economic concerns, there can be no doubt that it has imposed other significant costs on society. Among the most important of these are higher health care costs, political inequality resulting from the empowering of an articulate and rich medical political lobby, and major impediments to implementing reforms in the health care system that would enhance access to care for those currently unserved or underserved. In addition, the chief argument for according physicians a favored economic position is most compelling if it is construed as a justification for ensuring them a comfortable living; it cannot justify the extremely favored economic position physicians actually achieve in this country. On the contrary, there is the danger that the exceptionally high economic prospects enjoyed by U.S. physicians may attract those in whom the service commitment is not the dominating motivation.

7. If one element of the normatively adequate—or, as we might also say, the legitimating—conception of a profession is effective collective self-regulation, including sanctions to ensure compliance with authoritative, contentful norms, then the American medical profession does not exemplify such a conception. It follows that in the sense in which the medical profession could be said to be legitimate—that is, a justified, socially constructed inequality—there is no medical profession in this country. There is, instead a privileged occupational group whose defenders wrongly present it as exemplifying the normatively adequate conception of a profession.

8. Even if there is, strictly speaking, no medical profession in this country (in the legitimating or normatively adequate sense), there is still, to some extent, the public belief that there is a profession. One aspect of this belief—the allegiance to the myth of professionalism—is status trust: the assumption that a physician is entitled to significant trust simply because he is a member of the medical profession. The prevalence of status trust may have therapeutic benefits in some instances, but it also has serious social costs.

9. Among the social costs of the recognition of medicine as a profession, and of the concomitant status trust in physicians, is an inability to consider objectively the full range of options for coping with conflicts of interest.

It is worth emphasizing that I have *not* argued that the medical profession should be abolished or that the professional status of physicians should be revoked. Instead, I have only argued that the legitimacy of a profession, as a socially constructed inequality, requires a convincing showing that having a medical profession is a good bargain for society and that this burden of justification *has not* been borne. Strictly speaking, nothing in my analysis demonstrates that it is *impossible* to provide convincing evidence that the existence of the profession is a good social bargain. However, in arguing that the burden of justification has not been borne, I have, I believe, shown that providing the needed evidence will be hard indeed.

There are, it seems, three possible responses to my analysis. First, one might attempt to show that, despite appearances to the contrary, granting professional status to medical practitioners is a good social bargain. Second, proposals might be offered for improving the performance of the profession (especially with respect to collective self-regulation) so that the bargain would become a good one. Third, one might opt for a serious departure from the model of professionalism, and in particular from reliance on self-regulation, by developing other means for controlling conflicts of interest, including external regulation. My main objective in this chapter is to challenge the legitimacy of the profession so as to get these three options on the table.

Whether pursuing the third option would amount to the abolition of the medical profession depends on how malleable the concept of a medical profession is. We do speak of lawyers and financial advisers as professionals even though they are subject to much more substantial external regulation, especially with regard to conflict of interest, than physicians are.

The implications of these conclusions for the current debate about rationing, medical entrepreneurism, and professionalism are significant. The much-lamented erosion of professionalism in medicine may be better characterized as the disintegration of the myth of professionalism. We might well welcome this process of disillusionment as a recognition that the time has come for renegotiating the social bargain, if not for refusing to perpetuate it.

Early in this chapter, I distinguished between the ideal or normative conception of the medical profession and the sociological conception. The chief difference between the two is the sociological conception's emphasis on the special status, favored economic position, and relative freedom from external regulation of the medical profession. It is these features—these socially constructed inequalities— that call for justification. It is these features that cast doubt on the legitimacy of the profession if a convincing justification for its existence is not forthcoming. What must have struck the reader by now is how *separable* these problematic features are from the laudable characteristics that constitute the ideal conception of the profession. Indeed, from the standpoint of common sense, these two sets of features are not only separable but also conflicting, the danger being that the high status and exceptional economic reward of being a physician in this country undoubtedly will attract some people to the profession who are motivated by self-interest rather than the desire to serve others.

We have seen that the cost/benefit and social bargain justifications attempt—rather unconvincingly—to forge a necessary connection between the special advantages of the profession and the characteristics of the ideal conception, in particular, the service commitment and the commitment to excellent performance of the special activity of the profession. Once we realize the tenuousness of this connection, we may well conclude that our way of thinking about the medical profession requires a major revision. We should jettison the idea that it is somehow in the nature of the medical profession that this group should enjoy high status, economic privilege, and relative freedom from external regulation. We should then ask physicians and ourselves the following questions. How did we come to regard these problematic social inequalities as inextricably linked with an otherwise admirable conception of the profession? Why should we assume that a steadfast and overriding commitment to serve others can—much less must—be combined with high status and economic privilege? To what extent does this assumption reflect a particularly American cultural interpretation of the idea of a medical profession? Might it be the case that a society gets the medical profession it deserves?[46]

Notes

1. Examples of incentives for underutilization include pressures hospitals put on physicians (including the threat of revocation of hospital admitting privileges) to conform to the Diagnostic Related Groups (DRG) system for Medicare-reimbursed hospital charges and year-end "hold back" or bonus arrangements in which HMOs or other forms of managed care use financial penalties or rewards to discourage utilization.
2. For example, a financial interest in amortizing the debt on an expensive piece of diagnostic equipment, or an interest in a laboratory or dialysis center of which the physician is an owner, can encourage overutilization.
3. In some cases, the hospital's attempt to stay within DRG reimbursement ceilings can cause patients to be discharged from the hospital before they are able to care for themselves adequately. If family support is lacking when the patient is discharged, there may be a serious risk of injury or illness. Similarly, if, in order to stay within the utilization constraints of the HMO, a physician forgoes a test that would have detected a serious but treatable condition, the consequences for the patient may be grave.
4. Edmund Pellegrino, Trust and Distrust in Professional Ethics, in *Ethics, Trust, and the Professions: Philosophical and Cultural Aspects* 69–89 (Edmund Pellegrino et. al., eds., 1991).
5. An example of one who assumes that trust is unique to professionalism is Edmund Pellegrino. *Id.*, at 72–76.

6. *See* Robert Sokolowski, *The Fiduciary Relationship and the Nature of Professions, in Ethics, Trust, and the Professions, supra* note 4, at 23–39, 23–26, and citations therein. Note that there are other, less formal uses of the term "professional". Sometimes we refer to someone as a professional to indicate that he or she is not an amateur, meaning only that the person performs the activity in question to earn a living, not as a mere hobby or pastime.

7. Some analysts, such as Eliot Friedson, include the requirement that the special knowledge in question be formal. Eliot Friedson, Nourishing Professionalism, in *Ethics, Trust, and the Professions, supra* note 4, at 193–220, 194–95.

8. Some analysts distinguish an additional element in the ideal conception of a profession: a commitment to serve the public interest, as distinct from, and sometimes in opposition to, the interests of their clients or patients. *See*, e.g., Chapter 4 by Hazard in this volume, at "Civic Reponsibility". Although it may be true, as Hazard says, that professionals as such are liable to experience a conflict between their obligations to their patients or clients and their obligations to society, it is not so clear that the obligations of professionals to society are different from the obligations of other persons to society. For example, a physician may experience a conflict between his obligation to his patient (John Wilkes Booth) and his obligation to the public or the state as the agent of the public concerning the apprehension of a dangerous fugitive. But from this it would not follow that the obligation to the public good (as opposed to the conflict between this obligation and the professional's obligation to his or her client or patient) is peculiar to professions.

   In this chapter I will not take a stand on the issue of whether professionals as such have a peculiar obligation to the public, or to serve the public good, over and above their obligations to particular members of the public who are their clients or patients and over and above their obligations to preserve the distinctive knowledge of the profession, to maintain high standards, and so on.

9 . I am indebted to Christine Korsgaard for clarifying this point.

10. *See*, e.g., Uwe Rheinhardt in Arnold Relman and Uwe Rheinhardt, An Exchange on For-Profit Health Care, in *For-Profit Enterprise in Health Care* 212–213 (Bradford Gray, ed., 1986).

11. In his excellent book, Marc Rodwin documents in detail the medical profession's relative lack of external regulation compared with other professions, including lawyers, financial advisers, and government officials. Especially important is his observation that the law of fiduciary obligations, which is well developed for other professions, is almost nonexistent for physician. (Rodwin, *Medicine, Money, and Morals: Physicians' Conflicts of Interest,* Chap. Seven (1993).

12. There is a looser sense of the term "professional" according to which anyone who engages in an activity to earn a living is a professional. Moreover, sometimes we say that a particular task or job was "professional," meaning only that it was done according to high standards of performance.

13. There is little doubt that organized medicine, and many individual physicians, exaggerate both the objectivity and the certainty of medical expertise, as well as its inaccessibility to laypersons. One important aspect of a comprehensive critique of the myth of medical professionalism would be to define the pervasiveness of uncertainty and subjectivity in the exercise of clinical judgment. That task is, however, beyond the scope of this chapter.

14. For a concise explanation of the most basic concepts of principal-agent theory, see Allen Buchanan, Principal/Agent Theory And Decision-Making in Health Care, 2 *Bioethics* 317 (1988).

15. There is a growing literature, including public testimony before governmental groups, reports by health insurance groups, and scholarly articles, documenting not only the prevalence of

self-referral but also the fact that ownership biases clinical judgment regarding referral. The following is a selection of sources cited in Marc Rodwin, *Medicine, Money, and Morals: Physicians' Conflicts of Interest* (1993).

Issues Related to Physician "Self-Referrals": Hearings Before the Subcommittee on Health and the Subcommittee on Oversight of the Committee on Ways and Means, House of Representatives, 101st Congress, 1st Session, on H.R. 939. testimony of Richard P. Kusserow, March 2 and June 1, 1989. (Serial No. 101-58), at 124–1440.

State of Florida Health Care Cost Containment Board and Department of Economics and Department of Finance, Florida State University, *Joint Ventures Among Health Care Providers in Florida*, Vols. I–III (1990).

Jean Mitchell and Elton Scott, New Evidence on the Prevalence and Scope Physician Joint Ventures, 268 *JAMA* 80 (1992).

Jean Mitchel and Elton Scott, Evidence on Complex Structures of Physician Joint Ventures Under Existing Regulation, 9 *Yale L.J.* 489 (1992).

David Hemenway *et. al.*, Physicians' Response to Financial Incentives from For-Profit Ambulatory Care Center, 322 *N. Engl. J. Med.* 1059 (1990).

Bruce Hillman *et. al.*, Frequency and Costs of Diagnostic Imaging in Office Practice—A Comparison of Self-Referring and Radiologist-Referring Physicians, 323 *N. Engl. J. Med.* 1604 (1990).

Inspector General, U.S. Government, *Financial Arrangements Between Physicians and Health Care Business: Report to Congress* (0AI-12-88-01410) (1991).

Medical Affairs Division, Blue Cross and Blue Shield of Michigan, *A Comparison of Laboratory Utilization and Payout to Ownership* (1984).

Department of Health and Human Services, Health Care Financing Administration, Division of Health Standards and Quality, Region V, *Diagnostic Clinical Laboratory Services in Region V* (No. 2-05-2004-11) (1983).

Medical Services Administration, State of Michigan, *Utilization of Medicaid Laboratory Services by Physicians with/without Ownership Interest in Clinical Laboratories: A Comparative Analysis of Six Selected Laboratories* (1981).

Alfred Childs and E. Diane Hunter, Non-Medical Factors Influencing Use of Diagnostic X-ray by Physicians, 10 *Medical Care* 323 (1972).

Alfred Childs and D. W. Hunter, *Patterns of Primary Medical Care — Use of Diagnostic X-Rays by Physicians* (1972). *See also* Chapter 13 by Jean Mitchell in this volume.

16. It would be difficult to argue that legal regulation, when it has existed in this area, resulted from a request or demand from a united medical profession.

17. There is one situation in which something like the exchange model would be literally true: when the profession as an already organized corporate entity enters into negotiations with government concerning the conditions of practice (e.g., political bargaining between leaders of organized medicine and the leadership of Congress over ceilings for physicians' fees). The difficulty with extending the model beyond this particular situation is that the model cannot explain the creation of the profession if it assumes that a profession already exists as one of the parties to the exchange.

18. Eliot Friedson, note 7, *supra*, at 197.

19. Bernard Shaw, *The Doctor's Dilemma* (1954).

20. The average (mean) pre-tax, after-expenses income of U.S. physicians in 1991 was $170,600, while the median was $139,000. American Medical Association Center for Health Policy Research, *Socioeconomic Character of Medical Practice* (1993).

21. *See, e.g.*, Paul Feldstein, *Health Associations and the Demand for Legislation: The Political Economy of Health Care* (1977), and *Health Economics* (1979). See also Paul Starr, The *Social Transformation of Medicine in America* (1982).

22. Very recently, several medical specialties have begun to take steps to devise significant procedures for ensuring that their members continue to possess technical competence. However,
it is worth noting that even with these continuing competence requirements, those who fail to
meet them are still able to practice medicine so long as they do not represent themselves as
recertified specialists.

23. Russell Localio *et. al.*, Relation Between Malpractice Claims and Adverse Events Due to
Negligence, Results of the Harvard Medical Practice Study III, 325 *N. Engl. J. Med.* 245
(1991).

24. In many locales, state medical associations suppressed HMOs by blacklisting HMO doctors
from specialty organizations and revoking their admitting privileges in hospitals owned or
controlled by association members. In some cases, medical associations have lobbied to make
midwifery illegal; in others, they have succeeded in placing so many restrictions on the practice of midwifery as to make it economically unfeasible.

25. Rodwin, *Medicine, Morals, and Money*, especially chapter two.

26. *Id.*, at chapter 2.

27. *Id.*, chapter 2.

28. *See*, e.g., AMA Rules Against Self-Referrals, *Chicago Tribune*, N20 (December 9, 1992).

29. It is far from clear that organized medicine in the United States could take effective measures
to ensure a reasonable level of compliance with substantive standards concerning conflicts of
interest even if it did a much better job of articulating such standards than it hitherto has. Since
only about one-half of practicing physicians in the United States even belong to the AMA, the
threat of expulsion is somewhat less than devastating. Moreover, the AMA only has the power
to recommend policies to state medical associations, which may or may not ratify them.
Finally, it can be argued that antitrust laws in particular, as well as the general emphasis in our
legal system on individual freedom of contract, greatly restrict the feasible range of alternatives for ensuring compliance.

30. Uwe Rheinhardt makes this point in Arnold Relman and Rheinhardt, An Exchange on For-
· Profit Health Care, *supra* note 10, at 213.

31. Dan Brock and Allen Buchanan, Ethical Issues in For-Profit Health Care, in *For-Profit
Enterprise in Health Care* 242 (1987).

32. *See Socioeconomic Characteristics of Medical Practice*, Table 48 (Martin Gonzalez, ed.,
1992).

33. See Rheinhardt in Relman and Rheinhardt, An Exchange on For-Profit Health Care, pp. 209,
211, 212, 213. See also, Brock and Buchanan, *supra* note 31, at 241.

34. Rheinhardt in Relman and Rheinhardt. An Exchange on For-Profit Health Care, at 212.

35. For two discussions of data showing that the higher the average income of a given specialty
the more applicants there are for residency positions in that specialty, see letters to the editor
by Mark Ebell and by David Shulkin, 262 *JAMA*. 1630 (1989). The former analyzes data from
the National Residency Match Program (1988); the latter uses data from that source and from
the Medical Economics Earnings Survey (1988).

36. Paul Feldstein, *Health Associations and the Demand for Legislation: The Political Economy
of Health* 480–553 (1977).

37. Daniel Fox, *The Politics of Trust in American Health Care, supra* note 4, at 10–13.

38. Charles Beitz, *Political Equality* (1989); Joshua Cohen, Deliberation and Democratic
Legitimacy, in *The Good Polity* 17–34 (Alan Hamlin and Philip Pettit, eds., 1989); and
Thomas Christiano, Freedom, Consensus, and Equality in Collective Decision Making, 10
Ethics 151 (1990).

39. Richard Zaner, The Phenomenon of Trust and the Physician–Patient Relationship in *Ethics,
Trust, and the Professions: Philosophical and Cultural Aspects, supra* note 4, at 480.

40. I am not aware of empirical studies on this phenomenon, but can report from my own experience as a patient that it certainly does occur. For example, when I asked a urologist whether there were any risks of infection from the cystoscopy he had just ordered for me (without asking my permission and without explaining the costs and benefits), he was astonished at my impudence. When, after his reluctant admission that there was such a risk, I declined his recommendation, he terminated the relationship.

41. The strongest case presently available for this approach is found in Marc Rodwin's book. *See* note 16, *supra. See also* the discussions of fiduciary duty by Morreim in Chapter 11 and by Shimm and Spece in Chapters 3 and 14, respectively.

42. This alternative for legal control of conflicts of interest is considered, but not endorsed by Rodwin, note 15 *supra.*

43. *See* Chapter 10 by Mark Hall in this volume. See also supra note 14.

44. *Supra* note 14, at 317–333.

45. *See*, e.g., Ian MacNeil, *The New Social Contract: An Inquiry into Modern Contractual Relations* (1980).

46. I am indebted to the following people, who generously supplied astute comments on earlier versions of this paper: Thomas Christiano, Christine Korsgaard, Jean Hampton, Thom Hudson, John Rawls, Tim Scanlon, and Roy Spece. I also have benefitted from the perceptive comments of several members of the audience at a colloquium of the Center for Ethics and the Professions at Harvard University, where I presented this paper.

6

Screening

Charles W. Wolfram

This chapter will assess conflict-of-interest problems handled by practitioners in law firms and in the securities industry. In both areas, conflicts are heavily regulated. Yet those areas of professional and business practice are not normally thought of as notably parallel to medicine. My focus here will be on a particular subset of conflicts issues—those raised by the so–called Chinese wall,[1] or screening, defense to a charge of conflict of interest—that would also seem to have little practical application in medicine.

Why, then, should one think that a reader intent on studying conflicts of interest in the medical profession would profit from considering conflicts of interest, and a particular way of dealing with these conflicts, in other professions or lines of business? Will the comparison be useful because the problems in these professions or businesses, if not the same, are nicely analogous—because solutions to conflicts that have worked in one realm will work in the other? Or is the pay-off somewhat different? Although disparate accusations may share certain kinds of conflicts and responses to them, here, as in almost any other comparative study, the main lesson to be learned (actually, to be relearned) is that context matters, and it matters immensely. Insights gained by studying any one profession or area of business must be carefully placed in their relevant context when one considers whether the same or a similar insight might apply to the possibly unique circumstances of any other profession.

137

"Screens" are arrangements that have been set up within law firms and securities firms on the premise of successfully and regularly preventing the evils spawned by some kinds of conflict of interest. At least in law firms, however, screens do so without purporting to root out entirely the source of the conflict itself. What we will see is that, by and large, the bar associations, courts, and other institutions regulating the legal profession have been rather determined in their reluctance to allow lawyers to end conflicts routinely through screening, while the governmental and private institutions regulating the securities industry have been more receptive.

Why the difference in the two? Here I explore two possible explanations. First, as a matter of description, screens in securities firms turn out to be very different from those in law firms. Securities firms are also required to maintain complementary features—restricted lists and watch lists of companies in whose stocks and bonds they may not trade or may trade only with restrictions. In view of these features, screens within the securities industry will be seen to be an unpromising source from which to borrow regulation for the legal profession. I then turn to a set of larger considerations having to do with the differential social value of large size law firms and securities firms that might explain, if further explanation is required, why law firms have been notably reluctant to accept screening to deal with conflicts of interest, despite its general acceptance by the securities industry.

What this comparison across professional and business boundaries suggests is that devices such as screens are not readily transportable to different environments. What might work in one profession or industry for a problem that, on the surface, appears to be the same or similar may turn out, on closer inspection, to be quite different. Context, to repeat, matters.[2] For those focusing on conflict-of-interest issues in the medical profession, the lesson can be simply put: Beware of suggestions that the medical profession borrow wholesale and uncritically concepts, devices, institutions, or other substantial features from other professions or industries in dealing with conflicts of interest. Some such loans may, after careful analysis, be found likely to succeed in medicine; others will be found to be poor risks; and still others will work only after substantial modification to fit particular needs. All such possibilities should be considered before accepting the inter–professional loan.

Screens in Law Firms

An understanding of the operation of screening devices in U.S. law firms requires some appreciation of the background rules of conflicts of interest in the legal profession. For most of its history, the American legal profession has operated with conflict-of-interest rules that, for present purposes, can be described in the following oversimplified way. In general, the sweep of conflict-of-interest rules depends on whether the conflict relates to concurrent representations of the lawyer or to former representations; moreover, the rules provide for both a personal taint of an individual lawyer because of a conflict and an imputed taint of the lawyer's entire firm. Lawyers are not permitted to represent *concurrently* two or more clients with seriously conflicting interests, at least not without informed consent. Even if the representation of a client is over at the time the lawyer undertakes to represent a new client, the former client remains entitled to protection of his confidential information. This is accomplished through a rule that prohibits the later representation if it is substantially related to the former representation. In other words, it is permissible to sue (or otherwise litigate with) a former client, but only if the litigation is not substantially related to the work that the lawyer had formerly performed.

For law firms, however, the most important rule is the additional requirement, imposed on top of concurrent–representation and former client conflict rules, that lawyers most often call the rule of *"imputed disqualification."* ("Imputed prohibition" might be a better term, since disqualification of the lawyer by a court is only one of many remedies. These remedies may also include damage awards or fee forfeitures that a court might later impose. We will abide by the popular vocabulary here, which almost uniformly refers to imputed "disqualification.") The imputed disqualification rule, in effect, holds that if one lawyer in a law firm is disqualified, then all lawyers in the firm are disqualified to the same extent.

Let me illustrate, first with a concurrent representation. If Lawyer A in Firm represents Husband in ongoing estate–planning work, by force of the imputed disqualification rule Lawyer B in Firm cannot represent Wife in her action against Husband to dissolve the marriage. Consider, next, a former client conflict situation. If Lawyer A in Firm formerly represented Husband in the estate–planning work, even if the representation is now ended, Lawyer A cannot represent Wife in her dissolution action because the looming importance of property division in the divorce action would make the later representation "substantially related" to the former. Most germane to screening devices, Lawyer B in Firm is also prohibited from representing Wife by force, again, of the rule of imputed disqualification.

It is on that last point, imputed disqualification, that conflict-of-interest rules have worked some of their most stringent prohibitions on lawyers. Conflict-of-interest rules will occasionally put a crimp on the practice of even small–town lawyers in solo practice. But because of the rule of imputed disqualification, the impact of conflict-of-interest rules may increase as the size of the law practice increases. A newly formed firm of three lawyers formerly in solo practice who continue the same sort of law practice, now in a firm, will find that the conflict-of-interest problems of the firm have increased exponentially over the problems the three had as individual practitioners. Whereas each lawyer may have been conflicted out of three representations in a year, the new firm will find that an average of nine conflicts occur each year, and each of the nine will apply to *each* lawyer (the implications of the conflict rules for the economics of firm formation among small groups of lawyers are fascinating but little explored in the literature).

In fact, of course, the increase is not exponential in all firms by any means. As a general rule, the larger the law firm, the fewer the clients and the fewer the matters handled per lawyer. Large–firm lawyers thus function quite differently from their small–firm counterparts as far as the impingement of conflicts rules are concerned. Thus, it is conceivable that some of the largest law firms may actually experience less conflict–driven need to decline clients, per lawyer, than would be the case with some small firms and solo practitioners. On the other hand, turning down a million–dollar fee because of a conflict will occur commonly only in larger firms, making the consequences of the imputed disqualification rule somewhat more graphic, per episode, for larger firms. And as will be shortly seen, marketing strategies and lateral hiring of established lawyers, which may be concentrated among larger firms, may, after all, present a greater concentration of conflict problems for large firms.

For years, the American legal profession has functioned with basically the above set of arrangements for managing conflicts in law practice. But in recent years, at least two forces have combined to make the conflict shoe pinch in ways that it had not done in former times. The increased pain, in turn, has raised the number and volume of lawyer complaints about overly stringent conflicts rules, particularly the rule of imputed disqualification.

The first force is the revolution in lawyer liability litigation. That revolution, for lawyers, has trailed by approximately two decades the era of vastly expanded damage liability to which physicians have been subjected.[3] Once it began (in approximately the mid–1970s), the still rising increase in lawyer malpractice exposure has made the conflict–prohibition rules much more important to lawyers. Among other consequences, breach of the conflict rules can now provide the foundation for very large damages awards. Those rules have, to say the least, had a strong influence in the field of lawyer liability for damages. The professional rules on conflicts were developed primarily with an eye to their use in lawyer discipline proceedings. The concepts behind the rules emerged, however, primarily from law developed in dealing with lawyer–disqualification motions, that is, proceedings in which a client or former client of a law firm asks a court (usually early in the litigation) to disqualify the firm from representing an opposing party. In dealing with those motions, courts have been somewhat freer than in lawyer discipline proceedings to devise sensible rules that seem to fit the specific professional requirements of law practice. As with their flexible and creative approach in disqualification proceedings, courts in lawyer malpractice actions seeking the recovery of damages can also exercise some flexibility in defining the circumstances in which conflicting representation creates liability.

The second factor that has caused many lawyers to object to the traditional rules mandating conflict avoidance is the increase in the size of American law firms in recent decades.[4] Law firm growth is probably fueled by considerations of profit for law firm partners, although it may also reflect, perhaps only in part, the changing world of commerce and industry generally. In recent years, law firms have been increasingly inspired by what they perceive as business methods for conducting, and allocating financial rewards from, the practice of law. As professional parlance has it, firms have been increasingly fascinated with the bottom line, the firms' annual profit and partnership draw.

The result has been a significant increase in the number of very large law firms (measured in traditional terms)—the mega–firm with hundreds of lawyers, typically in offices in several major cities. Growth of law firms has been achieved in part with aggressive marketing. A traditional strategy of client–getting has been to accept a large, wealthy client on a small retainer in the hope of developing a more lucrative practice for the client. A companion strategy of marketing has been lateral hiring of lawyers with a client base established at another firm. On occasion, this has taken the form of wholesale firm mergers, as large firms become larger very quickly or expand rapidly into a new city or specialty–practice area through acquisitions of smaller firms by merger. Each of these growth strategies produces an increase both in conflicts and in the costs of conflict avoidance.

Thus, the last two decades have also witnessed a vast increase in the number of firms with hundreds of lawyers, many offices, and many clients. Some lawyers seek to explain at least part of this trend on the basis of service, not increased incomes: Law firms, it is argued, have been required to increase the number of lawyers and the number of branch offices because of the increasingly widespread nature of the activities and legal consequences of their clients with their far–flung business empires. Yet this explanation seems somewhat off target, because American industry spread nationally long before American law firms did so.

Whatever might explain the explosion in their size and organizational complexity, American law firms are unlikely to shrink significantly in the foreseeable future. Thus ever–growing firms with ever–increasing appetites for new clients have come up against the rigors of the imputed disqualification rule. As firms grow larger, the task of conflict avoidance becomes much more complex and produces its own tensions. Many firms now require computer–controlled conflict checks before a firm lawyer takes on any new client or new matters for an existing client. Legal malpractice insurers often require firms to install and scrupulously monitor elaborate procedures for conflict checking. Those systems, in turn, require extensive documentation of client intake, computer checking of incoming new matters, supplementary new–client memoranda to all partners, and conflicts committees of partnership–level lawyers to shepherd the system, deal with novel or otherwise problematical cases, and mediate disputes among firm lawyers.

The stakes can be considerable. In most law firms, a lawyer denied the opportunity to represent a client because of a conflict loses significant personal income because of the common "eat–what–you–kill" system of providing rewards for new business, even if the legal services are performed in whole or part by other firm lawyers. At the very least, being required to turn down a potential client for conflict reasons can injure professional pride and frustrate one's sense of duty to a former or existing client. In some firms, the resulting tumult among partners has been enormous as senior partners engage in titanic internal power struggles to determine which of them will refuse a retainer, sometimes of a long–time client, in order to save the firm from the gridlock of firm–wide conflict.[5] In some instances, a frustrated lawyer or group of lawyers will break away from their large firm with their own stable of clients to form a smaller firm or to merge with another firm in order to avoid the looming imputed–conflict problem. The reverse strategy is also sometimes, although rarely, used. Some firms have terminated a senior lawyer to avoid a conflict otherwise produced by that lawyer's clients or former clients.

In a fast–receding age (in fact, only a generation ago), law firms probably dealt with stress over some kinds of conflict by use of a strategy that today most managing partners would consider too risky: simply ignoring the conflicts and hoping that none of the affected clients would notice or complain. However, with the increasing threat of damage awards and occasional instances in which even prestigious firm lawyers have been ignominiously hauled before lawyer–disciplinary agencies for conflict violations, playing fast–and–loose with the conflict rules has become much riskier. Thus, as a new literalism about conflict rules has been visited on large–firm lawyers, they have become predictably insistent on amelioration of what they accurately perceive to be one of the chief impediments to ever–increasing firm growth: the imputed disqualification rule.

Until the mid–1970s, there seemed to be no good alternative. But at that point, the American Bar Association's ethics committee discovered the screening device.[6] At least, it had never been discussed or approved as a cure for conflict in any ethics opinion or judicial decision until that time. The ABA committee did so in a rarified context—conflicts produced by a new firm lawyer who was formerly in government service. Typically, the lawyer had returned from a government position, through the proverbial revolving door, to a much more lucrative practice in a private law firm. Many such conflicts were particularly painful because they included what lawyers call "benign" conflicts— those that occur when the lawyer's private–practice client is on the *same side* as the former governmental client–employer—as well as the more familiar "side–switching" conflicts, which are similar to those in private practice. As with other conflicts, the pain was particularly acute because of the threat of imputed disqualification of all firm lawyers. Without differentiating between the kinds of conflict involved, the ABA ethics committee put forward the idea of the screening device. With its use, the immunized former government lawyer, although personally disqualified, would not spread the conflict to other lawyers in the firm.

What most lawyers today forget is that the ABA committee authorized use of a screen only if the former government client consented to the arrangement. However, that severely limiting aspect of the ABA opinion has long since been ignored in the lawyer–code rules as well. Removal of the client–consent requirement was accomplished in the ABA's new lawyers code, promulgated in 1983. Rule 1.11(a) of the new code, which has been widely copied by the states, has dropped the requirement of consent and now provides uniformly for screening protection for firms containing former government lawyers, regardless of possible objections by former government clients.

The screening device for former government lawyers has served the objectives of those who pushed for such a rule, but it has also fired the imaginations of large–firm lawyers generally. The direction of thought is predictable: If screens are permissible for former government lawyers, why not allow them more generally for many, if not all, types of law firm conflicts? Were the ABA to review its ethics code today, it is possible that its governing body, which has a substantial and disproportionate representation of large–firm lawyers, would approve extensive private–practice use of screening devices. But there is no textual support in the present (1983) lawyer code for such acceptance. To the contrary, the fact that the lawyer code accepts screens for former government lawyers and says nothing about accepting screens in other private–practice arrangements strongly suggests that they are not acceptable in those other areas.

Courts, with some exceptions, have agreed on this restrictive view of screening devices. A majority of jurisdictions that have passed on the question have simply refused to accept screens outside the former–government–lawyer situation. Firms that practice in states adopting this anti–screening rule are, in effect, faced with the need to comply with the full panoply of conflict rules, including the prohibitions of the imputed disqualification rule.

Judicial acceptance of screens, to the limited extent it has occurred, has been grudging and guarded. The occasional accepting court has done so with sensitivity to the types of cases in which it is permitted. For example, no case, to my knowledge, has permitted one firm lawyer to sue a client defended by another firm lawyer in another matter simply because of a screen between the two lawyers.[7] Courts that have accepted screens have generally tolerated only minimal threats to the confidentiality interests of clients (in the event that the screen is accidentally or intentionally breached), which is the interest typically at stake in screening cases.[8] In other words, it is only where the personally disqualified lawyer possesses only unimportant information that most courts will show much interest in a screening defense.[9]

Higher courts that have accepted screens have typically not assured law firms that they would be available automatically, even in the limited areas and isolated jurisdictions in which they are sometimes accepted. The typical ruling has recognized that a lower court has discretion to accept or reject a screening defense based on the particular facts before the court. Most courts insist on screening at an early point in the conflicted representation and on the law firm establishing elaborate procedures to maintain and monitor the screen.

Moreover, the limited acceptance of screening has not meant smooth sailing for law firms in the minority of jurisdictions that have permitted them. Firms implementing screens have often found that they produce administrative, staffing, and collegiality challenges—problems which have led some firms to authorize them only in exceptional cases. Segregating lawyers, paralegals, secretaries, and files produces significant initial disruption and, during the often extended period when the screen must remain in place, seriously complicates normal collaborative working arrangements among firm lawyers.

A second problem with screens is whether they do any more than prevent disqualification of the firm. Most of the court decisions recognizing screening have involved disqualification motions, which, once again, are efforts in litigation to remove the lawyers for one side from further participation in the case. Even the few reluctant decisions accepting screening in disqualification cases do not necessarily mean that the same lawyers are also immune from professional discipline. Some courts, although denying disqualification, have referred the discipline question to the lawyer–discipline body in the jurisdiction. Thus, at least theoretically, a jurisdiction could decide that a screen provides protection only in disqualification motions, not in professional discipline. The refusal of a discipline system to enforce the lawyer code would require an interesting (I do not say impossible or even unlikely) exercise in reading the current code in force in the great majority of American jurisdictions. At least until jurisdictions resolve the question of immunity from professional discipline due to the screening defense, lawyers who construct screens may find that they have avoided one sanction only to become involved in litigating about another. On the whole, the screening device in American law firms offers only a begrudging, occasional, and problematic solution to firm–wide conflict-of-interest problems.

Screens in Securities Firms

Lawyers sometimes assert, although much more commonly in conversation than in published writing, that the rules regulating lawyers' use of screening devices are unduly strict. Some of these lawyers point to the expansive permission (or so it is claimed) for screens in the securities industry. Lawyers, they claim, should be trusted at least as much as investment bankers and enjoy at least equal freedom to protect themselves against disabling conflict by their own use of screens. On closer examination, however, the practices of the securities industry are neither permissive nor reassuring to lawyers on the use of screens. In the end, those practices hardly support permissive use of screens in the legal profession.

While the problems that screens seek to resolve in securities firms are complex, both in their transactional and organizational settings and in their legal implications,[10] the following seeks to capture the essence of the issue, if again in simplified outline. As with the use of screens in law firms (other than in the instance of former government lawyers), screens in securities firms are neither required nor explicitly warranted by legislation or regulation. Instead, they are devices that, the Securities and Exchange Commission and some court decisions have indicated, may provide a defense against criminal or civil liability. Importantly, however, their acceptance is by no means required, universal, or without reservations. Substantial doubt exists among "a respectable number of securities industry professionals" whether screens significantly deter insider trading.[11]

At bottom, the conflict issue is based on the fact that modern securities business is multifarious. Modern securities firms encounter most of their conflict-of-interest problems because they structure and market themselves as multi–service or integrated capital-transfer firms.

The service activity of securities firms most familiar to investors is trading securities for the accounts of retail customers. Those accounts are a high–volume source of capital that securities firms can put to other uses as well. One way this can be done is by making discretionary reinvestments of existing account shares (selling present account holdings and purchasing new ones) or making original investments of surplus funds in the accounts (from dividends, cash contributions, and the like). Another way of exploiting the capital potential of retail accounts is making buy–sell recommendations through the retail broker–salespeople who manage the accounts or through investment advisers who assist customers in managing their own portfolios.

Much hidden potential for conflict exists in handling retail accounts alone, but the combination of the retail–account activity with activities conducted in other areas of a multiservice securities firm provides the most graphic realization of the potential for conflict. To see how conflicts of interest can arise, take retail accounts as a starting point and consider another trading activity in which the securities firm may be engaged at the same time. Most securities firms trade for their own accounts, as well as for the accounts of retail customers. In their own–account trading activity, they expose to risk the portfolios and wealth of the firm and the firm's own principals, seeking profits that will also be shared only by the firm's principals. In the absence of conflict-of-interest rules prohibiting the practice, a securities firm's trader trading on the firm's own account will occasionally have economic motivation to favor the firm's fortunes over those of retail–account customers. For example, the trader could be motivated to dump the firm's holdings in shares of a company about which the firm had learned bad news, and to do so before it became public. (We will see in a moment that a third activity commonly allows the firm to acquire such material, nonpublic information.) The cash–rich account of an unwitting retail customer could be an attractive and available buyer for such shares.

But there is more. Securities firms engage in a wide range of financial transactions beyond securities trading, whether for themselves or for their customers. Prominent among such transactions is investment banking. With their ready access to investors and thus to potentially large accumulations of capital, securities firms may be well positioned to serve corporations, government entities, and similar organizations that need large infusions of funds. Those infusions take many forms, such as a leveraged buy–out, a government bond issue, an initial issue of corporate stock, corporate bonds, or (as with junk bonds) corporate non–equity debt, or any other form of capital accumulation that involves gathering together the funds of others.

Inevitably, in the course of investment banking, the securities firm will learn important confidential information about the plans of investment–banking customers, who seek the firms' access to the capital markets and who pay the firms' sizable fees. The law requires that such information must, for most purposes, be kept secret. To take an obvious example, a plan by an investment–banking customer, Corporation A, to accumulate capital to make a bid for a controlling interest in the shares of Corporation B must be kept secret until the last possible moment to maximize Corporation A's chance of success. Yet, the securities firm functioning as the investment banker for Corporation A may wish to purchase shares of Corporation B for the securities firm's own account or for the account of favored customers in order to profit from the almost inevitable run–up in share prices of the target company that greets the announcement of a takeover attempt.[12]

The legal complication in all such situations, of course, is that securities firms are not free to play both ends against the middle. The law does not define their relationship with their customers in the ordinary way—the so–called arm's–length relationship in which sharp practices are countenanced so long as they do not amount to fraud. Instead, the law defines the duties of securities firms as, at best, four–dimensional. Multiservice securities firms must respect the interests of at least two sets of customers (retail and investment banking) and those of the investing public, in addition to serving their own self–interest as own–account investors.[13]

The interest of customers is protected by legal rules requiring that securities brokers deal fairly with them. Thus, it is against the law to churn a customer's account (buying and selling shares in the account solely for the purpose of generating commissions on the transactions), to sell secretly the firm's own–account stock holdings to a customer's account (self–dealing), or to sell own–account holdings to a customer after identifying the shares as own–account but without revealing material nonpublic information adversely affecting their value (insider trading).

Similarly, beyond individual customers are the legally protected interests of the investing public. Those interests are elaborated primarily in federal and state securities laws seeking to maintain properly and fairly functioning securities markets. The working of those laws is, again, complex but can be grasped from the following. Take again the example of investment–banking activities in Corporation A's planned takeover of Corporation B. The law governing the relationship between the securities firm and its investment–banking customers requires that the securities firm keep confidential any material information it may have concerning the acquiring client's intended takeover. Agency law itself generally requires agents in such circumstances not to reveal the confidential information of their principals.[14] From this perspective alone, one might conclude that investments in the target company's shares by the securities firm for its own account (or for the accounts of retail customers) would be permissible so long as the investment was placed discreetly, so as not to alert others to the planned takeover. But other law goes further than agency law and prohibits even that activity.

As highly publicized prosecutions during the last several years have dramatically shown, federal securities law prohibits securities trading based on insider information. Stated simply, one who possesses insider information—such as the nonpublic information about the planned takeover possessed by the securities firm in our example—must either disclose or refrain. The firm must either publicly disclose the information before buying or selling the security, so as to make it available to other investors, or else it must refrain from any trading in the security until public disclosure is made (by anyone). But, of course, making the information public would directly violate the firm's duty to its investment–banking customer to keep the information secret. Equilibrium of obligation can be achieved only if the firm refrains from any own–account or retail–account trading in the stock, despite the strong temptation to do so.

The resulting clash of legal obligations and practical opportunities sets up the conflict-of-interest quandary for securities firms, and for those responsible for attempting to ensure the compliance of such firms with legal requirements. With the same multiservice securities firm investing for securities customers, investing for its own account, and assisting investment–banking clients with capital accumulation projects, the potential for conflict is rife. Leaving the remedy for violations of legal duties by the securities firm and its employees solely to after–the–fact prosecutions or civil suits for money damages (while available) would be too limited to protect adequately the legal interests involved. Among other things, persons bringing suits against a securities firm would face a stonily silent monolith. The defending firm would typically possess almost all the facts, and the incentives for all within the firm with knowledge of wrongdoing to form a united front of denial and obfuscation are strong.

A draconian legal solution would be to prohibit a securities firm from performing all but one of the conflict–producing activities, so that all securities firms would be in single–service, if different, lines of work. If such an unwise solution were ever put in place, securities firms would have to undertake dramatic downsizing. Although that solution might have appealed to some reformers at an earlier time, it is not conceivable, in the present context of intense global competition for capital services among investment–banking and securities firms, that American law would move in that direction. Even in an earlier time when competition was primarily national, large size was simply too important when performing capital–accumulation services, customers were too strongly attracted to a single–firm source of multiple capital services, and the resulting small and non–diversified firms lost the efficiencies[15] that can be achieved only if single firms provide related financial and securities services. Those considerations led to a variety of proposals to solve, or at least ameliorate, the conflict problems while permitting large, multiservice securities firms to continue their several lines of business.

If multiservice securities firms were to continue to exist in the legal environment described above, what was required was a mechanism that would permit the coexistence of different activities within the same firm, while at the same time achieving overall compliance with the sometimes conflicting legal obligations imposed on the firm and the practical incentives available to it. Obviously, the mechanism would have to *segregate* those functions somewhat while permitting as much *integration* of functions as possible consistent with legal requirements. The most likely solution would focus on information flow within the firm, for many (but not all) of the legal constraints dealt with misuse of confidential information. Finally, the mechanism would deal directly with less than all of the legal requirements involved, so long as its operation satisfied all of them. In other words, it might be possible to achieve multiple regulatory bird kills with fewer stones than birds.

The eventual device seized on was the screen. The screen could be constructed to isolate information within securities firms so that it would not pass to others in the firm who legally were not permitted to deal in the information. Initially, the simple and unadorned solution of the screen was greeted with enthusiasm. However, it was soon discovered that the problems of conflicting legal obligations and economic incentives required another mechanism to buttress the screen.

In brief, an initial response was the proposal to create screens in the multiservice securities firm. That would be done, for example, between the investment–banking department (with its "hot" insider knowledge of customers' intended takeover activity) and the trading and brokerage divisions (with their illegitimate thirst for such information). In that way, it was hoped, the firm would be in full compliance both with federal securities laws (because its trading and brokerage departments would not be trading on insider information) and with its obligation of confidentiality to its investment–banking customers (because it would not permit transfer of that information to its other divisions). At least for this problem, the mechanics of the screen were also fairly straightforward. The protective devices required were limited to the investment–banking division, whose employees would be strictly instructed to confine or eliminate the circulation of written and spoken information about target companies (or similarly attractive investment possibilities).

However, the foxes would guard the hen house. The proposal was not to constitute a body of independent and reliable "securities police" who would monitor intrafirm communications to ensure no breaches of the screen. Instead, at least initially, the idea was to insist on the scout's honor of securities participants that they wouldn't engage in forbidden communication. But accepting such simplistic screens would often put the investing public and regulators in the same can't–win situation as damage actions and criminal prosecutions: They would have to accomplish the undoable task of demonstrating, from evidence almost always controlled by the securities firm, that the screen had been breached.

Some commentators eventually noted that a simple addition to the screen could both eliminate the need to prove the unprovable and make screening a realistic method of compliance. This additional device was "restricted list." This consists of a list of the names of all stocks in which research, sales, or trading by the firm's employees is prohibited, so long as the stock continues to appear on the list. (Many firms also use "watch lists" to test whether screening restrictions are being honored within the firm. The firm's compliance officers monitor trades in the shares of a company about to be put on a restricted list to detect any prelisting surge in activity, which may indicate insider trading.) At the same time, the restricted list attempts to address a Catch–22 aspect of insider–trading enforcement: If an effective system of screens was indeed created, this would not ensure that, through serendipity, a division of the multiservice firm screened off from confidential information wouldn't guess right and make a dumb–but–lucky investment. Even though the investment would not have violated the spirit of the securities laws, a public and public agencies nervousness about insider breaches of self–imposed measures would rightly wonder how effective the screen was. A related anomaly of a screens–alone system is an investment adviser urging a customer to sell a stock at the same time that a screened–off investment banker in the firm knows that its secret plans make the stock a buy. With restricted lists, departments of the firm would simply be notified that the firm's employees were prohibited from trading (either buying or selling) or other activity in any listed security. Given the multiservice nature of the firm, the appearance of a name on the restricted list, it is hoped, won't necessarily signal whether to buy or sell, particularly as lists grow longer. With modern computer–driven record keeping, securing compliance could become both realistic and relatively inexpensive.

Note, however, what has happened. While the screen–insulating information remains important for a limited number of purposes, much of the assurance of law compliance by the screened–off divisions of the securities firm in fact comes from the restricted list. The important feature, for our present purpose, is that the temptation to succumb to a conflict of interest in securities trading is removed, not only by screening traders in the firm from insider information possessed by the firm's investment bankers, but also by prohibiting both of them and all other firm employees from trading in the security.[16]

That feature of the complete system of securities screen–plus–list regulation is what makes screening in securities firms such an inappropriate model for the very different device in law firms bearing the same name. For the analogy from the securities industry to hold in law firms, the latter would be required to do more than install screens. They would also be required to set up a system of restricted activities analogous to restricted lists. Perhaps the only sensibly analogous restriction would be to preclude the law firm from conducting activities in behalf of clients on the list. In effect, obviously, that would disqualify the firm from the conflicting representation! That is where we started, and that is what lawyers want screens to avoid. In the end, then, the screen–plus–list approach employed in securities firms would leave law firms no better off than they are under the present set of rules on conflicts of interest.

Screens in a Theoretical Context

The acceptance of screening devices in the securities industry and their rejection, by and large, for law firms can also be understood in terms of some fundamental aspects of conflict regulation. Briefly exploring those fundamental points requires a brief canvass of conflict regulation itself. As will be seen, what is arguably needed is equal solicitude about conflict avoidance in both the securities industry and law practice. What differentiates them at a fundamental level is a quite different justification for large securities firms to deal with capital accumulation, while no similar justification exists for large law firms. That differentiation may be important on a practical level—for example, should an imaginative device be suggested to implement screens–plus–lists in law firms in a way convincingly analogous to the way those protections operate in securities firms.

At the level of theory, the general disapproval of conflicts of interest is at least as old as the New Testament dictum that no person can serve two masters. And assuredly this concept, which resonates at the most basic level of trust, must be much older than that. To be sure, conflicts of interest in dealings between persons seem inescapable, and perhaps in some settings even desirable. Buyers and sellers often negotiate over limited resources and with decidedly conflicting aims; at least in many transactions, a good deal for one is a poor deal for the other. In the broadest sense of the term, conflicts of interest are presumably what drive nations to war, politicians and citizens to their separate political parties, and interested citizens to their lobbies and similar pressure groups (in their organized form we call the last "interest groups" in recognition of their conflicted interests with the interests of others, perhaps including the public at large).

Thus, much conflict exists in any social order and is tolerated, or even encouraged, by the legal system. A ready example is the way the law both subsidizes and protects markets where sellers and buyers can meet, negotiate, and carry out their conflicted, but socially useful, exchanges. Indeed, as small social units such as the family, church, and village have been replaced in modern mega–urban life with the formal and impersonal mechanisms of a more structured society, mediating conflicting claims has become more and more important in keeping the peace and has consumed a correspondingly increasing share of social and political resources. (Lawyers, for the many who are counting, have increased in number and importance to fill the widening social void.) For the most part, the law merely sets outer limits for the operation of those acceptable conflicts, leaving a vast plain for conflicting players to wrestle their differences to earth.

But social and legal tolerance for conflict is not infinite. All legal systems limit their acceptance of conflicting interests and recognize and enforce the private settlements that arise out of conflict. Certain conflicts or their manifestations are either discouraged or prohibited outright. Most often that is done categorically and without regard to the identity of the actors, such as in the definition of certain activities as crimes or civil wrongs (theft or fraud). Other conflicts are discouraged or regulated not because they are considered wrongs in themselves (e.g., business dealings) but because the participants in the transaction are seriously unequal (e.g., a business deal between lawyer and client). It is these conflicting interests, characterized by certain types of protected relationships, that we refer to in everyday popular and legal parlance by the otherwise overbroad term "conflict of interest."

Whatever the appeal of consumerism, it has never been imagined that the law would routinely intervene to micro–manage bargain relationships, investigating all situations in which one participant claims that he or she was at a disadvantage. The law is more discriminating in defining situations in which conflict-of-interest rules have real bite. Conflicts of interest between persons, when recognized in the law as a problem requiring a specific remedy to ameliorate abuses of power, almost always have two characteristics. First, the law imposes what its courts often refer to as a "fiduciary duty." Such duties are characterized by a clear definition of the obligation. The definition demonstrates an unusual solicitude for the direct victims of violations of the duty, often with strong and condemnatory moral overtones lurking just beneath the surface (and often rising above it), and remedies for breach of the fiduciary duty that are flexible, energetic, and otherwise unusual in the law. Second, the situations subject to special fiduciary duties usually involve long–term, and thus stable, but imbalanced power relationships of enduring social and political importance.

In protecting fiduciary relationships, a fiduciary duty can roughly be defined as a duty more demanding than mere crime and fraud avoidance, which are duties of all persons toward all others in a legal culture. The more exacting fiduciary duties are expressed in the law in two general ways: substantive rules imposing the higher obligations themselves and procedural rules that implement such duties or complement them in case the legal proceedings seeking enforcement of those duties ensue.

An example of the higher substantive standard is the common fiduciary obligation not to engage in self–dealing with entrusted property, such as occurs when a trustee purchases property from the trust. The fiduciary duty prohibiting the transaction expresses a policy against certain transactions in which, the law has concluded, the risk of self–interested or otherwise distorted favoritism is too great and the reasons for permitting the conduct are too flimsy to permit such activities. Presumably, the arguments in favor of permitting a trustee to purchase property from the trust estate in the normal way ("at arm's length," as the law says in its typically muscular disregard for moral niceties) would include such reasons as encouraging the liquidity of property holdings and upholding the finality of agreed–to bargains. Such policies are impaired in only trivial ways by prohibiting trustee self–dealing. A similar rule that binds lawyers as fiduciaries states that a lawyer may enter into a business deal with a client only if the deal is fair and reasonable to the client.

Beyond special substantive rules governing fiduciary duties are procedural rules that effectuate them. For example, complementing the fair–and–reasonable–terms rule for client–lawyer business transactions is a procedural rule applied if litigation concerning the transaction ensues between the lawyer and client. Every state places the burden of proof on the lawyer who enters into a suspect deal to demonstrate fairness and reasonableness. In litigation *not* involving fiduciaries—for example, a suit by a buyer of property, who is not owed fiduciary duties, to set aside the transaction because of the seller's fraud—the buyer must prove the fraud. The buyer thus will lose if witnesses with critical testimony are dead or otherwise unavailable to testify, if available witnesses report or actually have defective memories on matters that the buyer must prove, or if the jury ends up being uncertain about what happened.

Conflicts change those procedural rules. If, for example, the buyer is the seller's client, the burden is shifted to the lawyer–seller, who must present evidence demonstrating fairness and reasonableness. The lawyer–fiduciary is thereby made to bear the risks of absent evidence and the "fog of war" that afflicts many trials even when the jury conscientiously attempts to find the facts. Occasionally, a jurisdiction will articulate this concept, placing the burden of proof on the lawyer as a "presumption" that the lawyer has "defrauded" the client. But the net effect is merely rhetorical. The important meaning is more accurately captured by the procedural notion of shifting to the lawyer the burden of demonstrating that the deal is fair and reasonable.

The second hallmark of fiduciary relationships is that they tend to be situations that are long–term as well as relational, and are marked by a significant and stable imbalance of bargaining power between the person on whom the duty is cast and the person who receives greater protection from the duty. Indeed, this hallmark of fiduciary relationships is at the causal root of the law, for without such justification the duties of fiduciaries would not be created in the first place. The relationships last, or are expected to last in the typical case, for more than the time that random buyers and sellers, for example, encounter each other in markets to make simple exchanges. At least at the descriptive level, the relationships typically concern a need or want on the part of the protected person that is endemic and continuing in their situation. Legal clients have long–term problems requiring attention over a period of time. Investors in securities make substantial commitments to purchase securities that will often be held for substantial periods, and capitalists have long–term needs for liquidity in financial markets in which they seek to raise capital.

For lawyers, the legal system—speaking through courts and through lawyer codes—has determined that the inequality that typically or often characterizes the client–lawyer relationship requires broad and strict protection for confidential client information and for the loyalty interests of clients. That instinct has led most jurisdictions to be relatively restrictive about the extent to which law firms can minimize conflict–of–interest problems through the use of screening devices.

The law's regulation of the financial–services industry has shown a much greater tolerance for in–house arrangements that address the risks to customers and the investing public posed by the firms' possession of confidential, nonpublic information. Yet, the two fields are hardly distinguishable on the ground that the relationship between a securities firm and its customers is insufficiently long–lasting, dependent, and socially important to require fiduciary protection. Many of the hallmarks of fiduciary relationships exist there. The relationship often extends over a relatively long term. With many customers, it is also a one–sided, imbalanced power relationship favoring the firm. And although practitioners in the securities industry are less likely than lawyers to engage in what Supreme Court Justice Felix Frankfurter once derisively called self–congratulatory praise of the high–minded public nature of their work, it must be conceded that the securities industry is of enduring social, economic, and political importance.

The acceptability of screening devices in the securities industry cannot be based on the assurance that the screens prevent all unlawful exchanges of information. To the contrary, it is commonly believed that occasional leaks of critical information do occur and that huge (and often conflict–ridden) profits are sometimes derived. Many observers also believe that some of those violations are undetected and probably undetectable. Nonetheless, the risks involved in permitting screens in the securities industry, along with the buttress of restricted lists, are considered acceptable. Without screens or their equivalent, securities firms could not engage in the multiservice activities necessary to sustain their present size.

Thus, it may be that the differential treatment of law firms and securities firm with respect to screening devices comes down to different justifications for large size in the two industries. Law firms, at least historically, have been of modest size in comparison with securities firms. Particularly as securities firms have been drawn into international markets and international competition, the arguments for their large size have become increasingly compelling. These include some arguments, such as those based on the need to maintain international competitiveness and to provide methods of capital accumulation for even domestic financing, that have important public dimensions.

The arguments for large size in law firms are much less obvious and much less based on public interest. That some law firms include as many as 1,000 lawyers, and that almost all law firms wish to grow, may reflect nothing of broad public significance but only the internal, profit–generating dynamics of law practice and the profit–generated structure of law firms. Law firms are almost always structured as a profit pyramid. This arrangement requires a large number of aspiring nonpartner lawyers (usually called "associates") whose services are charged at fees far in excess of their compensation, thus leveraging the income of the (typically) smaller number of law–firm partners, who alone participate in profits. That pyramidal arrangement alone does not explain growth. At least in theory, a firm could maintain any particular size by advancing associates to partner status only as existing partners die or retire. What necessarily produces growth is that all partners remain partners but that additional partnerships—in excess of the number produced by vacancies—are made available to aspiring associates to give them enough incentive to work the horrendously long hours they are willing to put in to fuel the profit furnace.

The largest law firms may now have nearly their maximum size—given, among other factors, present conflict-of-interest regulations. Arresting growth at this point will doubtless cause important rearrangements in law firms, including perhaps wrenching changes in their profit structure, their hiring and promotion practices, and their tradition (until recently) of automatic retention of partners regardless of productivity. Whether those changes are too high a price to pay for present conflict-of-interest rules is part of a debate that will doubtless continue in the legal profession. Compared to the securities industry, however, lawyers simply cannot make out as compelling a case of need or public interest for more conflict tolerance.

In the end, then, the argument of lawyers for more protection through screening devices gains no support from the experience with screens in the securities industry. Given the additional requirement of restricted lists in securities firms, the analogy fails, either because it is inadequately descriptive or because it is self–defeating when the role of restricted lists is added to the comparative equation. Aside from this problem of inconsistency, the risks that a screening arrangement creates in the securities industry may be more acceptable simply because of the higher social and economic desirability of large securities firms. Preventing law firms from growing further, the chief impact of refusal to accept screening in the legal profession, may be a matter of interest only to lawyers, with consequences that are not at all socially compelling.

Notes

1. The term "Chinese wall" is sometimes used interchangeably with "screening." The former is a colloquialism that probably is meant to invoke the strength and impregnability of the Great Wall of China. *See* Charles Wolfram, *Modern Legal Ethics* 401 n. 65 (1986). However, one need not be an advocate of political correctness (I would say) to worry that the term might strike some as insensitive and perhaps racist. I have so worried (*id.*), as have others. *See, e.g.*, Grant Kolling, Sr., The "Chinese Wall": An Anachronism of Jurisprudence," 17 *Public L. J.* 10 (1993). Thus, despite some residual usage of the term in the literature, particularly that involving the securities industry, I employ here the widely used and surely inoffensive term "screening."
2. Perhaps the leading exponent of context-based analysis of ethical issues in the legal profession has been Prof. David Wilkins. *See, e.g.*, Wilkins, Legal Realism for Lawyers, 104 *Harv. L. Rev.* 468 (1990); Wilkins, Making Context Count: Regulating Lawyers After Kaye Scholer (limited circulation draft, 1992) (copy on file with author).
3. That is not to suggest, of course, that malpractice exposure is equal for lawyers and physicians. A rough, but roughly reliable, measure is comparable malpractice insurance premiums

rates for each profession. Lawyers pay a fraction of what physicians pay for comparable levels of insurance protection. My undocumented sense is that the fraction is on the order of one-fifth to one-tenth.

4. A fascinating and important book has recently reported a study of the growth of American law firms, indicating that the rate of growth has remained relatively constant since the early years of this century: Marc Galanter and Thomas Palay, *Tournament of Lawyers: The Transformation of the Big Law Firm* (1991). Even if growth has been constant, the increase from 20– to 40-lawyer firms is much less dramatic than the present increase from 500– to 1000-lawyer firms.

5. I here assume, blithely, that withdrawal from representing or declining to represent only one client will cure all conflicts. In truth, the matter can be much more complex.

6. ABA Legal Ethics Committee, Formal Opinion 342 (1976).

7. One must except Texas from this statement. Lawyers there operate under a rule, peculiar to that state, that permits even the same lawyer to sue an existing client if the lawsuit is not factually related to the lawyer's ongoing work on behalf of the client. *See* Texas Disciplinary Rule of Professional Conduct, Rule 1.06(b)(1). The Texas rule, which does not clearly state that proposition, has been explained by its drafters to have that effect. *See* Robert Schuwerk and John Sutton, Jr., A Guide to the Texas Disciplinary Rules of Professional Conduct, *27A Hous. L. Rev. 15,* 98–102 (1990). The much-relaxed Texas rule applies only in state courts. The federal appeals court with reviewing jurisdiction over all Texas federal courts has held that federal courts are to apply the much more familiar absolute bar against suing one's own client, including the imputed-prohibition aspect of that bar: *In re* American Airlines, 972 F.2d 605 (5th Cir. 1992). Other states are not as free-wheeling as Texas is said to be about concurrent-representation conflicts.

8. For example, perhaps the most widely cited case accepting the Chinese wall defense is Nemours Foundation v. Gilbane, 632 F. Supp. 418 (D. Del. 1986). The court there, however, noted that the lawyer in question had left his former firm. He thus had no possible opportunity to gather additional information. Moreover, while there he had functioned as a junior associate, and he had only limited contact with the matter, and in a context (preparing an expert witness to testify) that the court may have considered unlikely to involve significant secrets.

9. Such a minimal-risk test for Chinese walls has been tentatively approved by the American Law Institute (ALI), a private organization of lawyers, judges, and law professors who develop nonbinding, but hopefully influential, restatements of the law on various subjects. See ALI, *Restatement of the Law Governing Lawyers*, section 204(2) (tent. draft no. 4, 1991). The author serves as chief reporter for the Restatement, which is still in the process of development. Professor Hazard, another contributor to this work, serves as Director of the ALI. The question of Chinese walls has been, by far, the most controversial of the subjects yet encountered in formulating the Restatement.

10. *See* generally 8 Louis Loss and Joel Seligman, *Securities Regulation* 3618-31 (3d ed., 1991). A recent and comprehensive review of the range of legislation and compliance devices is Harvey Pitt and Karl Groskaufmanis, Minimizing Corporate Civil and Criminal Liability: A Second Look at Corporate Codes of Conduct, *78 Geo. L. J.* 1559 (1990). On the specific subject of Chinese walls and similar devices in the securities industry, see *id*, at 1617–1623.

11. 8 Louis Loss and J. Seligman, *supra* at 3630, citing Norman Poser, Chinese Wall or Emperor's New Clothes? Regulating Conflicts of Interest of Securities Firms in the U.S. and the U.K., 9 *Mich. Y.B. Int. Legal Stud.* 91, 127–134 (1988).

12. I ignore here a complication that can be important in many such scenarios—the possibility that the securities firm's investment in the stock of its investment banking customer or its

intent target will be great enough or will be accompanied by related market effects to raise the costs of the customer's intended stock offering, or will tip off the target or the world at large of the intended takeover. That also, of course, would be an effect of a conflict of interest prohibited to the securities firm.

13. Some writers on the subject have referred to the "triangular" nature of the conflict in the securities industry. *See, e.g.,* the editorial note introducing one of the watershed articles in the field: Martin Lipton and Robert Mazur, The Chinese Wall Solution to the Conflicts Problems of Securities Firms, 50 *N.Y.U. L. Rev.* 459 (1975). In fact, however, and as explained in the text, one should also keep in mind a fourth set of interests: those of the public or their regulatory surrogates.

14. Restatement (Second) of Agency, section 395 (1958).

15. As only one example, the research division of a multiservice securities firm can develop information and analysis that is directly relevant to investment decisions for trading customers (and for the firm's own-account trading activities) and that may be important for assessing and making recommendations on proposed takeovers by capital-service customers.

16. Skeptics note that the effectiveness of the walls-plus-lists system has not eliminated insider trading but has moved it outside the firm. The game now must consist of finding a complicit colleague outside the firm who will be willing to share the proceeds of market killings achieved through information gained from an insider within the firm. Many of the highly publicized recent prosecutions involving insider trading have involved such schemes.

Editors' Postscript: Screens In The Medical Setting

While one rarely hears of screens in the medical profession, it may be instructive to consider their possible relevance. Consider a partnership among several psychiatrists, Counseling Partners (CP). CP distributes a brochure to each patient explaining that information shared with one's therapist will be held in the strictest confidence, and will be disclosed to others only under compulsion of a court order or in similarly extraordinary circumstances. Any intended disclosure will be revealed to the patient, with an explanation of the reason for it. This brochure approximates the legal rules that would apply to CP and its partners by common law or statute. Much as with lawyers and their clients, the law protects confidential information in the medical setting primarily to foster the therapeutic relationship by encouraging patients to reveal all information pertinent to the medical provider's decision–making processes.

Mary and John Doe have been undergoing individual psychotherapy, Mary with Dr. A and John with Dr. B. A and B are partners in CP. Mary and John decide to divorce, and a custody dispute arises concerning their six–year–old daughter. John has told Dr. B that he had been having affairs with other women, which he financed with thousands of dollars Mary had given him from extra consulting work she had done. The money was supposed to be saved for a "dream trip" John and Mary were going to take on their tenth anniversary. Is there any conflict of interest for Dr. B?

Arguably there is. Just as a conflict of interest is presented when a lawyer might share confidential information about a former client with present law firm partners or when an investment adviser might use confidential information obtained through representation of a client to the investment firm's benefit, there is arguably a conflict of interest when a psychiatrist in a partnership breaches the confidentiality of one patient to assist a same–group psychiatrist who is treating another patient with directly adverse interests. If Dr. B were to share the information about John's affairs with Dr. A (arguably a very useful disclosure, considered from Mary's point of view), there would not be a conflict of interest, but rather a breach of an obligation of confidentiality owed to John. However, the situation of dual representation of patients by CP, which might tempt Dr. B to undertake such a breach of obligation, arguably constitutes a conflict of interest.

Suppose that John has told Dr. B that he has had sexual contact with his daughter. This particular aspect of the situation does not present a conflict of interest because Dr. B would have a statutory obligation to disclose this child abuse to the proper authorities. All physicians, including Dr. B, might be tempted not to report this situation because of the political, social, and economic ramifications of such disclosure. However, there is nothing unique about such a slight temptation, or about the situation generally, that would mark it as creating a conflict of interest. If Dr. B had special fondness for John or dislike for Mary or John's daughter, and was therefore strongly tempted not to report, that mental state would probably qualify as a conflict of interest.

Would a formal screen prohibiting partners in CP from discussing each other's patients and imposing monetary penalties help in either hypothetical case (that is, involving either John's affairs or his child abuse)? In the law and investment firm settings, a screen is a technique used to ameliorate a conflict of interest and thereby avoid a prohibition of certain relationships. In the case of CP, the screen would simply provide an additional incentive, beyond civil liability and professional discipline, for each psychiatrist to resist any temptation to share confidential information. This additional incentive would perhaps ameliorate the conflict of interest concerning the information about John's affairs. It would not apply to the child abuse because the statute would limit Dr. B's confidentiality obligation in that setting.

Now suppose that John reveals to Dr. B that he has tested positive for the HIV virus and that John and Mary occasionally cohabit and have sex despite their pending divorce petition. Dr. B asks John to share the information about his HIV status with Mary, but John adamantly refuses and boasts that he will continue to have an active sex life "just as before." Suppose further that the state where CP is located has a statute forbidding the disclosure of HIV status to any person other than health authorities and that it is widely known that the health authorities do not contact sexual partners. The legal prohibition against disclosure could be characterized as a screen between the physician, patient, and health authorities, on the one hand, and the rest of the world, on the other hand. In this situation, determining whether there is a conflict of interest that requires Dr. B to cease treating John might bring into view different legal and moral perspectives.

Assume, for purposes of argument, that the statute restricting disclosure of HIV status is clear, constitutional, and not otherwise subject to attack. There would then be no conflict of interest from the legal perspective, even if Dr. B strongly believed that spouses should be warned regarding HIV status. Dr. B would breach a legal obligation by informing Mary. Unless Dr. B's opposition to the statute's restrictions was strong enough to tempt him to violate it, the temptation to disclose to Mary created by her sympathetic and vulnerable situation would not seem to constitute a conflict of interest. It would not exceed the usual or basic temptation one might expect in the normal course of human conduct.

However, one moral perspective is that a physician has an obligation to warn sexual partners about a patient's HIV status if the patient refuses to cease risky conduct or to make the disclosure. Assuming that Dr. B agrees with that moral perspective, notwithstanding other obligations, there might be a conflict of interest posed by the screen. Dr. B is prevented by both a legal restriction and an instruction by his partnership not to disclose. These would likely be perceived as a substantial temptation not to act on the moral obligation founded in proper ethical analysis and in Dr. B's conscience. It would be odd (but not incorrect?) to view the legal prohibition as creating a conflict of interest, but the screen voluntarily imposed by CP would be easier to characterize as such a conflict.

This brief exploration of screens in the medical setting helps illustrate the distinctions among legal and moral obligations, breaches of obligation, and conflicts of interest. It also suggests that screens might be useful in dealing with conflicts of interest and moral problems in medical as well as other settings. Finally, it illustrates that conflicts of interest will sometimes be tolerated because their vitiation would be too costly. For example, it would be unreasonable to recommend a rule that counseling groups never see spouses because of the potential for conflicts of interest. The convenience to patients and access to possibly limited numbers of qualified counselors in certain communities are probably too valuable to sacrifice because of the remote risk of conflicts of interest.

One more aspect of the preceding problem might add to the understanding of conflicts of interest. Although in general there is automatically a criminal sanction for disclosing information made confidential by statute (usually a fine), the legal analysis is different in the civil system. Here the victim generally must prove that the medical provider was unreasonable and deviated from professional standards. When the alleged negligence also constitutes breach of a criminal statute, the civil law approach varies according to the jurisdiction. One approach holds that the violation of a statute constitutes negligence per se and automatically gives rise to liability for damages thereby caused. Another approach presumes that violation of a criminal statute constitutes negligence, but it allows the defendant to attempt to prove that his action was reasonable or consonant with the standards of his profession.

The different civil law approaches to violation of criminal statutes can be seen as the law's attempt to modulate the weight persons, in this case professionals, give to various interests. In the typical civil case, the risk of error in decision-making is placed on the plaintiff by giving him the burden of proof. From the legal perspective, the risk of error in the HIV disclosure hypothetical is that the physician will give too much weight to the interests of third parties. Under the per se approach, this risk is maximally ameliorated by not allowing the disclosing party to even attempt an explanation. Even under the presumption approach, the burden is still placed on the defendant provider who chooses to disclose information. However, he is at least allowed to attempt an explanation.

The existence of these approaches may signal different views regarding conflicts of interest. Under the presumption approach, the civil system can be seen as attempting to maximize the chance that persons, in this case professionals, will make the best decision in individual cases. Thus, although a physician might be liable for a nominal criminal fine for disclosing information, he might escape a much greater civil judgment by convincing a jury that his disclosure was the reasonable and professional action to take. This approach encourages consideration of competing interests. In the per se approach, on the other hand, the temptation to consider other interests can be seen as a conflict of interest that must be maximally discouraged.

Whether these different approaches are considered as ways of dealing with conflicts of interest or only as methods of adjusting the baseline for determining whether conflicts of interest exist, they certainly are examples of attempting to control behavior with a view to maximizing the performance of legal or moral obligations. Just such control is a major function of conflicts of interest.

With medical practice changing, so that there are increasingly situations where ever larger groups of physicians are treating growing groups of patients who might have conflicting interests, potential conflicts of interest and breaches of confidentiality are increasing. Nevertheless, no one is likely to recommend a prohibition similar to the presumption against dual representation applicable to lawyers in certain situations. This is because of the utility seen in large, managed practices. Moreover, although much is written about the concern for confidentiality, there are few substantial judgments that reflect societal concern about such breaches. Nobody has even lobbied for the sort of screen discussed here, but such screens might be useful to reduce the growing potential for breaches of confidentiality, including those caused by or associated with conflicts of interest.

Part II

CLINICAL PRACTICE

7

An Introduction to Conflicts of Interest in Clinical Practice

David S. Shimm and Roy G. Spece, Jr.

The chapters in this part focus on the entrepreneurial activities of practicing physicians and their financial incentives. Such activities and incentives have proliferated because of changes in the health care industry, and they have led to increased governmental, professional, and societal concern about conflicts of interest. Focusing on the entrepreneurial activities and financial incentives of physicians enables us to offer competing perspectives on a common set of problems and to array the empirical evidence bearing on those problems. It further makes possible a comparative analysis between law and medicine because there has been a surge in entrepreneurial activities of professionals in both fields. The insights in this part and in part I should equip the reader to analyze conflicts of interest—pecuniary or not—presented in clinical practice.

In Chapter 8, Nancy Moore compares physicians' and lawyers' ancillary business activities. She explains that various social and economic forces have led to greater ancillary business activities by lawyers and physicians and to increasing perception of the legal and medical professions as mere businesses. Both professions have addressed ethical and professional issues raised by these activities. The arguments made by those for and against such activities in both professions are similar and reveal deep divisions among their members. Both professions can learn from the other's problems and solutions, but, as Charles

Wolfram cautions in Chapter 7, each must be aware of the factors that might limit the transfer of lessons from one profession to the other. Since vague concerns about destroying the public perception of law and medicine as professions have in the past masked vested interests of at least certain segments of the professions, regulation of ancillary business activities in both professions should be based on specific ethical concerns. The primary question in both professions is *who* should do the regulating. Moore explains that the legal profession has enjoyed unprecedented autonomy, and that it should not abuse or threaten that autonomy by overreaching in its attempt to regulate ancillary business activities related to nonlegal clients. Professionals should learn from empirical studies and from persons outside the professions to help insulate themselves from the insidious influence of self-interest. They should undertake rigorous training to equip themselves to deal with the increasing complexities of conflicts of interest and ethical dilemmas. Finally, Moore observes that although disclosure is often an effective method to regulate conflicts of interest in the legal profession because of the sophistication of many clients and the alternative suppliers of services outside the legal profession, disclosure is often not efficacious in the medical profession because of the less sophisticated nature of most patients and the limited number of options available to them.

Mark Rodwin argues in Chapter 9 that although fee-for-service medical practice creates a conflict of interest encouraging overutilization of services, the "deflationary incentives" that have been created to counter overutilization do not obviate the conflicts of interest, but rather create new and more harmful ones. These deflationary incentives fit under the umbrella of managed care. The essence of managed care is to obtain the best patients (i.e., those who can pay and are likely to require relatively little care) and to limit utilization of services by those patients. Managed care entities share risks and benefits with physicians, mainly through primary care providers ("gatekeepers") whom they use to limit access to specialists and expensive diagnostic and therapeutic interventions. The basis of this risk/benefit sharing is to reward physicians by sharing with them the cost savings that result from limiting utilization of care and to punish physicians by forcing them to bear some of the costs associated with heavy utilization of services. Rodwin recognizes the limited empirical data on the effect of such incentives, but he concludes that the limited data available and logic coalesce to demonstrate their nefarious nature. He discusses federal laws that limit direct incentives to physicians by managed care providers and prohibit the same by hospitals, and argues that these laws should be significantly strengthened. He explores several indirect means—such as purchase of physicians' practices—by which hospitals encourage physicians to limit utilization of care. Rodwin argues that both direct and indirect deflationary incentives have a perverse effect on the physician–patient relationship by pitting the physician's financial interests against the best interests of his patients. He asserts that quality assurance and peer review activities are not sufficient to blunt the deleterious effects of deflationary incentives because standards of care are too nebulous to allow reviewers to document inappropriate limitations on care. Therefore, these deleterious effects must be dealt with through prohibition or careful administrative regulation. On the other hand, Rodwin contends that certain incentives—such as bonuses for providing quality care—can have a beneficial effect on physicians' behavior.

Although he generally rejects rationing, he accepts the notion of physicians serving as neutral referees to allocate services among a group of patients under budgetary constraints. In these circumstance, physicians cannot act as ideal fiduciaries, giving every patient precisely what is in his best interest.

Much of Rodwin's case seems to rest on the symbolic significance of direct financial inducements. Recall Moore's point that regulation of lawyers' and physicians' ancillary business activities must rest on specific ethical concerns rather than symbolism. "Symbolism," in this context, refers to the inculcation or reinforcement of attitudes in society and physicians. Moore argues that regulation of lawyers' and physicians' ancillary business activities cannot be justified by unregulated activities' supposedly deleterious effects on those professionals' benevolent attitudes. It might be argued that, similarly, regulation of direct financial incentives cannot be justified by those incentives' supposedly negative effects on society's and, ultimately, professionals' attitudes.

We agree with Moore that symbolism has been misused by professionals to justify selfish fee fixing and prohibitions on advertising. In the setting of such business regulation, symbolism has been misused because of physicians' conflicts of interest. On the other hand, where symbolism or professionalism serves to encourage, albeit perhaps inadvertently, responsible behavior on the part of physicians, to that extent each should be fostered. Rodwin and others who are troubled by physician incentives are not likely to overstate the importance of symbolism because of any vested financial interest. We agree with Rodwin that symbolism is a powerful argument in the setting of direct financial incentives. Shapiro has argued "regulation is language."[1] When we regulate financial incentives, we send a powerful message about what is expected from professionals. We agree with Rodwin that if we regulate such incentives weakly, we send the terrible message—to professionals and their patients—that it is permissible for professionals to favor their own financial interests over individual patients in a broad range of decisions. Even if we cannot empirically demonstrate the existence or deleterious effects of such a message, and even though it would be practically impossible or unethical to construct a study that would enable us to test our hypothesis, we know from logic and history that regulation is a powerful voice.

Mark Hall discusses deflationary conflicts of interest in Chapter 10. He argues that "the fundamental problem of public policy that must be resolved before this country can construct a respectable system for financing health care is how best to ration limited medical resources among competing beneficial uses, both within health care and among other societal needs." Hall asserts that agency cost theory is the best way to choose among the various mechanisms through which physicians can be encouraged to perform the necessary rationing.

Developing agency cost theory, Hall argues that there are two basic risks that a principal must manage when entering into a principal–agent relationship: that the agent will not understand the wishes of the principal, and that the agent will act in his own interests. The methods used to minimize these agency risks can be broken into two categories: external monitoring and internal incentives. An agency cost is the cost of reducing or bearing agency risks, and there are two categories of agency costs—those of over- and of underprotecting against agency risks. Control of agency risks and costs can be imposed through one or a combination of three mechanisms: (1) assumption by the agent, (2) imposition by the principal, or (3) legal imposition by society. Bonding is an example of self–regulation. In the professions, ethical codes are the equivalent of bonding. The principal can impose limitations on the agent through contractual agreements. Legal rules such as those applied to fiduciaries are an example of society imposing rules. *Relational contract theory* is an extension of agency cost theory that looks at the transaction costs involved in choosing among the ways of controlling agency risks.

Applying agency cost theory and relational contract theory to the physician–patient relationship, Hall argues that patients have dual agency problems. The *medical agency problem* is making sure that the physician as agent makes *appropriate medical choices*. Incentives here include fee-for-service reimbursement to encourage optimal patient care (possibly), bonding through physicians' adherence to ethical codes, and malpractice and fiduciary laws imposed by society. However, fee-for-service reimbursement to solve the medical agency problem creates an *economic agency problem* by distorting physicians' spending decisions so that they fail to reflect what patients would have decided was cost effective were they willing and able to pay out–of–pocket.

One might respond to the economic agency problem by imposing categorical rules about noncoverage of certain care. However, categorical, rule-based rationing imposes costs of inaccuracy and lack of individualization. It is also open to political pressure. Moreover, categorical rules cannot reach the vast domain of discretion inherent in medical practice. These shortcomings are exemplified by the Oregon rationing plan, which Hall characterizes as a "meat ax" approach to rationing that reflects the political bias of special interest groups.

Hall next observes that, when made in absolute terms, the argument that physicians should not be induced to play a rationing role via financial incentives is trivialized by agency cost theory. It views financial incentives as one of a menu of motivational techniques. The only question is what techniques, in what combination, and in what strength work best. Agency cost theory takes seriously the risk that financial conflicts will erode trust and confidence, but it allows a modulated and differentiated response depending on the actual strength and pervasiveness of this concern. Economic incentives must be limited by some categorical rules. However, these rules can be opted out of contractually, depending on the particular situation.

Hall concludes that agency cost theory indicates that deflationary incentives can be beneficial, that other mechanisms alone are inadequate, and that the HMO industry and the legal apparatus under Medicare have acted responsibly in setting the outer limits of financial motivation while leaving room for creative experimentation. Given the theoretical effectiveness of financial incentives, the lack of empirical evidence of negative effects, and the concession by some ethicists that physicians can ration for the benefit of groups or society, Hall asserts that physician rationing is permissible even when there is a limited personal financial incentive potentially deleterious to individual patients.

Hall argues that Rodwin's acceptance of physician participation in rationing within a group of patients logically commits him to general acceptance of rationing. Rodwin disagrees, arguing that, in the former context, the physician acts to maximize benefits to his patients as a class. In the latter context, he rations for his own benefit.

Rodwin and Hall share the belief that some limitations on health care can be relatively painless by eliminating wasteful or marginally beneficial care. Rodwin insists that this is not rationing because rooting out waste is, by definition, something other than rationing. Hall expects the limitation of marginally beneficial care—which he openly characterizes as rationing—to be accomplished by financial incentives, while Rodwin wants this to be done by administrative regulation.

Questions that we believe require further consideration include the following: (1) Will clearly beneficial care be rationed? (2) If so, which method—deflationary incentives, administrative regulation, a mixture of the two, or some other approach—is the best way to ration? (3) What should be considered marginally beneficial care?[2] (4) Is there enough of it so that its elimination would have a significant impact on health care costs? (5) Are patients less likely to be familiar with, and therefore on guard against, deflationary as opposed to inflationary incentives? and (6) Is one way to explore the possible benefits and costs of direct financial incentives to consider implications of the data on physician self-referral—discussed by Mitchell in Chapter 13—for HMO incentive plans?

For example, how much do physicians make through single acts of self-referral, and how does this compare to profits from single acts of rationing patient care? How do the magnitude of self-referral arrangements and HMO incentives compare on a monthly or yearly basis? Are there differences in the way physicians might react to self-referral as opposed to HMO incentive plan inducements?

Rodwin does not address the argument that patients could be protected by disclosure of deflationary incentives. He has argued in another forum, however, that such disclosure would simply weaken the physician–patient relationship.[3] Hall seems to agree that disclosure must take place,[4] but he does not address any of its possible costs. In Chapter 11, E. Haavi Morreim adamantly disagrees, while in Chapter 12 Katz agrees that disclosure is not an appropriate remedy. Morreim contends that the question of whether disclosure is an adequate way to protect patients from the dangers of physician self–referral fundamentally misconceives the issue. The issue should be: Is there adequate justification to prevent patients from using the services of physicians who engage in self–referral? This issue assumes that patients are competent agents who must make their own decisions about health care. To support this perspective, Morreim points to the informed consent case law and doctrine.

Her second major point is that there are common law principles, regulations, and statutes that adequately deal with the dangers of self-referral. Morreim identifies three levels of abuse in self–referral: (1) failure of informed consent, (2) breach of fiduciary duty, and (3) fraud, kickbacks, negligence, and bad faith. As to failure of informed consent, she strongly argues that it *is* inappropriate for a physician to refer a patient to a facility without obtaining the patient's fully informed consent. She implies that the law of informed consent and state consumer protection laws can guard against any dangers of nonprovision of information. As to the dangers of breach of fiduciary duty, she implies that the common law doctrine developed in the *Moore* case, discussed in Chapter 3, can be used to police sufficiently breaches of fiduciary duty involved in abusive self-referral. As to the third level of serious abuses, in which a physician flagrantly exploits his patient for personal gain, Morreim argues that powerful legal tools already exist to combat such abuses: the Medicare and Medicaid Patient and Program Protection Act of 1987, the Office of the Inspector General's Safe Harbor Guidelines, the common law doctrines of bad faith breach of contract and negligence, and antitrust law.

Morreim's chapter is devoted primarily to developing the possible use of federal antitrust laws to police abusive self-referral practices. She carefully demonstrates how these antitrust laws' prohibitions on tie-ins, exclusive dealing arrangements, and group boycotts might well apply to certain *abusive* self-referral practices. Self-referral accompanied by *appropriate* disclosure would be safe from prosecution. She observes that patients or competitors harmed by abusive self-referral would have the right to sue under such laws.

In Chapter 12, Jay Katz develops the argument that disclosure does not address adequately the dangers of physician self-referral because the nature and quality of informed consent, even in its traditional context of consent to diagnosis and treatment, are grossly deficient. Katz recognizes that the Institute of Medicine and the AMA (at times) have taken the position that patients should be made aware of the conflicts of interest in self-referral arrangements so that they can respond "appropriately." Faced with such disclosure, patients basically have two choices: (1) acquiesce or (2) ask questions and implicitly impugn their physicians' integrity. Katz states: "It may be the greater part of wisdom if the profession were to take the unprecedented step of prohibiting—to the extent consistent with existing legal mandates—all commercial practices beyond fee–for–service except under the rarest and most carefully defined circumstances." As long as this policy recommendation cannot be implemented, he believes that means other than informed consent must be found to curtail exploitation of patients (through unnecessary procedures) and of the state and other third-party payers (through unnecessary costs). He feels that the invocation of informed consent as a suitable mechanism is "a political ploy to stave off federal regulations and maintain physician autonomy" rather than a viable alternative.

In the last chapter of Part II, Jean Mitchell reviews the empirical data—including several of her own studies—on the impact of physician self-referral arrangements, as well as research on physicians' responses to other financial incentives. She argues that physicians' responses to these other financial incentives support data showing that they respond directly to self-referral incentives. Mitchell recognizes arguments in favor of self-referral, but rejects them and argues that such arrangements are anticompetitive and lead to "cream skimming" of well-heeled patients, overutilization, increased costs, and perhaps poorer quality. Although Mitchell contends that the studies show that physicians respond to within-office and extra-office self-referral, as well as to a variety of other financial incentives, she argues that within-office self-referral should not be banned. She implies that many of these arrangements are for the convenience of patients and argues that there are, in any event, better ways to deal with any abuses in the within-office setting: "denial of payment for self-referred within-office service, reimbursement of self-referred imaging or physical therapy at a lower rate than paid for referred diagnostic imaging or physical therapy, or bundling the payment for clinical lab tests, diagnostic imaging or physical therapy as part of the reimbursement for an office visit."

Mitchell summarizes the findings from a study of joint ventures in free-standing facilities and self-referral to these facilities that she and Elton Scott performed under a mandate from the Florida legislature in 1989. There were no apparently negative effects on access, cost, charges, or utilization in acute care hospitals and nursing homes. The opposite was true for clinical laboratories and for diagnostic imaging, radiation therapy, and physical therapy-rehabilitation facilities.

Mitchell also notes the extremely complex business arrangements that physicians have employed. She cautions that any legislation must be designed to prevent avoidance of regulation through lawmakers' failure to untangle these complexities or anticipate additional avoidance maneuvers.

We close with a few comments suggested by Mitchell's chapter. More work needs to be done on the within-office/free-standing self-referral distinction, on the distinction between deflationary and inflationary incentives, and on the finding that self-referral led to no negative effects in the acute care hospital and nursing home settings.[5]

As to inflationary versus deflationary incentives, Mitchell refers to studies showing both that (1) fee-for-service can lead to more utilization and that (2) HMO structure and capitation generally, and the deflationary incentives discussed by Rodwin and Hall in Chapters 9 and 10, specifically, can lead to less utilization. However, the ultimate conclusion on whether these differences represent over- or underutilization cannot be made without a standard of optimum utilization. Since these studies do not offer such a benchmark, they all, in a sense, beg the question. The only valid point one can draw from these studies is that physicians respond to financial incentives. One possible explanation for the fact that Mitchell and Scott found no deleterious effects in physician investor-owned acute care hospitals and nursing homes is that, with prospective payment and utilization review, they may be regulated well enough to prevent abuse.

Having reviewed the various chapters in this part, and their many astute observations about physicians' entrepreneurial activities and the effects of formal incentives, we urge the reader to keep in mind how the insights offered in this part might apply to conflicts of interest presented by other activities of, and incentives working on, physicians.

Notes

1. *See* Michael Shapiro, On Not Watering All the Flowers: Regulatory Theory in the Funding of Heart Transplantation, 28 *Jurimetrics* 23–31 (1987).
2. Compare our discussion of "proportionate care" in Chapter 3 of this volume.
3. Marc Rodwin, *Medicine, Money and Morals: Physicians' Conflict of Interest* (1993).
4. *See* Chapter 10 of this volume, notes 26 and 27.
5. Morreim addresses the within-office versus extra-office distinction in Chapter 11 of this volume.

8

Entrepreneurial Doctors and Lawyers: Regulating Business Activities in the Medical and Legal Professions

Nancy J. Moore

Increasingly imbued with the entrepreneurial spirit, doctors and lawyers have moved beyond professional advertising and are diversifying into business activities outside the traditional practices of medicine and law. For doctors, the new entrepreneurialism[1] includes physician self–referral, that is arrangements by which physicians refer their patients to health care facilities in which they have an economic interest.[2] These investments generally consist of ownership of corporate stock or partnership interests (including limited partnerships) in entities operating clinical and physiological laboratories, durable medical equipment suppliers, home health agencies, and ambulatory surgical centers, as well as hospitals and nursing homes.[3] For lawyers, the new entrepreneurialism includes lawyers and law firms making significant investments in their clients' businesses, as well as providing nonlegal services to both clients and nonclients. In particular, the "ancillary business" phenomenon typically refers to law firms, especially large firms, acquiring or forming nonlegal businesses such as investment banking, financial consulting, advertising, engineering, and real estate development.[4] These business are typically structured as separate subsidiaries to be managed and staffed by nonlawyers, with customer bases overlapping the law firm's clients, although in some instances the nonlegal services are provided by law firms with nonlawyer partners or employees.[5]

The rapid growth of new forms of medical entrepreneurialism is primarily the result of the radical restructuring of the health care industry that began in the 1980s.[6] Cost–containment policies implemented by insurers and other third–party payers (mainly the federal government)–combined with a growing surplus of physicians and the aggressive development of for–profit health–care corporations and alternative health delivery systems–have produced a competitive environment similar to that in the economy generally.[7] One effect of the new "medical–industrial complex"[8] has been to decrease the physician's ability to generate primary income while simultaneously increasing the physician's ability to generate secondary income (i.e., income from sources other than professional services provided by the physician or attorney).[9]

For example, cost containment policies have caused a shift in the delivery of health care from inpatient to outpatient settings. This shift has reduced professional fees resulting from hospitalizations; however, it has also produced new opportunities for physician investment in the newly created free–standing entities in which outpatient care is offered.[10] Physician fees are also being constrained by containment strategies aimed directly at physicians, such as Medicare's 1991 freeze on fees[11] and the prohibition on physician billing for independent laboratory services.[12] At the same time, the rapidly developing technologies that are increasingly important to medical practice–such as magnetic resonance imaging (MRI)–are now capable of being delivered outside the hospital setting.[13] Finally, if need and opportunity were not themselves sufficient to prompt more investment activity, physicians have also been receiving a direct message from hospitals, insurers, and the government itself that the response to economic incentive is *precisely* the behavior now being encouraged under the present policy of cost containment through competition.[14] Given this background, it can hardly come as a surprise that, as of 1989, at least 12 percent of physicians billing Medicare had ownership or investment interests in entities to which they made patient referrals or that approximately 25 percent of clinical laboratories and 27 percent of independent physiological laboratories were owned by referring physicians.[15]

There is no analogy in the legal profession to the role played by the federal government and other third–party payers in prompting the recent transformations in the medical profession. Nonetheless, the last two decades have witnessed profound changes and innovations in the legal community, including a dramatic increase in both the number of lawyers and the size of law firms, the rise of specialization and "boutique law firms,"[16] and the increased use of legal advertising.[17] As in medicine, the hallmark of many of these changes has been increased economic pressure and aggressive competition for clients. Moreover, rising costs and lower profit margins are forcing lawyers to place more and more emphasis on generating additional fees by either billing more hours or bringing in new business.

This competitive environment is particularly intense in the elite corporate law firms.[18] Their spectacular growth in recent decades spawned a similarly spectacular rise in costs–including associates' salaries–which, in turn, produced enormous pressures to increase billings.[19] At the same time, growth in the size and power of corporate in–house counsel, who are increasingly sensitive to legal costs, has meant that the elite law firms are losing business to corporate legal departments and competing with other elites for the available outside work, which is no longer concentrated in a single firm.[20] The elite firms were also hard hit by the reduced level of corporate activity generally and the decimation of traditional practice areas such as regulated industries and antitrust law during the recent era of deregulation and relaxed antitrust policies.[21]

The economic needs of lawyers in large law firms may not be more intense than those of other lawyers, nor is it clear that large–firm lawyers are more active in business transactions with their clients. What is apparent, however, is that the opportunity to tap new revenue sources by diversifying into ancillary business activities seems tailor–made for the large elite law firms, that is those with corporate clients large enough to need (and be able to afford) a multidisciplinary approach to problem solving. Thus, many large firms throughout the country are running investment banking ventures, energy and environmental consulting, and management services, as well as employer benefits consulting services, real estate development services, and at least one full–service consulting firm for the financial industry.[22] Not surprisingly, these businesses are competing in some areas with similarly diversified management advisory services offered by large accounting firms, as well as by advertising agencies and investment bankers.[23]

The professional–entrepreneur's ability to generate secondary income[24] has caused consternation among more traditional members of both professions. Citing potential harm to clients and patients, as well as a general loss of professionalism,[25] the traditionalists favor vigorous regulation of these new forms of income production.[26] Some have even urged a ban on virtually all ancillary business activities that potentially pit the financial interests of professionals against the interests of their patients or clients.[27] Meanwhile, the entrepreneurs themselves insist that any potential harm to the public is clearly outweighed by the potential benefits, and thus that only minimal regulation (if any) is warranted.[28]

The major professional organizations–the American Medical Association and the American Bar Association–have attempted to address the issues; however, their efforts so far have been stymied by deep divisions among their respective members. Thus, while delegates of both organizations recently voted to support the traditionalists' call to ban most ancillary business activity, they reversed their votes the very next time the issues were presented.[29] Indeed, the AMA's House of Delegates reversed itself yet again within six months, approving a resolution condemning the practice of self–referral with only two exceptions.[30] Nor has the question been finally laid to rest. Yet another flip–flop by the physician delegates is not out of the question, although, the AMA's Council on Ethical and Judicial Affairs insists that its opinion declaring most self–referral activity unethical is unaffected by any of the delegates' recent votes.[31] As for the ABA, the vote to reject the ban was as narrow as the initial vote in its favor, suggesting that the issue is likely to surface again.[32]

Even if there were consensus within the AMA or ABA, considerable dissent would likely exist among the substantial number of professionals who do not belong to these organizations. Only about 50 percent of physicians belong to the AMA, and an even smaller percentage of attorneys belong to the ABA.[33] Both organizations are perceived by many professionals to represent primarily the elite or conservative elements of the professions, and many professionals typically oppose the formal positions of both bodies. Moreover, both bodies are limited in their ability to discipline even those professionals who are members. Both organizations can expel members, but that is seldom done and it does not connote drastic consequences. The ABA has slightly more power indirectly, since some bodies with jurisdiction over lawyer discipline, typically state courts, have adopted the ABA model code.

This chapter explores similarities and differences in the debates in both the legal and medical professions on the assumption that, as doctors and lawyers continue to ponder the question, each group may benefit from considering how the other is handling the ancillary business phenomenon. As the chapter demonstrates, there are numerous similarities, particularly in the types of arguments and counterarguments that emerge from debates over the pros and cons of the current activities–entrepreneurs citing the potential benefits of the new business orientation, while traditionalists in both professions invoke a variety of ethical and professionalism concerns.[34] Balancing potential benefits against potential harms, it is concluded that despite recent efforts by both the AMA and ABA to stress the importance of professionalism, any targeting of ancillary business activity probably is justified only by a need to satisfy more specific ethical concerns regarding the well–being of individual patients and clients.[35] It is here, in assessing these ethical concerns, that significant differences between the two professions begin to emerge, both in the nature of the conflicts of interest presented[36] and in the regulatory framework in which these conflicts are addressed.[37] The chapter concludes that the disclosure and consent process probably offers sufficient protection for the vast majority of clients of law firm ancillary businesses; however, there is good reason to believe that it will be insufficient to prevent abuses in physician self–referrals.[38] In any event, both lawyers and doctors need to continue to stress professional training in identifying and dealing with a broad spectrum of conflicts of interest and other ethical concerns if the professions are to survive (in their present favored status) the ever–changing environments in which law and medicine are now practiced.[39]

The Pros and Cons of Ancillary Business Activities: Similarities in Argument and Counterargument

Both physician and lawyer entrepreneurs view their efforts as "one type of innovative response to the new business orientation [which] may produce positive, pro–competitive effects in the industry."[40] Certainly traditional practice has often been uneconomical,[41] and thus some change in incentive structure is long overdue. Indeed, the "new business orientation" has already had some beneficial effects: for example, price reductions attributable to both competitive advertising and more efficient practice management.[42] Nonetheless, as to the present ancillary business activities in both professions, there is fundamental disagreement regarding the significance of any potential benefits in relation to potential harms.

Legal entrepreneurs argue that recent multidisciplinary efforts are driven primarily by the needs of clients in an increasingly complex corporate environment, and that the law firms' response to client demand is but an aspect of rigorous competition ultimately benefitting consumers who are themselves increasingly conscious of their needs.[43] Thus, by offering the nonlegal services of an affiliate entity, a law firm can offer its clients the convenience of "one–stop shopping" while simultaneously reducing the cost of finding nonlawyer experts.[44] Moreover, diversified law firms can offer a distinct and creative approach to solving legal problems, often by focusing on nonlegal solutions beyond the range of the traditional law firm.[45] The case for self–referring physicians is more difficult to make, since it is by no means obvious how allowing physicians to invest in entities to which they will refer patients benefits anyone but the investors themselves.[46] Nonetheless, entrepreneurial physicians and their supporters contend that (1) the newly formed free–standing entities make services and equipment available in less expensive, more convenient settings,[47] and (2) because practitioners in the community are in a unique position to detect and respond to the health care needs of the community, their capital and their willingness to take risks are often essential to successfully launching these entities and keeping their costs low.[48] Prohibiting self–referrals might dry up a valuable source of capital; and, in any event, investing physicians who also make referrals have both the incentive and the motivation to monitor the quality of patient care.[49]

In opposition to the entrepreneurs, traditionalists in both legal and medical practice argue that whatever the benefits of the ancillary businesses might be,[50] they are far outweighed by the potential for harm — to individual patients and clients, to the professions themselves, and to society at large. The dangers typically cited fall into two categories: ethical concerns and professionalism concerns.

The primary ethical concern in both professions is conflicts of interest. At the most obvious level, when professionals make referrals to entities in which they have a financial interest, the danger exists that the professionals' independent judgment will be compromised, that is, that either consciously or unconsciously, the professionals will place their own interests above patients' or clients' interests.[51] As a result, the quality and cost of care or representation will be compromised–for example, through questionable recommendations that ancillary services are necessary at all and through questionable choices regarding the quality and cost of the particular entity selected. Indeed, there is already evidence in the medical profession of a direct relationship between physician ownership and utilization of some ancillary services.[52]

This danger is compounded in the legal profession by the possibility of conflicting interests between clients of the law firm and customers of the ancillary business, in which case there is also the potential for misuse of confidential client information.[53] Lawyers worry that customers of the business entity will be confused and fail to understand the inapplicability of either the attorney–client evidentiary privilege or professional rules of conduct, including rules relating to conflicts of interest and confidentiality.[54]

In addition to these ethical concerns, traditionalists in both law and medicine are concerned that the ancillary business phenomenon will contribute substantially to a serious decline in "professionalism," by which they mean a special orientation of the professions to public service, in contrast to business's orientation toward the bottom line.[55] To some extent, these broader concerns are merely another variation of the primarily *ethical* concern that an orientation towards profit will cause professionals to act in ways that harm their patients or clients–for example, the argument that professional-entrepreneurs will be so caught up in the business enterprise that they will not act competently or diligently in their professional practices.[56] What is different, however, about the professionalism concerns is the potentially far–reaching effects of a radical change in orientation. Thus, critics claim that negative press from financial scandals—or other breaches of professional integrity—will result in a loss of public trust that is not easily regained.[57] Similarly, they argue that the professions will lose their distinctiveness and, along with it, their right of self–regulation.[58]

Of course, the benefit to society of maintaining public trust in the professions (and professional self–regulation) is not self–evident.[59] Thus, the traditionalists argue not just that the professional–client relationship is itself a public good, but that also professionals serve society even more directly. For example, it is commonly thought that the legal and medical professions are committed to serving the poor, or at least improving their access to legal and medical services.[60] In addition, lawyers may portray themselves as "an independent force for preserving government under law,"[61] while physicians cite their fiduciary responsibilities to oversee institutional quality of care[62] and to disseminate freely and share medical knowledge.[63] Both professions also acknowledge a fiduciary duty to assist in societal decision-making in regard to health care and law reform issues.[64] According to this view, then, society has a great deal to lose if the ancillary business phenomenon does in fact contribute to an unfortunate trend away from professionalism.

Not surprisingly, this litany of dangers has provoked strikingly similar responses and counterresponses by entrepreneurs and their critics in both law and medicine. For example, the entrepreneurs point to a long history of entrepreneurial activity in both professions, including physicians owning hospitals, pharmacies, nursing homes, and office testing equipment,[65] and lawyers providing nonlegal ancillary services such as escrow and title search and examination services, as well as lobbying and mediation.[66] They also note that conflicts of interest and other ethical issues are pervasive in legal and medical practice, not just in ancillary business activities but in all aspects of professional practice, including fee–for–service and referrals among lawyers in law firms and physicians in group practice.[67] While not disputing the historical facts, the traditionalists nonetheless argue that the dimensions of the present business activity present a potential for harm on an unprecedented scale,[68] and that this potential is exacerbated by the significant role now played by nonprofessionals in the delivery of ancillary services.[69]

As for the fear of declining professionalism, the entrepreneurs' primary response is that the complaints are far too speculative.[70] Indeed, in one of the few instances of cross–fertilization in the ancillary business debate, the Federal Trade Commission argued to lawyers opposed to ancillary services that other professionals, *notably physicians*, increasingly practice in a wide variety of organizational structures without no apparent decline in professionalism,[71] a claim that is (not surprisingly) vigorously disputed by some physicians.[72] In any event, the entrepreneurs further argue that the traditionalists' view of professionals and professionalism represents, at best, "pathetic nostalgia"[73] and, at worst, a dangerously "narrow and rigid view of what it is to be a lawyer"[74] or physician.[75]

Resolving the Dilemma: Professionalism versus Ethical Concerns and the Emergence of Significant Differences in Professional Situations of Physicians and Lawyers

Under pressure to finally resolve the issues being debated, significant groups within both the AMA and the ABA favor banning most ancillary business activities.[76] Although official reports supporting the bans cite both ethical and professionalism concerns, in the final analysis, it is the latter that appears to have been most persuasive. Thus, despite its stated belief that "physicians in general can be trusted to deal appropriately with the conflicts presented by self–referral," the AMA Council opted to eliminate that practice because of its strong conviction that in order to demonstrate their "commitment to professionalism," physicians must avoid "some activities involving their patients...whether or not there is evidence of abuse."[77] Similarly, the ABA's Section of Litigation, official sponsor of a proposed rule banning ancillary business, devoted the entire conclusion of its final report to the "threat to professionalism brought about by law firm diversification," ending with the solemn warning that if such diversification is not stopped, "the unique professionalism of the law will become indistinguishable from the mores of any other businesses."[78]

However, the connection between ancillary business activity and professionalism concerns seems remote.[79] As for popular opinion, the public is already so disenchanted with doctors and lawyers that any additional negative press is unlikely to contribute significantly to a further erosion of public trust. In addition, the ancillary business phenomenon is sufficiently peripheral to the core functions of both law and medicine that it is simply implausible that it will cause these professions to lose their distinctiveness and, along with it, their right to self–regulation.[80] There may indeed be an important "symbolic significance" to ancillary business activity in regard to alternative conceptions of lawyer and doctor roles as those of a professional or entrepreneur;[81] however, these alternative conceptions involve the entire spectrum of changes associated with the growing commercialization of the professions. Given the harm that has already been done in the name of professionalism—such as absolute bans on lawyer and physician advertising and promulgation of minimum fee schedules[82]—more than symbolic significance should be required before professional organizations impose significant restrictions on the autonomy of the affected individuals, including both members of the public and the professionals themselves.[83]

If ancillary business activity is to be singled out for special regulation, a more appropriate justification would be the ethical concern for safeguarding the well–being of individual clients and patients.[84] Here, however, what must be avoided is the essentially circular reasoning used by some traditionalists, in which these important *ethical* concerns are thought to be supported by unsubstantiated presumptions about *professionalism*: that is the apparent belief that doctors and lawyers who are involved in ancillary businesses are less likely than their more "professional" peers to fulfill their fiduciary duties.[85] Thus, physicians who voted to reverse their original vote banning self–referrals apparently did so because they were angered by the implication that they could not be trusted to act professionally in caring for their patients. These physicians understand that it is unethical to recommend unnecessary procedures or to refer patients to inappropriate facilities; however, they "object to the implication that every physician that [sic] is involved in investing in some kind of facility is guilty of a violation of ethics."[86] To them, it is just as likely that a fee–for–service physician will recommend unnecessary service (or that a physician with expensive in–office equipment will overutilize it), and yet it is self–referral that has been targeted for special treatment.[87]

Ethical Justifications for Prophylactic Rules Banning Self–Referral

Given that the medical profession lacks a strong tradition of regulating conflicts of interest in medical practice,[88] it is not surprising that physicians have difficulty understanding when a prophylactic ban on certain activity might be justified or how lines between similar sorts of practices might be drawn. Here the more extensive experience of the legal profession in addressing a wide range of conflicting interests[89] might be useful in resolving the ancillary business dilemmas in both professions.

Under the current legal ethics regulatory framework, conflicts of interest arise whenever there is a substantial risk that the representation of a client[90] will be materially and adversely affected by the lawyer's own interests or by the lawyer's responsibilities to another client, a former client, or a third person.[91] Regardless of whether the conflict is actual or merely potential, representation is prohibited in such cases when the affected parties do not give adequately informed consent or when the conflict is deemed by law to be nonconsentable.[92] Lawyer codes sometimes specify prohibited transactions, such as agreements giving the lawyer literary or media rights to client information before the representation ends.[93] More often, the conclusion that a conflict is nonconsentable is reached by applying a general standard–for example, that it is not obvious that the representation will be adequate[94] or that the lawyer does not reasonably believe that the representation will not be adversely affected.[95] Regardless of which standard is applied, the rationale underlying a determination that a conflict is nonconsentable–thereby restricting the autonomy of both clients and the affected lawyer–is that a client who gives informed consent in such a case has not truly understood or appreciated the significance of the risk (in relation to the potential benefit) or has not felt entirely free to reject the representation.[96]

Under this framework, lawyers are already required to disclose significant financial interests in ancillary businesses to which they refer their clients.[97] Similarly, at a minimum, disclosure should also be required whenever a self–referring physician has a significant economic stake in the facility in question,[98] since there is unquestionably a substantial risk that the decision to refer will be affected–either consciously or unconsciously–by the physician's own financial interest.[99] Indeed, the need for such disclosure has been recognized by most physicians, even those opposing further restrictions.[100] For both doctors and lawyers, then, the more difficult question is whether disclosure is sufficient or whether the conflict should be deemed to be nonconsentable.[101]

Those who favor banning physician self–referrals argue that disclosure is inadequate because of "the typical patient's reliance on the physician and the lack of consumer knowledge concerning medical services."[102] This argument, however, is vulnerable to a charge of excessive paternalism;[103] after all, the informed consent doctrine in medical malpractice jurisprudence already presumes that a patient is competent to make decisions regarding the medical choices covered by that doctrine, regardless how difficult those choices might be.[104] Of course, informed consent doctrine typically applies only when a doctor proposes a significant bodily invasion, that is, procedures where there is usually a risk of serious bodily harm to the patient.[105] Faced with this risk, patients are likely to give the matter serious thought, carefully weighing the extent to which they consider the risk worth taking. Moreover, if in fact patients end up simply deferring to a trusted physician, there is little cause for concern, since absent some identifiable conflict of interest, the physician's recommendation can be assumed to conform to standard medical practice.[106]

As for self–referrals, if disclosure occurs in a case in which the informed consent doctrine already applies,[107] then physician self–interest is simply an additional factor for the patient to weigh, along with other important information regarding the risks and benefits of the proposed procedure. However, the more typical self–referral involves either a procedure to which the informed consent doctrine does not otherwise apply (i.e., there is no significant bodily invasion)[108] or one in which the doctrine applies but the risk of serious bodily harm is either nonexistent or so low that the only factor likely to be taken seriously is the cost.[109] And in these cases, the cost of a single referral tends to be relatively small to the patient, either because it is low in comparison with other costs incurred or because it is covered in whole or in part by a third–party payer, such as the government (in the case of Medicare or Medicaid) or a private insurer.[110] As a result, unlike decisions regarding major surgery or risky diagnostic procedures, patient decisions on whether to permit self–referral for an x–ray, a blood test, or even an MRI are unlikely to prompt patients to ask probing questions or seek a second opinion before deferring to the physician's judgment.[111]

This is apparently not the case in the most recent examples of law firm self–referrals. As noted earlier, the volume of ancillary business activity prompting the ABA ban is concentrated in the large, elite law firms whose corporate clients are large enough to need and afford a multidisciplinary approach to legal problem solving.[112] Not only are these corporate clients sophisticated and experienced in the selection of legal counsel; they are also increasingly sensitive to both conflicts of interest and legal costs, forcing the law firms to compete actively with each other for even a piece of a corporation's legal business.[113] As a result, there is little support for the conclusion of the ABA Litigation Section that a "law firm's client may feel impelled to use the firm's ancillary business...for fear of insulting a firm's attorneys and becoming a second–class citizen on legal matters."[114]

Another factor relevant in the determination of whether a conflict should be consentable is whether it is likely that clients are assuming the risk in order to reap significant benefits.[115] Motive aside, law firms offering one–stop shopping through their expansion into such areas as investment banking and real estate development do seem to be offering services tailored to meet the specific needs of clients and other customers.[116] Indeed, the market is now occupied not only by law firms and their multidisciplinary ventures, but also by large accounting firms, advertising agencies, and investment bankers.[117] Thus, it is hardly accurate to say of lawyers, as it is sometimes said of doctors, that the practitioners are in a position to create their own demand[118] for the services being provided.

As for physician self–referral, the expected benefit to patients is certainly questionable, particularly in light of empirical information strongly suggesting overutilization of ancillary business services by physicians.[119] Unlike law firm clients, for whom the close connection between the firm and its ancillary business is part of what makes the business attractive, medical patients receive no direct benefit from physicians' investment in a medical facility. Rather, patients benefit only if these facilities offer services and equipment in less expensive, more convenient settings and, in addition, only if the facilities would not otherwise exist if doctors were not free to invest and refer patients.[120] Given the profitability of many of these facilities,[121] it seems implausible that, in general, only physicians in a position to make self–referrals will detect and respond to community needs.[122] It may be true that investors will profit *more* if they include physicians with both the ability and the incentive to refer their own patients; however, this is not to say that the facilities would not otherwise be available if a general ban on self–referrals were to be enacted.[123]

Regulatory Options: Further Differences Between the Professions

In the preceding section, it was argued that a conflict should be deemed nonconsentable only when clients or patients are unlikely to give informed and voluntary consent, as seems to be the case in physician self–referrals. Even then, it is arguable that a per se ban is not justified if there are feasible alternatives that are less restrictive of individual autonomy. For example, lawyer codes generally do not ban business transactions between lawyers and clients–despite the serious threat of overreaching[124]–but instead require certain additional protections for clients (e.g., that the terms of a transaction be fair and that the client have an opportunity to consult independent counsel).[125]

A number of proposals have been made to regulate the practice of physician self–referral without banning it entirely, including such alternatives as "investment side regulation" (which focuses on the type of investor, distribution of funds and profits, and amount invested)[126] and "referral side guidelines" (which regulate physician referral patterns to the facility).[127] In addition, some commentators have suggested mandated disclosure to third–party payers, who are often in a position to monitor inappropriate utilization and refer cases to local peer review organizations.[128] Others have recommended banning self–referrals to certain types of facilities and services that may be more susceptible to abuse than others.[129]

Perhaps more important than choosing among the competing proposals (including the proposal to ban physician self–referral entirely) is deciding which institution should do the choosing. The AMA understandably prefers to avoid further incursions on professional self–regulation; however, there are a number of reasons why, in the case of physician self–referral, it might be more appropriate to leave the decision-making to legislative and administrative bodies.

For example, many of these proposals require a degree of fine–tuning that is not typically available either in a professional code or in the more expansive interpretations sometimes given by authoritative professional bodies like the AMA Council.[130] Moreover, the AMA probably does not have the expertise to determine whether and when physician investment is needed to meet the health care needs of a particular community. Finally, the AMA has little ability to enforce its own regulatory proposals. Not only is it is ill–equipped to determine exemptions based on medical need; it does not have the disciplinary authority to sanction those physicians who clearly fail to comply with AMA guidelines.[131] Given the extent to which legislative and administrative bodies have come to regulate the medical profession[132]–particularly when the public has an obvious and substantial interest, such as containing the cost of health care[133]–physicians might be better advised to use their expertise to influence the course of any proposed legislation (or administrative regulations), rather than resisting such efforts entirely.

As for the legal profession, the preceding section suggests that additional protection for law firm clients may be unnecessary. Clients aside, however, there may be some danger that nonclient customers of the ancillary businesses will be confused and fail to understand the inapplicability of certain protections afforded clients of a law firm (e.g., in such areas as conflicts of interest and confidentiality).[134] Thus, the ABA Standing Committee on Ethics and Professional

Responsibility at one time proposed an amendment to the lawyer codes that would require lawyers to treat such customers as if they were clients, unless they had been clearly advised that the relationship was not one of lawyer and client.[135]

Unlike physician self–referral, there are no legislative or administrative bodies presently contemplating alternative regulatory proposals for law firm ancillary businesses. This is at least partially attributable to the lack of any public outcry. Perhaps a more important explanation, however, is the lack of a tradition of external regulation of the legal profession, at least by legislatures or administrative bodies. Indeed, ultimate authority over the legal profession is typically vested not in legislatures–which oversee all other professions, often through administrative agencies–but rather in state courts.[136] Moreover, these courts are comprised of judges, who are not only members of the broader legal profession but also former (and often future) practicing lawyers. As a result, the legal profession has achieved a degree of self–regulation unparalleled among the other professions.[137]

Of course, the status quo is always subject to change. If the public becomes sufficiently dissatisfied with the manner in which the legal profession chooses to regulate itself, then it may reclaim for itself the right to control the conduct of lawyers.[138] It is unlikely that the ancillary business phenomenon alone will cause this to happen;[139] however, the manner in which lawyers choose to regulate this (and other phenomena) is a possible source of concern.

In particular, the ABA Standing Committee's proposal is vulnerable to criticism on the ground that it attempts to regulate in areas beyond the proper scope of lawyer disciplinary codes. That is, it is one thing to caution lawyers involved in ancillary business activities to avoid confusing nonclient customers and even to discipline them if their conduct fails to comply with applicable guidelines. However, the ABA Standing Committee's proposal goes further, extending protections to nonclient customers that are not typically available to clients of accountants or investment bankers,[140] thus giving law firm ancillary businesses a potential advantage over their competitors.[141] In this respect, the proposal is subject to the same charge that has recently been leveled at other provisions of lawyer codes–that it is part of a continuing effort by lawyers to *supplant* rather than *supplement* other law, thus impermissibly elevating lawyers above all other citizens.[142] Of course, professional codes have always been subject to the criticism that they elevate the professionals' own interests above the interests of both their clients and the general public;[143] however, this conflict of interest is significantly reduced when the sphere of professional self–regulation is narrowly confined.

Perhaps part of the problem is that in an increasingly complex world, it becomes more and more difficult to tell which proposals favor the professionals' own interests at the expense of other important interests. In this respect, lawyers may have something to learn from the experience of physicians. Like the AMA, the ABA has limited expertise in some areas. Moreover, there will be times when solutions to difficult problems demand a degree of fine–tuning unavailable either in lawyer codes or in ABA or other authoritative interpretations. Finally, while courts have the authority to enforce lawyer codes, their practical ability to do so is limited.[144] If lawyer codes need at times to be supplemented by other law (or by remedies other than lawyer discipline),[145] then lawyers, like physicians, should be prepared to devote their expertise to influencing the development of that law rather than resisting such efforts entirely.

Conclusion

Until recently, there has been little effort to examine a profession's ethics in relation to what is being done in other professions.[146] As the various chapters of this book clearly demonstrate, there is much to be gained from such comparisons, as well as from recent scholarship by historians, sociologists, and philosophers of the professions.[147] Even the study of a single phenomenon–here, the emergence of ancillary business activities among doctors and lawyers–can produce insights concerning the ethics and situations of the professions of law and medicine, insights that can, in turn, be extended to other ethical issues and even to other professions.

For example, the primary lesson for physicians might be the extent to which their lack of any tradition of regulating conflicts of interest has left them ill–equipped to deal with the ancillary business phenomenon as it has manifested itself in medical practice. Moreover, to the extent that physicians can learn from the lawyers' more extensive experience in regulating conflicts, that learning can then be applied not only to the ancillary business phenomenon, but also to other situations involving conflicts of interest, including physicians employed in nontraditional forms of practice.[148]

As for lawyers, the primary lesson might be that their continued right to self–regulation depends not on their willingness to resist any and all forms of commercialization, but rather on their ability to examine issues and fashion regulations that are genuinely designed to foster the public interest rather than the interest of the lawyers themselves. Moreover, to the extent that lawyers sometimes lack either the expertise or the perspective to separate the two, they may need to rely on both empirical data–such as the utilization studies conducted on physician self–referral[149]–and the views of respected nonlawyers (as well as the experience of other professions) in order to ensure that their own positions have not been determined by even unconscious rationalizations of self–interest. After all, because lawyers are typically regulated by courts, and not by legislatures or administrative agencies,[150] they are often insulated from the views of anyone other than their fellow lawyers (and judges, who are themselves former and sometimes future practicing lawyers). Finally, if self–regulation is to continue, lawyers should be careful not to attempt to expand their authority beyond the limited arena in which self–regulation is appropriate.[151]

Perhaps the most important message for both lawyers and doctors is the need for enhanced professional training in identifying and dealing with the wide range of conflicts of interest and other ethical problems they will encounter in the continually changing environments in which law and medicine are now practiced. Medical students are not currently trained in conflicts-of-interest doctrine, primarily because such a doctrine has not yet been systemically developed by either physicians or medical ethicists.[152] Law schools typically require a separate course in legal ethics in which conflicts of interest doctrine is routinely covered; however, the difficulty of applying the doctrine in myriad different circumstances suggests the need for enhanced training, including discussion of conflicts in substantive law courses and in continuing professional education.[153] That is, rather than bemoaning the new business orientation, the professions should be equipping themselves and their students with the necessary tools to meet the challenges of an increasingly demanding public, including the challenge of maintaining both ethical standards and a sense of professionalism in a highly competitive environment.

Notes

1. The 1984 Annual Health Conference held by the Committee on Medicine in Society of the New York Academy of Medicine was entitled "The New Entrepreneurialism in Health Care." *See, e.g.*, Bradford H. Gray, Overview: Origins and Trends, 61 *Bull. N.Y. Acad. Med.* 7 (1985). Of course, entrepreneurial activity in medicine is not itself new; what is new is the "more openly entrepreneurial" forms it has recently taken. Bradford H. Gray, Introduction to the Volume, in Institute of Medicine, Committee on Implications of For-Profit Enterprise in Health Care, *For-Profit Enterprise in Health Care* xvii (1986) (hereafter "For-Profit Enterprise").

2. *E.g.*, Theodore N. McDowell, Jr., Physician Self Referral Arrangements: Legitimate Business or Unethical "Entrepreneurialism," 15 *Am. J. Law Med.* 62 (1989). *See also* David Hyman and Joel Williamson, Fraud and Abuse: Regulatory Alternatives in a "Competitive" Health Care Era, 19 *Loyola U. L. J.* 1131 (1988), and Hyman and Williamson, Fraud and Abuse: Setting Limits on Physicians' Entrepreneurship, 320 *N. Engl. J. Med.* 1275 (1989). For a thorough description and analysis of other forms of the new entrepreneurialism—investor-owned health care providers, particularly hospitals—see generally For-Profit Enterprise, *supra* note 1.

3. McDowell, *supra* note 2, at 62–63. The most controversial structure is the limited partnership, in which physicians purchase an equity interest and, at the same time, limit their potential liability. *Id.*

4. *See, e.g.*, Is Ancillary Business the Future?, 1 *Prof. Law.* 1 (1989). For a discussion of some of the other aspects of lawyers engaged in business activities, including lawyers loaning

money to or investing funds in clients' enterprises, see Justin Stanley, Lawyers in Business, 8 *No. Ill. U. L. Rev.* 17 (1987).

5. *See generally* ABA Section of Litigation, *Report to the House of Delegates on Ancillary Business Activities of Lawyers* (June 1991) (hereafter *ABA Section of Litigation Report.*

6. *See, e.g.,* McDowell, *supra* note 2, at 62–65.

7. *Id.* The analysis in the medical setting is complicated by the uncertain nature of medical markets. Some commentators argue that medical markets should not and cannot be like competitive markets; other contend that they should be regulated so as to be more like standard markets; and still others assert that although medical markets are different, their competitive aspects make them amenable to fairly traditional economic analysis and regulation. *See Competition in the Health Care* Sector ix–xvii (W. Greenberg, ed., 1978).

8. Arnold Relman, The New Medical-Industrial Complex, 303 *N. Engl. J. Med.* 963 (1980). While Dr. Relman refers here to the for-profit sector of health care providers, others see similarities in the behavior of for-profit and nonprofit hospitals, including the formation of multi-institutional arrangements to gain economies of scale and greater access to capital, aggressive marketing and vertical integration to increase market share, and heightening cost control. *For-Profit Enterprise, supra* note 1 at 9. *See also* Arnold Relman, Practicing Medicine in the New Business Climate, 316 *N. Engl. J. Med.* 1150 (1987) (many nonprofit hospitals behaving like profit-oriented businesses). This entrepreneurial behavior, even among nonprofits, includes offering financial incentives to physicians to comply with general cost containment strategies. *Id.* at 156–157. *See also* Linda Burns and Douglas Mancino, *Joint Ventures Between Hospitals and Physicians* (1987).

9. *See, e.g.,* Norman Fost, Ethical Considerations of Hospital–Physician Joint Ventures, in Burns and Mancino, *supra* note 8, at 44.

10. *See* Office of the Inspector General, Department of Health and Human Services, *Financial Arrangements Between Physicians and Health Care Businesses* 1–3 (May 1989) (hereinafter *OIG Report*).

11. *See, e.g.,* The Limits of Medicare, *New York Times* A18 (November 27, 1989).

12. 42 U.S.C. 1395nn (1991) (effective for referrals made on or after January 1, 1992).

13. *OIG Report, supra* note 10, at 2.

14. McDowell, *supra* note 2, at 64. According to some, government polices are contradictory, and thus the message being sent is a mixed one. *See* AMA Council on Ethical and Judicial Affairs, Conflicts of Interest: Physician Ownership of Medical Facilities, 267 *JAMA* 2366, 2367 (1992) (hereafter "AMA Council Opinion").

15. *OIG Report, supra* note 10 at iii. A recent survey of health care businesses in Florida indicates that at least 40 percent of Florida physicians involved in direct patient care have an investment interest in a health care business to which they may refer their patients. Jean Mitchell and Elton Scott, New Evidence of the Prevalence and Scope of Physician Joint Ventures, 268 *JAMA* 80 (1992). Legislation regulating or prohibiting self-referral will continue to affect these numbers.

16. "Boutique" firms are highly specialized, small firms that cultivate their competitive advantage in selective specialties, such as health care and microcomputers. *See* Marc Galanter and Thomas Palay, Why the Big Get Bigger: The Promotion-to-Partner Tournament and the Growth of Large Law Firms, 76 *Va. L. Rev.* 747, 808–809 (1990).

17. *ABA Section of Litigation Report, supra* note 5, at 3–9.

18. *See generally* Symposium: The Growth of Large Law Firms and Its Effect on the Legal Profession and Legal Education, 64 *Ind. L. J.* 423 (1989).

19. *See* ABA Communication on Professionalism: "In the Spirit of Public Service": A Blueprint for the Rekindling of Lawyer Professionalism, 243 *F.R.D.* 243, 259–260 (1986).

20. *See, e.g.*, James Jones, The Challenge of Change: The Practice of Law in the Year 2000, 41 *Vand. L. Rev.* 683, 684–686 (1988).
21. *See, e.g.*, *ABA Section of Litigation Report, supra* note 5, at 5–6.
22. *See, e.g.*, James Fitzpatrick, Legal Future Shock The Role of Large Law Firms by the End of the Century, 64 *Ind. L. J.* 461, 467 (1989). A review of the *National Law Journal's* survey of the nation's 250 largest firms showed that 33 of them were involved in 48 ancillary businesses. The controversy over ancillary business activities discussed in the text at notes 25 to 32 has perhaps chilled the expected quick growth of ancillary business activities. In 1991 only two new businesses were established by the large firms and in 1992 only three. Conversely, eleven were started in 1990. Thom Weidlich, Ancillary Business Prospering Quietly, *National L. J.* 1 (December 21, 1992).
23. *Id.*, at 466.
24. See *supra* note 9 and accompanying text.
25. By their use of the terms "professional" and "professionalism," traditionalists typically mean to invoke what they view as the essence of the professions—a devotion to public service as opposed to "the bottom line." *See* AMA Council Opinion, *supra* note 14; *ABA Section of Litigation Report, supra* note 5, at 16–25; 36–37. This concept of professionalism is problematic: indeed, a wealth of recent scholarship by historians and sociologists, as well as by critics within the legal profession itself, argues that "professionalization" is a historical process representing the selfish efforts of certain occupations to obtain a state-sanctioned monopoly for their services. *See* Nancy Moore, Professionalism Reconsidered, 1987 *Am. Bar. Found. Res. J.* 773, 780. For a description of recent efforts to "reformulate" a concept of professionalism that recognizes and deals with the evidence amassed by critical historians and sociologists, see Nancy Moore, Professionalism: Rekindled, Reconsidered, or Reformulated?, 19 *Cap. U. L. Rev.* 1121 (1990). See also Buchanan's chapter (5) in this volume. For a more sympathetic scholarly view of the usefulness of professionalism in the medical profession, see Eliot Friedson, The Centrality of Professionalism to Health Care, 30 *Jurimetrics* 431 (1990).
26. *See, e.g.*, McDowell, *supra* note 2, at 76–106 (discussing various regulatory responses to physician self-referral, including (a) complete prohibition; (b) disclosure requirements; (c) percentage of ownership limitations; and (d) structural guidelines); ABA Rejects Ancillary Business, Inroads on Client Confidences, *ABA/BNA Lawyers' Manual on Professional Conduct*, Current Reports 256 (August 28, 1991) (summarizing different regulatory approaches presented at the American Bar Association's 1991 annual meeting). For a discussion of the varying approaches taken by the AMA Council and AMA members, see *infra* notes 29–31 and accompanying text.
27. *See* authorities cited at *supra* note 26.
28. *See infra* notes 40–49 and accompanying text.
29. In December 1991, the AMA House of Delegates voted to accept an opinion of the AMA Council on Ethical and Judicial Affairs, which said that physicians should generally not engage in self-referral. Six months later the delegates reversed their vote. See AMA Votes to Ease New Curbs on Physician "Self-Referral," *The Washington Post* A20 (June 24, 1992). Shortly thereafter, they reversed themselves yet again. See *infra* note 30 and accompanying text. In August 1991, the ABA House of Delegates voted to add a new rule to the ABA Model Rules of Professional Conduct making it unethical for law firms to offer nonlegal services to customers who are not clients of the firm. ABA Rejects Ancillary Business, *supra* note 26. The ABA delegates similarly reversed their vote at the next annual meeting. *See* ABA Rule on Ancillaries Doesn't Survive First Year, *ABA/BNA Lawyers' Manual on Professional Conduct, Current Reports* 261 (August 26, 1992).

30. *See, e.g.*, AMA Rules Against Self-Referrals, *Chicago Tribune* N20 (December 9, 1992). The resolution says that it is unethical for physicians to own centers used for self-referral except to meet a special medical need for a community or if the only way the center could be established is through involvement by doctors who would refer there. For a discussion of the difficulties the AMA will face in enforcing this resolution, *see infra* note 130 and accompanying text.

31. AMA Softens "Self-Referral" Stance, But Officials Say Vote Won't Alter Ethics Code, *Chicago Tribune* C1 (June 24, 1992).

32. *See* ABA Rule on Ancillaries Doesn't Survive First Year, *supra* note 29.

33. Telephone interview of Jill Hirt of the AMA by David Shimm, September 27, 1993; telephone interview of Karen Gruenke of the ABA by Roy Spece, August 15, 1994 (351,911 out of 865,615 attorneys belong to the ABA).

34. *See infra* notes 40–75 and accompanying text.

35. *See infra* notes 76–83 and accompanying text.

36. *See infra* notes 102–123 and accompanying text.

37. *See infra* notes 124–137 and accompanying text.

38. *See infra* notes 90–123 and accompanying text. The debate about the efficacy of disclosure is carried forward by Morreim and Katz in their chapters (11 and 12) in this volume. The position here is that the relatively small consequences to individual patients and the pressures on them not to question the ethics of their physicians (described by Katz) make disclosure an inadequate approach.

39. See text following note 151 *infra*.

40. McDowell, *supra* note 2, at 107. *See also, e.g.*, Fitzpatrick, *supra* note 22.

41. *See, e.g.*, George Annas, Sylvia Law, Rand Rosenblatt, and Kenneth Wing, *American Health Law* 125–126 (1990) (experts from a variety of disciplines agree that inflation in health care prices derives from the manner in which health care was traditionally financed and organized, including insulation of both providers and patients from the costs of the services delivered); FTC Staff Report, *Improving Consumer Access to Legal Service: The Case for Removing Restrictions on Truthful Advertising* (1984) (lawyer advertising has the effect of bringing down the price of legal services).

42. *See, e.g.*, Linda Burns, Changing Hospital–Physician Relationships: Joint Ventures as Strategic Alliances, in Burns and Mancino, *supra* note 8, at 13; Fost, *supra* note 9, at 49; FTC Staff Report, *supra* note 40.

43. *E.g.*, Jones, *supra* note 20, at 684–686. *Cf.* Duncan MacDonald, Speculations by a Customer About the Future of Large Law Firms, 64 *Ind. L. J.* 593 (1989) (in-house corporate counsel on benefits to client of commercialization of legal practice).

44. Fitzpatrick, *supra* note 22, at 465. This term has been picked up by traditionalists and used to deride the entrepreneurs. *See, e.g.*, *ABA Section of Litigation Report, supra* note 5, at 8, n.28 ("[t]his practice is also called, in New Age lingo, practicing 'holistic law' or maintaining a 'synergistic' practice").

45. *See* Fitzpatrick, *supra* note 22, at 470–471. *See also* FTC Unit Lauds Law-Firm Diversification, *Legal Times* 14 (April 18, 1991) (excerpt of a letter from the director of the FTC Bureau of Competition commenting on a proposed ban on law firm ancillary services).

46. Even the FTC concedes that the benefits of self-referral are less obvious than those of alternative delivery systems such as health maintenance organizations and preferred provider organization. Bureau of Competition, Consumer Protection and Economics, Federal Trade Commission, *Comments Concerning the Development of Regulations Pursuant to the Medicare and Medicaid Anti-Kickback Statute* 14–15, (December 18, 1987) (hereafter *FTC Comments*).

47. *E.g.*, *For-Profit Enterprise*, *supra* note 1, at 155.
48. *E.g.*, McDowell, *supra* note 2, at 71–72 (summarizing FTC position set forth in two different letters).
49. *Id.*
50. Traditionalists in the medical profession are particularly anxious to dispel the notion that physician self-referral has any appreciable benefit to the public. *See, e.g.*, Arnold Relman, Conflicts of Interest and the Physician Entrepreneur, 314 *N. Engl. J. Med.* 252 (1986) ("[h]ospitals, private corporations, and venture capitalists seeking to start new facilities don't really need physicians' capital. What they want is their patronage, which they seek to ensure by giving physicians a financial stake in the enterprise"). *See also* McDowell, *supra* note 2, at 72, n.54 and n.57. And, indeed, these arguments are quite persuasive. *See infra* notes 119–123 and accompanying text.

    Some lawyers have argued that the provision of ancillary services by law firms may in fact be anticompetitive. *See, e.g.*, Philip O'Hara, Will Title Agents Go the Way of the Buffalo?, *New York L. J.* 2 (April 10, 1990) ("[i]f lawyers and lenders can 'steer' the title insurance of their clients and borrowers to their own title agencies there is no open competition"). These arguments are less persuasive. *Cf. infra* notes 105–107 and accompanying text.
51. *See, e.g.*, McDowell, *supra* note 2, at 68–70; *ABA Section of Litigation Report*, *supra* note 5, at 9–11. For a more extensive analysis of the conflicts of interests presented, see *infra* notes 90-122 and accompanying text.
52. *See* McDowell, *supra* note 2, at 6 (discussing a number of recent studies that document the overutilization problem, including the OIG report cited at *supra* note 10). *See also* Mitchell's chapter (13) in this text. On the contrary, no evidence of actual harm to clients arising from lawyers' participation in the recent ancillary business activities has been documented. *See* ABA Standing Committee on Ethics and Professional Responsibility, *Recommendation and Report to the House of Delegates* (August 1991) (hereafter *ABA Standing Committee Report*).
53. For example, a corporation represented by the law firm might be planning a takeover of an ancillary business customer. If retaining the ancillary business customer is economically important to the health of the law firm, the law firm might be tempted to advise the customer to take anticompetitive measures, thus violating both duties of loyalty and confidentiality owed to the law firm client. On the other hand, if retaining the law firm client is more important, the law firm (or its ancillary business) might act in a way that harms the ancillary business customer. While present conflict-of-interest rules require disclosure of the conflict of interest to the law firm client (*see infra* note 96 and accompanying text), they do not protect ancillary business customers who are not also clients of the law firm.
54. For this reason the ABA Standing Committee on Ethics and Professional Responsibility, which was unwilling to support a ban on ancillary business activity, proposed treating ancillary business customers as if they were law firm clients, unless the business matter is unrelated to legal representation and the law firm clearly communicates to the customer that the relationship is not that of lawyer and client. *See ABA Standing Committee Report*, *supra* note 51, at 3. *See also infra* notes 135–143 and accompanying text (discussing the ABA Standing Committee proposal).

    In addition, there may be concern that the ancillary businesses will engage in forms of advertising and solicitation that would be unethical if done by lawyers. *See ABA Model Rules of Professional Conduct*, Rules 7.1–7.3 (1983). Of course, if done with the primary goal of producing new clients for the law firms, such conduct might violate present rules of professional conduct. *See id.*, Rule 8.4.

55. *See supra* note 25. "Public" can be construed to apply to special regard for clients *and* the general public. In chapter 5 of this volume, Hazard addresses the possible conflict between regard to clients and the public generally. On professionalism generally, see also the authorities cited by Shimm and Spece at note 1 of chapter 3 of this volume.

56. *See* L. Harold Levinson, Independent Law Firms That Practice Law Only: Society's Need, the Legal Profession's Responsibility, 51 *Ohio St. L. J.* 229, 242 (1990); *ABA Section of Litigation Report, supra* note 5, at 11–13.

57. *See, e.g., ABA Section of Litigation Report, supra* note 5, at 13–16.

58. *Id.*, at 16–25; cf. AMA Council Opinion, *supra* note 14, 267 *JAMA* at 2367 ("[t]he medical profession's ability to preserve autonomy...ha[s] largely succeeded in large part due to the profession's lack of tolerance for 'commercialism' in medicine").

59. *See generally*, Moore, Professionalism Reconsidered, *supra* note 25.

60. *See, e.g.*, Fost, *supra* note 9, at 46–47; Levinson, *supra* note 55, at 242.

61. *ABA Section of Litigation Report, supra* note 5, at 37.

62. *See, e.g.*, "The Changing Nature of Physician Influence in Medical Institutions," in *For-Profit Enterprise, supra* note 1, at 171.

63. *E.g.*, Fost, *supra* note 9, at 47.

64. *See, e.g.*, Relman, The New Medical–Industrial Complex, *supra* note 8, at 968 (public responsibilities of the medical profession in evaluating drugs, devices, diagnostic tests, and therapeutic procedures in the public interest); ABA Communication on Professionalism, *supra* note 19, 243 F.R.D. at 281–283 (when not representing clients before legislative bodies, lawyers should support legislation in the public interest).

65. *See, e.g., For-Profit Enterprise, supra* note 1, at 154.

66. *See, e.g.*, FTC Unit Lauds Law-Firm Diversification, *supra* note 45. Although mediation can be considered a legal service—i.e., when performed by a lawyer as part of a legal representation, typically representation of both parties—it is more often considered a nonlegal service, particularly when performed by nonlawyers, such as marriage or divorce counselors.

67. *See, e.g.*, FTC Comments, *supra* note 46, at 15–16.

68. *See, e.g.*, Arnold Relman, Dealing with Conflicts of Interest, 313 *N. Engl. J. Med.* 749 (1985); *ABA Section of Litigation Report, supra* note 5, at 4–5.

69. *See, e.g.*, Levinson, *supra* note 56, at 242; *cf.* Arnold Relman, Practicing Medicine in the New Business Climate, 316 *N. Engl. J. Med.* 1150, 1150–1151 (1987) (to protect professional independence, physicians should avoid direct individual employment by a for-profit corporation; physicians practicing in health maintenance organizations should be either self-employed or part of a self-managed medical group that contracts with the company).

70. *See, e.g., ABA Standing Committee Report, supra* note 51, at 9 ("the postulation of speculative harms resulting from lawyers' ancillary business activities—a decline in professionalism, or a loss of self-regulatory authority—cannot justify a prohibition [on ancillary business activity]"); *cf.* Fost, supra note 9, at 52–53 (skeptical of traditionalists' claim that a "more contractual relationship between physician and patient" will result in loss of trust; indeed, this trend may result in improvement in physician–patient relationships).

71. FTC Unit Lauds Law-Firm Diversification, *supra* note 45.

72. *See, e.g.*, Arnold Relman Salaried Physicians and Economic Incentives, 319 *N. Engl. J. Med.* 784 (1988) (including accounts of salaried practice from a physician in a for-profit walk-in clinic and a physician employed by a health maintenance organization).

73. Simon Rifkind, Professionalism Under Siege, 58 *N.Y.S.B.J.* 66 (February 1986), in *ABA Section of Litigation Report, supra* note 5, at 18, n.56 (traditionalist characterizing critics' attack on those who speak in favor of professionalism).

74. Note, Altering People's Perceptions: The Challenge Facing Advocates of Ancillary Business Practice, 66 *Ind. L.J.* 1031, 1045, n.79 (1991) (telephone interview with James Fitzpatrick).

75. Like their counterparts in the legal profession, medical entrepreneurs argue that change is inevitable and that "physicians should promote entrepreneurialism or else nonphysicians will control the market completely." McDowell, *supra* note 2, at 74.

76. *See supra* notes 29–32 and accompanying text.

77. AMA Council Opinion, *supra* note 14, 267 *JAMA* at 2367–2368.

78. *ABA Section of Litigation Report, supra* note 5, at 37.

79. As noted earlier, certain aspects of what is sometimes referred to as "professionalism" concerns are in fact merely another way of stating what is actually an ethical concern that an orientation toward profit will cause professionals to act in ways that harm their patients or clients. *See* note 56 and accompanying text. *See also infra* note 85 and accompanying text. Whether ancillary business practice causes such harm is discussed *supra* at note 52 and in the accompanying text.

80. Even if it is true, as the ABA Section of Litigation suggests, that law firm ownership of ancillary businesses ultimately may lead to a relaxation of rules now prohibiting lawyers from working for entities owned in whole or in part by nonlawyers, this does not necessarily mean that lawyering will become "indistinguishable from any other profit-seeking enterprise" or that "legal practice will be under tight state regulation." *ABA Section of Litigation Report, supra* note 5, at 37. After all, rules regulating the delivery of legal services are clearly evolving; indeed, the Kutak Commission, which had been appointed by the ABA to draft the Model Rules, initially recommended getting rid of the ban on nonlawyer interest in law firm ownership. Note, Altering People's Perceptions: The Challenge Facing Advocates of Ancillary Business Practice," *supra* note 74, at 1037–1038. Indeed, at least one jurisdiction has adopted a significant relaxation of the rule. *Id.* at 1049–1052 (discussing rules recently adopted for lawyers practicing in Washington, D.C.).

81. AMA Council Opinion, *supra* note 14, at 2367.

82. *See, e.g.*, Moore, Professionalism: Rekindled, Reconsidered, or Reformulated?, supra note 25, at 1125:

> Even the United States Supreme Court has recognized the harm that has been done in the professionalization process. As noted in the [report of the ABA Commission on Professionalism], the Court has struck down as unconstitutional such monopolistic practices as absolute bans on lawyer advertising, prohibitions and restrictions on lawyer participation in group legal service plans, and promulgation of minimum fee schedules. *In each instance, a practice which was in fact harmful to the public interest was sought to be justified by bar associations, all in the name of "professionalism."* (Emphasis added; footnotes omitted.)

83. As already noted, there are empirical studies that strongly suggest that doctors are overutilizing ancillary business services; see *supra* note 51 and accompanying text. However, this evidence of actual harm is more properly considered under the rubric of ethical as opposed to professionalism concerns, since any such overutilization would be a direct violation of ethical obligations owed by physicians to their patients.

84. *See supra* notes 51–54 and accompanying text.

85. *See supra* note 56 and accompanying text.

86. Michael Abramawitz, AMA Votes to Ease New Curbs on Physician "Self-Referral"; Financial Interest in Labs Was Seen as Possible Conflict, *The Washington Post* A2 (June 24, 1992).

87. One physician asks, "Why is it ethical for a physician to purchase an electrocardiographic machine for $3,000 and perform electrocardiograms in his office, but unethical for him to organize with other physicians to purchase equipment for $100,000 to perform blood chemistry

tests in a common location?," Stephen Goldman, To the Editor, 314 *N. Engl. J. Med.* 251 (1986).

88. Until recently, the position of the AMA and its Judicial Council seemed to be that although physicians must always place the welfare of their patients above their own financial interests, there is nothing inherently improper in physicians' owning or investing in health care businesses. If they act on their financial interest by overusing services or through kickbacks and rebates, that would be considered improper; *but only actual abuses are of concern, not hypothetical or potential conflicts of interest.* Relman, The New Medical–Industrial Complex, *supra* note 8, at 97. As Dr. Relman notes, the AMA's recently revised Principles of Medical Ethics contains no statement whatever about economic conflicts of interest. *Id.*

89. *See generally* Charles Wolfram, *Modern Legal Ethics* 312 (1986) (a thorough discussion of conflict-of-interest rules in the legal profession).

90. Legal conflict-of-interest doctrine refers almost entirely to potential harm to clients themselves, not to the potential for harm to other affected parties or to the public. *See infra* note 109. But see *infra* note 95 (recognition of the institutional interest of the justice system in ensuring that each party's interest is presented vigorously).

91. *See* American Law Institute, *Restatement of the Law Governing Lawyers* (Tent. Draft No. 4), Sec. 201 (1991) (hereafter *ALI Restatement*). *See generally* Wolfram, *supra* note 89.

92. *See ALI Restatement, supra* note 91, Sec. 202.

93. *See* ABA Model Rules of Professional Conduct, Rule 1.8(d) (1983).

94. *See* ABA Model Code of Professional Responsibility, DR 5-105(C) (1969).

95. *See* ABA Model Rules of Professional Conduct, Rule 1.7(a) and (b).

96. *See* ALI Restatement, *supra* note 91, at Sec. 202, Comment (b). *See also* Nancy Moore, Conflicts of Interest in the Simultaneous Representation of Multiple Clients: A Proposed Solution to the Current Confusion and Controversy, 61 *Tex. L. Rev.* 211 (1982). A separate ground for prohibiting some conflicts in litigated matters is the institutional interest in ensuring that each party's interest is presented vigorously. ALI Restatement, *supra*, at sec. 202, Comment (b).

97. For example, under the conflict-of-interest rule adopted in most jurisdictions, "a lawyer shall not represent a client if the representation of that client may be materially limited by...the lawyer's own interests" unless "the lawyer reasonably believes the representation will not be adversely affected" and "the client consents after consultation." ABA Model Rules of Professional Conduct, Rule 1.7(b). Given the obvious danger that a lawyer's significant economic interest in an ancillary business may affect the lawyer's independent judgment in recommending the use of that business to a client, *see supra* note 50 and accompanying text; it is clear that, at the very least, the lawyer's interest must be disclosed *to the client*. The Rules of Professional Conduct, however, do not require lawyers (or nonlawyers with whom they are affiliated) to make similar disclosure to customers of the ancillary business. Thus, the ABA Standing Committee on Professional Ethics proposed extending current protections to such customers. *See supra* note 54. *See also infra* notes 135–143.

98. Of course, there is no easy way to determine what constitutes a "significant" interest. Various federal and state statutes prohibit physician self–referrals only when the physician has a "significant" ownership interest, which is variously defined as direct or indirect ownership of 5 percent or more of an agency, 10 percent, $5,000, or sometimes a "controlling" interest. McDowell, *supra* note 2, at 88. Percentage–of–ownership levels are also used in such legislation as a threshold to trigger more extensive protective mechanisms, such as disclosure. *Id.* The difficulty with all of these rigid definitions is that they ignore the fact that an investment return on a small percentage interest may be sizable and may create powerful economic incentives. *Id.* Perhaps for this reason, conflict-of-interest rules for the legal profession do not attempt to define rigidly what constitutes a significant interest.

99. Under the legal ethics framework, it is not necessary to assume deliberate disregard of fiduciary duties, since it is assumed that it is just as likely that a professional's independent judgment will be unconsciously influenced by a predisposition to view the client's interests as compatible with the professional's own interests.

100. *See* AMA Softens "Self-Referral" Stance, But Officials Say Vote Won't Alter Ethics Code, *Chicago Tribune* C1 (June 24, 1992). *See also* Relman, Dealing with Conflicts of Interest, *supra* note 68 (prior AMA rule requiring physicians to disclose their financial interest in a referral facility). Unlike rules of legal ethics, rules of medical ethics such as those promulgated by the AMA are not typically enforceable as rules of law. See infra note 131 & accompanying text. However, in cases involving the traditional informed consent doctrine (*see infra* notes 104–111 and accompanying text), courts are beginning to recognize an independent basis for physician disclosure. *See, e.g.,* Moore v. Regents of the University of California, 51 Cal. 3d 120, 793 P.2d 479 (1990) (a physician was held liable for failure to inform a patient that cells from the removed spleen would be used to develop a new cell line in which the physician had a substantial economic interest).

101. An additional concern is the *extent* of any disclosure given.

102. McDowell, *supra* note 2, at 87.

103. *See, e.g.,* E. Haavi Morreim, Conflicts of Interest; Profits and Problems in Physician Referrals, 262 *JAMA* 390 (1989).

104. *See, e.g.,* George Annas, *The Rights of Patients* 89 (2d ed., 1989) ("the law presumes every adult is competent").

105. *See, e.g.,* Marjorie Schultz, From Informed Consent to Patient Choice; A New Protected Interest, 95 *Yale L.J.* 219, 223 (1985) (criticizing the limitations of the current doctrine). The requirement of a physical touching originated in battery actions but has been carried over to the negligence arena as well. Id. If there is an inherent risk of death or serious bodily harm, then the requirement may be stretched somewhat. *Cf.* Annas, *supra* note 103, at 87–88 (informed consent is required for administration of drugs, performance of diagnostic tests, and performance of major or minor surgical procedures when there is an inherent risk of serious harm, when the probable success is low, or when alternatives exist).

106. Thus, an action under the informed consent doctrine exists separate and apart from any action based on physician incompetence. *See generally* Schultz, *supra* note 105.

107. For example, patients referred to ambulatory surgical centers will certainly be asked to give informed consent to whatever major or minor surgical procedure is contemplated. *See supra* note 104. The informed consent doctrine also applies to radiation oncology treatments and alternative treatments for kidney stones. *See, e.g.,* note 33 in chapter 11 of this volume.

108. For example, patients referred to clinical and physiological laboratories will often be taking routine tests, such as blood tests, which typically do not require informed consent because the risks are minimal and generally well known. *See* Annas, *supra* note 104, at 89. An exception might be an HIV blood test, in which the risk of at least psychological harm is quite high. *Id. See also supra* note 107 (the informed consent doctrine applies to such procedures as radiation oncology and alternative treatments for kidney stones).

109. Again, while this is the typical case, there are certainly instances in which procedures are *both* invasive and potentially harmful. Here physician self–interest will be an additional factor to consider, along with information regarding the risks and benefits of the proposed procedure. *See supra* notes 107–108 and accompanying text.

110. Indeed, the primary risk of harm in physician self–referrals may not be to the individual patient but rather to the public, which suffers from aggregate increases in the cost of health care. *Cf.* McDowell, *supra* note 2, at 87 (discussing the suggestion by some that "patient disclosure requirements should be supplemented with mandated disclosure of ownership inter-

ests to third-party payers"). Thus, it is not surprising that the AMA initiative to ban the practice came only after it became increasingly apparent that federal and state legislatures were moving to enact regulations of their own, making further inroads on the ever-shrinking autonomy of the medical profession. *See, e.g., id.* at 76-106 (discussing various federal and state proposals to curb abuses of physician self–referral). Unfortunately, the conflict-of-interest doctrine, as it is commonly understood in the legal profession, does not address conflicts between professional self-interest and the public interest in the cost and quality of professional services.

111. Fear of harming the physician–patient relationship is an inhibiting factor affecting many patients in situations involving *both* risky invasive procedures and the more typical instances of physician self-referral. Such fear is more likely to inhibit patients in the less risky self-referral cases, because what is at stake for the patient often seems trivial in relation to the importance of maintaining a relationship of trust and confidence.

112. *See* text following *supra* note 21.

113. *Cf. supra* note 20 and accompanying text.

114. *ABA Section of Litigation Report, supra* note 5, at 11.

115. *See* Moore, *supra* note 96, at 226.

116. Profits, not selfless devotion to clients, may indeed be the "chief impetus behind law firm diversification." *ABA Section of Litigation Report,* supra note 5, at 7. Nonetheless, if law firms have detected an important client need that they are in a position to meet, and if they can market themselves accordingly, then motive should be irrelevant.

117. *See supra* note 23 and accompanying text.

118. McDowell, *supra* note 2, at 87.

119. *See supra* note 52 and accompanying text.

120. *See supra* notes 47–49 and accompanying text.

121. *See, e.g.,* Robert Pear with Erik Eckholm, When Healers Are Entrepreneurs: A Debate Over Costs and Ethics, *The New York Times* A1 (June 2, 1991).

122. *See supra* note 50.

123. What is more likely is that there may be particular communities where failure to permit physician investment will result in an absence of adequate facilities or financing. In such cases, the AMA Council Opinion provides that physicians who can demonstrate "plain medical need" will receive an exemption from the ban on self–referral. AMA Council Opinion, *supra* note 14, at 2368.

124. *See generally* Wolfram, *supra* note 89, at 479–485.

125. *See* ABA Model Rules of Professional Conduct, Rule 1.8(a) (1983).

126. McDowell, *supra* note 2, at 103.

127. *Id.* at 103–104.

128. *Id.* at 87. For a discussion of some of the practical objections to this proposal, see, e.g., *OIG Report, supra* note 10, at 29.

129. *See* McDowell, *supra* note 2, at 76–81 (discussing federal and state prohibitions, *e.g.,* in the context of home intravenous therapy, clinical laboratories, ambulatory surgery centers, and pharmacy permits). Morreim and Mitchell describe the many laws that have been recommended or adopted to regulate physician self-referral and entrepreneurial activities in their chapters (11 and 13) in this volume. The definite trend is toward prohibition of self-referral.

130. For example, the AMA Council proposes an exemption for physicians who can demonstrate community need; however, it sets forth neither substantive nor procedural criteria for determining which physicians will qualify for this exemption. *See* AMA Council Opinion, *supra* note 14.

131. All the AMA can do is urge "state, county, and specialty societies, through their grievance and discipline committees, to actively investigate reports of abuse or non-compliance with the Council's opinion." AMA, Statement of the Council on Ethical and Judicial Affairs 2 (September 4, 1991). However, even local societies have no formal sanctioning authority, since physicians are licensed and regulated by administrative agencies established by state legislature. *See generally* Randolph Reaves, *The Law of Professional Licensing and Certification* (1984).

Of course, the AMA can expel physicians from its membership; however, since the AMA is a voluntary organization—i.e., membership is not required to practice medicine—this sanction alone is unlikely to deter large numbers of physicians from engaging in prohibited practices.

132. As of 1991, there were more than thirty bills pending in Congress concerning reform of the health care system. For a recent summary of these proposals, see generally Health Care Reform: Major Legislative Proposals, Report of the House Ways and Means Committee, reprinted in *Medicare and Medicaid Guide* (CCH), Report No. 674, pt. II (October 24, 1991).

133. *See supra* note 110.

134. *See supra* note 54 and accompanying text.

135. *See ABA Standing Committee Report, supra* note 52.

136. *See, e.g.*, Wolfram, *supra* note 89, at 22–31. Under the "inherent powers doctrine," courts have claimed the affirmative power to regulate the conduct of lawyers, including the power to promulgate a lawyer's code, to admit lawyers to practice, to discipline admitted lawyers, and to define the unauthorized practice of law. *Id.* at 24. The negative aspect of this doctrine, followed by a large number of states (but not by the federal government), invalidates any legislative action deemed by courts to conflict with their own inherent authority and is said to be justified by the state constitutional law doctrine of separation of powers. *Id.* at 27.

137. See Nancy Moore, The Usefulness of Ethical Codes, 1989 *Ann. Surv. Am. L.* 7, 14–15.

138. *See* Moore, Professionalism Reconsidered, *supra* note 25, at 784, 787. In states that have adopted the negative aspect of the inherent powers doctrine (*see supra* note 135), this would require an amendment to the state constitution—a formidable but not insurmountable barrier to direct public regulation of the legal profession.

139. *See supra* notes 79–83 and accompanying text.

140. *See supra* note 53 and accompanying text.

141. Law firms might well argue that these restrictions also pose disadvantages, such as pushing up the costs; however, it is noteworthy that law firms have not objected to the fact that lawyers are covered by the attorney–client evidentiary privilege, while accountants doing similar work are not.

142. *See, e.g.*, Susan Koniak, The Law Between the Bar and the State, 70 *N.C. L. Rev.* 1389 (1992); and Roger Cramton and Lisa Udell, State Ethics Rules and Federal Prosecutors: The Controversies Over the Anti-Contact and Subpoena Rules, 53 *U. Pitt. L. Rev.* 291, 311–315 (1992). This charge has been leveled at code provisions that seek to exempt lawyers from laws of general application, such as the law of fraud, and those that attempt to regulate lawyers performing outside traditional lawyer roles, such as public prosecutors in their performance of executive rather than representative functions. *See* Cramton and Udell, *supra*, at 313–314; Nancy Moore, Intra-Professional Warfare Between Prosecutors and Defense Attorneys: A Plea for an End to the Current Hostilities, 53 *U. Pitt. L. Rev.* 515, 524, 539 (1992).

143. *See, e.g.*, Thomas Morgan, The Evolving Concept of Professional Responsibility, 90 *Harv. L. Rev.* 702 (1977).

144. *E.g.*, American Bar Association Commission on Evaluation of Disciplinary Enforcement, *Report to the American Bar Association House of Delegates* (1991) (on continuing inadequacies in the regulatory process).

145. Of course, additional remedies already exist in the form of criminal proceedings, as well as legal malpractice and other civil actions against lawyers. The limitations of these existing remedies should be obvious.

146. *See* Nancy Moore, Limits to Attorney–Client Confidentiality: A "Philosophically Informed" and Comparative Approach to Legal and Medical Ethics, 36 *Case W. Res. L. Rev.* 177, 181, n.19 (1986).

147. *See, e.g.*, Moore, Professionalism Reconsidered, *supra* note 25.

148. *See, e.g.*, Arnold Relman, Salaried Physicians and Economic Incentives, 319 *N. Engl. J. Med.* 784 (1988).

149. *See supra* note 52.

150. *See supra* note 136 and accompanying text.

151. *See supra* notes 142–143 and accompanying text. This is not to say that lawyers should not make their views known and attempt to influence the development of other law that affects them, but rather that they ought not attempt to *preempt* other law by improperly characterizing the issue as one that is exclusively a matter of self-regulation. *Id.*

152. *See supra* note 88 and accompanying text. Thus, there is a crying need for a volume such as this one.

153. *See* Moore, The Usefulness of Ethical Codes, *supra* note 137, at 18–20.

9

Physicians' Conflicts of Interest in HMOs and Hospitals

Marc A. Rodwin

Much scholarly attention has been paid in recent years to physicians' conflicts of interest that arise from incentives to increase services. One familiar example is physician self-referral.[1] Congress has even started to regulate such conflicts. But much less attention has been given to conflicts of interest arising from incentives to decrease services. This is a newer problem, but in an era of cost containment it promises to be potentially more significant. This chapter examines the origins and significance of incentives for doctors to decrease services in HMOs and hospitals and documents how these incentives operate. It shows that such incentives are becoming pervasive and create serious conflicts of interest. It explores their dangers and argues that they can and should be dispensed with, both because they place patients at risk and compromise physicians and because existing institutions and laws are an inadequate safeguard.

My argument assumes that physicians have an obligation under medical ethics since they take the Hippocratic Oath to act in the interest of patients, indeed to make the patient's interest their first consideration.[2] It also relies on the concept of conflict of interest as used in the law, which has two ingredients: (1) an individual with an obligation, fiduciary or otherwise, and (2) the presence of conflicting interests that may undermine fulfillment of the obligation. Physicians have a conflict of interest when their interests or commitments compromise their loyalty to patients or the exercise of independent judgment on their patients' behalf. Two main types exist: (1) conflicts between a physician's personal interests (often financial) and the interests of the patient and (2) conflicts that divide a physician's loyalty between two or more patients or between a patient and a third party (or society).[3] My focus is on financial conflicts of interest.

As defined in law, conflicts of interest are distinct from breaches of obligation. Although law or ethics may require not entering into conflict-of-interest situations, this is done only to prevent acts wrong in themselves. Conflicts of interest can influence action, but they are not acts and do not ensure disloyalty. They do, however, increase the risk that physicians may abuse their trust. The least serious possible breach entails professional neglect: A compromised physician may not perform at his or her customary high level of competence, diligence, or effectiveness. At worst, physicians may knowingly exploit their position or harm patients. Extreme disloyalty obviously presents the more dramatic danger and is easier to identify. Situations that compromise independence, loyalty, or judgment more subtly or even unintentionally occur more frequently and are harder to recognize. Yet even compromised clinical judgment can bias physicians' advice and imperil patients.

Withholding Services: An Emerging Problem

Many policies that give physicians incentives to withhold services originate from private institutions and government agencies as responses to the distortions of fee-for-service medical practice.[4] A simple syllogism has governed policy: Giving physicians incentives to perform services produces undesirable effects. Ergo, eliminate these problems by giving physicians incentives to refrain from performing services—overuse of services. Only one thing was overlooked: Rewarding physicians for using resources frugally does not eliminate financial conflicts of interest. It creates new conflicts with different effects.

Attempts to limit services are often born of good intentions: to eliminate waste and to limit expenditure on medical care, thereby making it more affordable. We need to limit medical care expenditures because we seek goals besides health, and we do have budget constraints. But when we need medical care, we generally don't want our limited personal income to keep us from it. Most people do not want to pay for medical care out of pocket. Likewise, providers would prefer to avoid depending on out of pocket payment. So we spread the responsibility and financial risk through private insurance and government programs. This third-party involvement weakens incentives for individuals to monitor the costs of medical care and for providers to use or recommend services in a frugal way.[5]

Insurers and government programs now bear most of the direct financial burden of health care. As health care expenditures rise, they must raise premiums or taxes to pay the costs. And here, as everywhere, there are limits. As costs rise, more employees and employers limit their insurance coverage or do not purchase or provide insurance. And if taxes rise too much, the public will exert pressure on government.

These trends have prompted insurance companies and third-party payers to limit the outlays to HMOs and hospitals. Medicare now pays most hospitals a set fee per inpatient patient, depending on the diagnosis.[6] Sometimes Medicare pays HMOs through a similar fixed-payment system. In such arrangements the entity bears a portion of the financial risk.

HMOs and hospitals often pass the buck. They force physicians to carry some of the financial risk for recommending tests, performing medical procedures, and making referrals. Proponents say these incentives will persuade physicians to cut out wasteful tests and procedures, so everyone will benefit, even patients.[7] But the incentives discourage use of resources in general, resources that can also benefit patients.[8] Paying physicians to act as cost-control agents for third parties pits the interests of physicians against those of patients. It gets physicians to consider their own financial interests in balancing the concerns of the payers and patients. And it compromises the ability of physicians to offer patients disinterested professional advice.[9] Yet HMOs and hospitals now do precisely that. To see how this occurs, consider some of the incentive plans that HMOs and hospitals now use.

HMOs and Financial Incentives

HMOs provide comprehensive medical care to subscribers, using a closed panel of physicians. Members pay a fixed monthly premium and only nominal fees for services rendered (copayments).[10] HMOs perform two distinct functions: They insure subscribers by guaranteeing comprehensive medical care, and they deliver these services. Medical providers that charge for each service have an incentive to perform many services. HMOs do not. They incur costs by performing services but do not increase their revenue. They have an incentive to minimize services. Federal law and policy have promoted HMOs to increase public access to reasonably priced medical care; to reduce excessive, inappropriate ordering of medical services; and to reduce unnecessary federal spending.[11]

The first HMOs, now called "staff model HMOs," owned medical care facilities and employed a group of physicians on salary. But changes in health care markets spawned several variations. For example, group model HMOs contract with an organization that employs the physicians. "Network model HMOs" contract with two or more physician groups. Independent practice association (IPA)

HMOs contract with the IPA, which, in turn, contracts with physicians who have their own practices, offices, and non-HMO patients. Usually their primary care physicians are paid either a fee-for-service or by "capitation," that is, a set fee for each member for which the physician is responsible.[12]

The preferred provider organization (PPO) is a hybrid between IPA HMOs and traditional indemnity insurance plans that reimburse beneficiaries up to a set level for medical expenses they incur. Subscribers have the choice of receiving medical care from a closed panel of physicians, as in an IPA-style HMO with only nominal copayments. They can also receive treatment from any other physician they choose, as in indemnity insurance, if they make a significant copayment (usually about 20–30 percent of the fee). Insurance coverage kicks in only after the patient has paid a deductible.[13]

HMOs and PPOs are managed-care providers. They attempt to control standards of practice and referrals to specialists and to hospitals. The term "managed care" refers to HMOs, PPOs, and, increasingly, to most indemnity plans with management structures that control practice standards and referrals.[14] Managed-care providers attempt to organize systematically the use of medical care and the manner in which it is delivered in order to achieve explicit objectives. The objectives can range from reducing expenditure and the use of services to expanding the range of services provided or improving patients' quality of life. Managing care requires restricting patients' choice of providers and medical options and physicians' clinical autonomy. Both the physician and the patient are managed.

The management is usually done by physicians, nurses, and trained administrative staff. It involves the use of medical protocols to assess clinical decisions, the use of primary care physicians as gatekeepers to control referrals to specialists, individual case managers to coordinate medical care in complex and expensive cases, the use of retrospective reviews of utilization of services and denial of payment for inappropriate services, and a host of other devices. The crucial factor is that choices traditionally made exclusively within the patient–physician relationship are explicitly controlled by organizational and institutional arrangements.

Staff model HMOs are a classic example of managed-care providers because such HMOs can effectively exercise control over all physicians they employ in a single location. However, the advent of utilization review, which allows insurers to monitor the behavior of physicians, now makes it possible to manage care in other ways as well. Insurance companies now offer preferred provider plans that give patients some choice of physicians, with discounts if they choose preferred providers. To be preferred, a physician must practice in what the insurance company deems to be a cost-effective manner. Here we focus on HMOs. But physicians working for other managed-care providers often face similar conflicts of interest.

Over time, physicians have developed practice styles based on fee-for-service incentives that encourage high utilization of medical services.[15] These practice styles are now deeply ingrained; many people believe they persist even when physicians are paid by salary. To counter them and reduce inappropriate use of medical services, HMO managers use several administrative techniques. They make primary care physicians gatekeepers who coordinate medical treatment and approve referrals to specialists. They monitor physicians' clinical decisions, determine their appropriateness, and deny payment for unnecessary medical care. And doctors often need to receive administrative authorization before admitting patients to hospitals.

HMOs and Physician Risk Sharing

Most HMOs also use payment incentives to tie the interests of physicians to the financial goals of the organization. They frequently make physicians—particularly primary care physicians—bear part of the financial risk for providing services, so that their incomes decrease as the cost of treating patients rises.[16] HMOs and physicians carry two kinds of risk for the cost of medical care: one for the clinical decisions physicians make and another for the health status of their patients. They can reduce their exposure by reducing the amount of services provided or by choosing healthier patients (who are less expensive to treat). Such incentives encourage physicians to ask themselves "How much will this cost me?" before providing or recommending medical services. As a result, physicians may recommend too little medical care.

Physicians can bear financial risk in an almost unlimited number of ways. But all risk-sharing plans rely on common approaches. One way is to compensate physicians by capitation. In this system, doctors' incomes are fixed by the number of patients they have; providing additional services to these patients reduces their time and resources.

HMOs often link risk-sharing payment to the primary care physician's role as a gatekeeper. Gatekeepers are supposed to coordinate medical care to eliminate unnecessary services and properly channel appropriate ones. They determine what specialty care patients receive, and some HMOs will not pay for or provide services without their approval. Many HMOs make primary care physicians responsible for part of the costs of specialty care, laboratory tests, and hospital care. This gives them an incentive to reduce their referrals. Without such incentives, primary care physicians, paid by salary or capitation, have an indirect incentive to substitute treatment by specialists for work they could perform themselves.

HMOs can, and often do, make primary care physicians bear risk for referrals whether they are paid by capitation, salary, or fee-for-service. Many HMOs withhold part of the basic payment to primary care physicians and make them forfeit the payment if HMO costs exceed targets. HMOs also often pay a bonus to physicians who refer frugally. Frequently HMOs use both bonuses and financial penalties. These two approaches are often contrasted as a payment and a penalty, a carrot and a stick. In both cases, physicians can increase their income by making clinical decisions that reduce services and lower the costs of the HMO. Sometimes the HMO looks only to the use of services and referrals of physicians individually. At other times, HMOs base their bonus payments on the performance of a group of physicians or on the HMO's profitability.[17]

Risk-sharing is the norm in HMOs.[18] A 1987 study by the Group Health Association of America, an HMO trade association, found that 85 percent of HMOs used financial incentives for physicians. Approximately two-thirds withheld part of physicians' fees, salary, or capitation payments—usually not more than 20–30 percent of the base pay—and returned all or part of the funds withheld later, depending on the amount and cost of referrals.[19]

A study of HMOs in Medicare's risk-contracting program found that 29 percent shared both profits and losses with physicians, 21 percent shared only profits, and 20 percent shared only losses.[20] Most studies estimate that 13–18 percent of HMOs distribute funds based on individual physician performance. But one study found that at least 60 percent of HMOs used individual physician performance, at least in part, to determine the level of incentive payments.[21]

Elements of Risk Sharing

Five features of risk-sharing plans limit the financial risk and resulting incentives: (1) the risk pool size; (2) whether physicians risk loss or stand to profit; (3) the services for which physicians bear risk; (4) the extent of risk sharing and whether there is any cap on potential profit and loss; and (5) how profits or losses are distributed among physicians.

Risk Pool Size. HMOs can force physicians to bear risk for their use of medical referrals alone or pool the risk among other physicians in their department, health center, or some other unit. Physicians who bear the risk individually sustain the consequences of their clinical decisions. Those who bear the risk collectively see the consequences of their actions spread among the group and share the consequences of their colleagues' actions. The greater the number of physicians in a risk pool, the smaller each one's pro rata share. The larger the group, the less financial risk physicians bear for their own decisions.

Some HMOs spread financial risk based on a combination of individual and collective risk pools. For example, they may create two risk pools: one collective and one for each physician. A surplus in the collective risk pool will be distributed, but only to physicians who have a surplus in their individual risk pools.

Profit and/or Loss Sharing. HMOs can share both loss and profit. Many HMOs reduce physicians' income when the volume of the services and referrals exceeds a target. A typical arrangement is to set a base payment (either salary, capitation, or fee-for-service) and to hold a portion of this payment (typically about 20 percent) in an escrow account. The funds set aside are released to physicians at the end of the year only if the individual physician or the physicians as a group did not provide more than the projected number of services. If physicians used more services than expected, the HMO draws on the withheld funds to cover the increased costs. The greater the amount by which services performed exceed the target, the greater the proportion of the withheld funds the HMO uses to cover its costs.

HMOs use similar strategies for sharing profits. They often provide bonuses when the volume of physicians' clinical tests and referrals falls below a target. HMOs frequently rely on both carrot and stick approaches. They establish a base pay and set aside a percentage that will cover losses from high use of services. If use of services is lower than targeted, they also pay bonuses.

Risk Sharing for Different Services. HMOs can make physicians bear risk for the cost of several different types of services: primary care, diagnostic tests, specialty care, drugs, hospitalization, and nursing facilities. Some HMOs give physicians the option of assuming risk for certain services.[22] HMOs usually place physicians at risk for the cost of some services but not others. They can also establish one kind of risk sharing for one service and a different kind for another service. The more services for which a primary care physician is responsible, the more risk born and the stronger the incentive to reduce services.

Limiting Risk and Profit. Usually HMOs limit the risk born by physicians, establishing a threshold for loss and placing caps on the profits that can be earned. Stop-loss and profit-cap provisions help temper the effect of incentives. The aim is to prevent the cost of caring for seriously ill patients from placing undue financial pressure on physicians and to prevent physicians' desire for personal gain from unduly tempting them to reduce medical services. Typically, HMOs limit the risk of loss or profit to 20 percent of the base income, but policies vary. One approach is to set a cap on the loss for each patient. Another caps each doctor's financial loss for his entire pool of patients. A third varies each physician's upper limit on financial risk for different kinds of services, setting one limit for referral services, another limit for hospital services, and so forth.

Distribution of Profit and Loss. HMOs can distribute the profit or loss to physicians in several ways. Most risk-sharing plans concern primary care physicians. However, specialists can share in the savings or deficits.[23] Risk-sharing plans can distribute the profit or loss based on individual or group performance, or a combination of both. Distributions may also reflect the number of patients, the physician's seniority in the HMO, or stock ownership. Profits are distributed quarterly or yearly, or on retirement, as part of a deferred compensation plan.

The more frequently HMOs evaluate and reward physicians, the fewer clinical decisions and patients are involved. And this links financial reward closely to individual clinical choices. In addition, when physicians receive payments soon after taking specific actions, there is also a clear link between performance and reward. The more directly rewards are linked to action, the stronger the inducement.[24]

Some Risk-Sharing Plans

As an example of an HMO risk-sharing plan, consider United Healthcare in Seattle, Washington, operated by the Safeco Insurance Company.[25] United Healthcare paid each primary care physician a set monthly fee for each patient to compensate them for providing or arranging all medical care. At the end of the year, the doctor shared any remaining funds with Safeco and was partially responsible for any deficit. But risk sharing was limited. Depending on the size of the physician's practice, the risk of loss was capped at 5–10 percent of reimbursed charges. Profit sharing was limited to 10–50 percent of reimbursed charges. In addition, to prevent distortions due to a few patients needing unusually expensive medical care, each physician's risk was limited to $5,000 per patient per year. Physicians paid on a fee-for-service basis (i.e., specialists) had a separate incentive plan. If United Healthcare ran a deficit, payment could be lowered to 85 percent of the ordinary fee. With a surplus, payments would be adjusted upward to 105 percent of ordinary charges. In 1979, slightly over half of physicians realized year-end surpluses. The average was $413 and the highest surplus was $5,000. The average deficit was $169 and the highest was $1,833. Despite these financial incentives, the HMO was unsuccessful and eventually went out of business.

Another such plan is Bluechoice, owned by Blue Cross/Blue Shield of Missouri.[26] As of 1988, Bluechoice made primary care physicians gatekeepers, responsible for coordinating all specialty care. It paid primary care physicians by capitation, and provided financial penalties and rewards to encourage them to reduce the amount of services they provide. Bluechoice withheld 20 percent of each physician's capitation payment and placed it in a pooled risk fund (PRF). The PRF was used to fund a portion of catastrophic patient care (i.e., care costing over $50,000). It was also used to fund unanticipated costs of hospital and specialists' services. Unused funds were returned to contributing physicians.

Bluechoice created a specialty comprehensive referral fund (CRF) for each physician's office. This fund was used to pay for the cost of each office's services provided by hospitals, specialists, and laboratories. The funds placed in the CRF were based on the anticipated usage of these services by each physician's patient group calculated using the patient's age, gender, and other factors. If a physician exhausted his CRF, the 20 percent withheld from that physician's office, set aside in the PRF, was used to cover the costs. If the sum was exhausted, remaining PRF funds, contributed by other physicians, were used. If a surplus existed in the CRF at the end of the year, primary care physicians split the surplus with Bluechoice, up to a maximum bonus of $50 per patient per year.[27] Depending on the HMO's finances and the clinical decisions made by physicians, Bluechoice paid primary care internists between $55,334 and $185,426.[28] The clinical decisions made by physicians on the scope and amount of services and referrals provided to their patients could increase their net income more than threefold.

The Physician's Perspective

In effect, doctors paid under risk-sharing arrangements participate in a joint venture with HMOs. By keeping costs down for the HMO, doctors promote their own financial well-being. Dr. Robert Berenson, an internist, explained the effect well: "Long accustomed to providing too much . . . medical care, physicians now have powerful incentives to withhold [it]."[29] This is because risk sharing offers doctors no economic incentive to be aggressive in providing services and even reduces their income as they increase the number of tests and procedures they order. Doctors make daily clinical decisions that can reduce the medical risk to patients but increase the costs of HMOs. Under risk-sharing arrangements they may be reluctant to do so. From the doctors' perspective, they are paying for part of every consultation, test, ancillary service, or hospital care a patient receives. Their share may be small, but the incentive can change perceptions.

Berenson recounts the change in attitude he underwent in caring for an elderly woman with a rare form of cancer when he was paid under risk-sharing arrangements. She represented an economic loss, and he "ended up resenting the seemingly unending medical needs of the patient and the continuing demands . . . [of] her distraught family."[30] The problem was not the patient's requests or performing the work. But under the risk sharing system, very sick patients devastated his accounts. Risk sharing makes "patients who come in often for care from me . . . or who want a referral for specialty care begin to look like abusers."[31] Many doctors adjust to these new financial rules, but others don't. Dr. Devra Marcus, a Washington internist, left her HMO practice just after joining. Her first two patients were diabetic, and she referred them to an ophthalmologist to check for retinal changes because diabetes can lead to blindness if not treated. Following these referrals, a colleague told her that her use of specialists would reduce her referral fund and could reduce her salary. "I pulled out. I didn't want to think about whether I would be losing money if I ordered an ophthalmologic consultation. I wanted to think about what was best for the patients."[32] Something is perverse in a payment system when it makes well-intentioned physicians consider sick patients they treat as a drain on their income.

Gauging the Effect of Financial Incentives

There is little hard data linking the effects of financial incentives to physicians' clinical decisions. One study found no relation between distribution of risk-sharing bonuses and physicians' referral decisions. But paying physicians by capitation led to lower rates of hospitalization, and placing physicians at financial risk was associated with lower rates of outpatient visits.[33] HMO managers generally believe that withholding funds and bonuses affects doctors' clinical decisions. A 1989 survey of the managing directors of 643 HMOs found that nearly four-fifths believed that withholding 5–30 percent of payment would affect the volume of tests ordered and elective hospitalization, and nearly one-half believed that bonuses of 5–15 percent would also affect clinical choices. Over one-third expressed concern at withholding payments between 15–30 percent. But managers in general believed that the incentive payments used by other HMOs were more worrisome than the incentives they used.[34]

As we shall see in more detail later, several patients have sued HMOs, claiming that risk-sharing incentives led physicians to withhold necessary services to their detriment. And many anecdotes suggest cause for concern. In an article on HMOs "earning more for doing less," the Associated Press reported the example of Dr. Denise Hart, a nephrologist. She recalls a patient who had kidney failure and spent the night in a hospital without dialysis or seeing a nephrologist because the HMO primary care physician denied authorization even though the emergency room physician informed him of the urgency. During the night the patient suffered from cardiac arrest and had to spend a week on a respirator.[35]

The *Chicago Tribune* reported the case of Daniel Bohnen, who was accidentally shot in the face with shotgun pellets. Shortly before he was scheduled for emergency surgery to repair his right eye, the HMO business office called and insisted that a consultant confirm the need for surgery. The surgeon warned the HMO that a delay would endanger Daniel's vision, but the HMO insisted on the second opinion, in the consultant's words, "to save money." The result: Daniel lost vision in one eye, and the HMO later paid Daniel's parents $1.2 million to settle the malpractice suit they brought.[36]

Presumably, HMO doctors serving as consultants, reviewers, and gatekeepers will place the patient's interest first, but the payment mechanism can define loyalties. Dr. J. Kristin Olson-Garewal, former medical director of University Family Care, an HMO in Tucson, Arizona, told of her role convincing doctors to substitute less costly medications. Asked if this might conflict with her obligations as a physician she replied, "When I became the medical director, I represented the payment entity."[37]

In the absence of definitive data on the effect of risk-sharing incentive payments, we must draw inferences from what we know about the effects of incentives in general. In theory, plans with strong financial incentives for reducing services are more likely to compromise physicians' loyalty to patients than plans with weak incentives. Physicians face greater temptations from strong incentives. And incentives are strong in several circumstances: when physicians bear risk individually or in a small risk pool, when they are at risk for expensive services, when stop-risk protection starts at a high level, when HMOs link penalties and bonuses directly to individual clinical decisions, and when physicians risk losing or gaining a large percentage of their baseline income.

While it is relatively easy to isolate factors that affect the financial risk of physicians, it is hard to determine the dollar value to a physician of any incentive arrangement. Dollar value depends on several factors noted earlier: the size of the risk pool, the extent of risk sharing and stop loss, the services for which physicians bear risk, how the profit or loss is distributed, and whether there is profit and/or loss sharing.

Another reason why dollar value resists definition is that risk-sharing incentives do not reward physicians each time they forego a service or referral. Indeed, it is impossible to identify all the possible services physicians avoid. Nor do risk-sharing plans penalize physicians for each service they use. Rather, they pay out benefits or impose penalties only if doctors perform more than a specified number of medical procedures or make more than a specified number of referrals. Even under incentive plans in which physicians bear risk individually, physicians cannot know whether or not they will be penalized until after tallying all their referrals, their patients hospitalized, their orders for tests, and so forth.

Even when a physician's utilization of services exceeds a threshold that triggers the financial incentive, the cost to the physician of a decision depends on the total volume of utilization. The same clinical decision has different financial implications, depending on the choices the physician makes for all patients before and afterward. When risk-sharing plans spread risk among a group of physicians, it is very difficult, if not impossible, for physicians to predict the cost to them of performing a service. Together, these factors make it hard to determine precisely how strong an incentive there is for physicians to withhold a particular service.

Still other factors—for example, the fees, salary, or capitation rate paid by an HMO—can affect how physicians will respond to risk sharing. If the base level is low, physicians will be more sensitive to financial incentives than if the base level is high and allows them to earn a comfortable income without profit sharing or despite any financial penalties.[38] Some physicians also work exclusively for an HMO, while others do so only part-time and earn income from outside practice. The more a physician relies on an outside practice for income, the smaller the bonus or penalty he will receive from the HMO and the less sensitive he will be to the HMO's financial incentives.

Despite the complexities of determining the effects of particular clinical choices under risk-sharing plans, physicians know that it is generally in their financial interest to limit the number of procedures, tests, and referrals. And even when the risk borne by individual physicians is small, incentives may create group pressure to use resources frugally, with ripple effects that spread beyond those caused by the financial incentive alone.[39] Most HMOs inform physicians when they deviate from the norm and use services heavily. The message is reinforced, explicitly and implicitly, on a regular basis. Physicians are also aware of the total amount of income they can gain or lose. One suspects that doctors contracting with or employed by an HMO will, over time, develop an intuitive sense of what style of medical practice best serves their interest. Their practice style will reflect the incentives offered by the HMOs.

Although economic theory suggests that strong incentives to reduce services place patients at greater risk than weak incentives, the effect of small incentives may outweigh their size, especially when applied to every clinical decision physicians make. Even small rewards can shift perceptions and attitudes. Payment also has symbolic value. It can bond physicians to payers, producing commitments disproportionate to the sums of money involved.

Hospitals and Financial Incentives

Until recently, hospitals had strong incentives to increase the number of services they provide and to disregard costs, since they were paid based on their cost of providing services. Medicare was particularly generous. In reimbursing hospitals for their costs, which included overhead and capital, Medicare fueled expansion and high utilization of services and technology.

But that has changed. Since 1983, Medicare has paid hospitals a set fee per patient, depending on the principal diagnosis. This prospective payment system uses what are called "diagnosis related groups ("DRGs")" to determine fees. The DRG payment is based on the average cost of treating the patients in each group of diagnoses.[40] Medicare makes an exception for unusually high-cost patients, paying one-half of the cost beyond the DRG payment. But in general, hospitals are at risk for the full costs of medical care. If their costs are, on average, higher than their revenues, they will run a deficit. If, on average, hospitals keep their costs lower than revenues, they will profit. These changes reverse previous incentives and make it in hospitals' interest to use resources frugally. Medicaid and private insurers have not yet adopted similar fixed payment systems. But they now monitor hospital charges closely and refuse to pay for services they believe are inappropriate or could be just as well delivered at lower cost outside the hospital.

The economic interests of hospitals and physicians are often at odds with each other.[41] Most physicians are still paid for each service and have an incentive to increase services. Physicians are not responsible for hospital costs, although they contribute to them by using hospital facilities and ordering tests. Routine clinical decisions, such as when to discharge patients, also affect costs. In response, hospitals now encourage physicians to take account of the hospitals' financial interests in practicing medicine. Hospitals often inform physicians of treatment costs, especially when physicians make clinical decisions that cost the hospital more than the average amount.[42] When they do, studies show, doctors order fewer and less costly diagnostic tests.[43] Hospitals monitor physicians and use persuasion to encourage frugality.

Hospitals have also devised programs that encourage physicians to reduce the services they provide. These include physician investment and self-referral in joint ventures, hospital purchases of physicians' practices, and physician recruitment and bonding programs. Variations of these practices include plans that make direct incentive payments to physicians, joint ventures with hospital staffs, physician ownership of hospitals through limited partnership, and economic credentialing.[44]

The most infamous hospital incentive plan is one devised for doctors by the Paracelsus Healthcare Corporation at its Hollywood Community Hospital in 1985. The hospital shared with physicians the difference between hospital charges, based on costs, and the Medicare DRG payment. What made the Paracelsus strategy different from others is that any resulting profit was shared with the physicians if they provided less treatment and discharged patients earlier. The greater the hospital profit, the larger the physician incentive payment. Critics charged that the Paracelsus plan provided too strong an incentive to withhold appropriate medical care, and it was discontinued after government investigations.[45] Congress later enacted legislation that prohibited hospitals receiving Medicare funds from making payments that gave physicians an incentive to reduce medical care for an individual patient.[46]

A number of other hospitals have become interested in incentive plans. Central DuPage Hospital in Infield, Illinois, made plans to develop a deferred compensation plan using incentives for reducing care. The hospital planned to pay physicians additional compensation based on their performance and several other criteria, including average length of patient stay and use of ancillary services for each patient. Each physician's "efficiency" performance would be compared to the revenues generated by treating patients. Physicians using fewer resources than average, or discharging patients earlier than average, would receive credit. The compensation was to be invested by the hospital and paid on each physician's retirement; however it was never put into effect.

Under another physician incentive plan—the so-called Medical Staff Hospital (MeSH) joint venture—the hospital would make incentive payments to physicians. As proposed, the medical staff would form a joint venture with the hospital. The hospital would make incentive payments to physicians if the cost of treating Medicare patients was less than a certain percentage of costs.[47] The incentive for reducing services would be spread across the medical staff, presumably diluting the incentive for each physician individually.

Hospitals and medical staff often undertake joint ventures. Such ventures have certain common features. They "harmonize the economic interest of hospitals and physicians," according to Robert Rosenfield, a lawyer who specializes in these issues.[48] Hospitals use these ventures to acquire or "capture" the loyalty of local physicians who control admissions and utilization of medical services.[49] One wonders how patients will fare if their interests conflict with those of physicians and hospitals once the latter two are "harmonized."

Hospitals also try to influence physicians by hiring medical staff organizations as part of a utilization review program. The organization reviews records to determine the appropriateness of admissions and treatment and to help teach physicians how to reduce unnecessary use of resources. Sometimes hospitals pay physicians on the basis of their cost savings, thus giving physicians an incentive to reduce their use of resources.[50]

Another trend is for privately owned hospitals to syndicate themselves and sell shares to local physicians.[51] Physician investment takes several forms. Frequently, a hospital corporation will retain a majority share in the facility and sell off the remainder as limited partnerships to local physicians. At other times, hospital employees own shares through employee stock ownership plans.[52] Physician owners have an incentive to admit patients to the hospital but also to reduce the services they provide to Medicare patients because their payment is fixed in advance.

Still another emerging trend is for hospitals to deny or revoke the admitting privileges of physicians based on the expense to hospitals of their clinical decisions.[53] Though an indirect measure, the power to cut off the means to a livelihood is a serious economic threat. In the past, hospital bylaws only authorized the administration to grant and revoke medical staff privileges on the basis of clinical competence and the quality of medical care. Now many hospitals are evaluating physicians in financial terms. Some lawyers recommend that hospitals revise their bylaws and credentialing process to give them the power to deny, limit, or revoke privileges to physicians whose clinical decisions result in hospitals losing or earning little money under Medicare's prospective payment system.[54] The lawyers suggest that hospitals develop economic profiles of physicians by compiling information about patients' average lengths of stay. Hospitals could conceivably terminate physicians who deviate from an acceptable standard.[55]

An American Hospital Association (AHA) study indicates that a negligible number of hospitals—only 1 percent—have bylaws that require physicians applying for admitting privileges to submit information on the cost effectiveness of the medical care they provide. Slightly more hospitals use financial profiles based on cost of treatment in renewing physician privileges. But some commentators believe these programs are destined to grow significantly in the future. The programs typically look at patients' length of stay, the number of medical tests the physician ordered, and the use of other resources that affect hospitals' costs. Despite the label "cost-effective," the programs generally do not examine the clinical impact of resource decisions. In effect, they evaluate physicians for behavior that reduces costs with little attention to benefits.

Hospitals also provide incentives for physicians to use resources frugally through their "bonding programs." Bonding programs include recruitment incentives, income guarantees, rent subsidies, advertising, patient referral programs, and in-kind services, and they are called bonding programs because they seek loyalty from physicians with admitting privileges. Although bonding programs do not specifically reward physicians for reducing medical services, they indebt physicians to hospitals for income and thereby encourage them to promote the hospitals' goals. Bonding programs have traditionally been used to induce patient admissions, but this situation is changing. In some cases, such as patient referral programs, hospitals already explicitly exclude so called high-cost physicians.[56] With the increasing emphasis on containing hospital costs, physicians indebted to hospitals are apt to provide fewer services to Medicare patients and to discharge them earlier.

The Dangers of Financial Incentives

The Corrosive Effects of Risk-Sharing Incentives

The practice of risk sharing poses a danger. Society makes a statement about the role of physicians when it provides incentives for them to help government or health care organizations reduce their costs, especially if there are no equivalent financial incentives for physicians to improve the quality of care. By using financial incentives to change the clinical practice of physicians, society endorses and calls forth self-interested behavior. In asking physicians to consider their own interest in deciding how to act, we alter the kinds of responses and attitudes we want physicians ideally to have. For if physicians act intu-itively to promote their patients' interests, we will worry less that they will behave inappropriately. But if their motivation is primarily self-interest, we will want their behavior to be monitored more carefully.

Incentives also undermine other values, such as informed consent. Law and ethics now require physicians to inform patients of the risks and benefits of any proposed treatment, alternatives, and nontreatment. To fulfill this role, physi-cians must provide patients with disinterested assessment and advice. They must explain the major choices and their implications in a manner understand-able to the layperson. But rewarding physicians for reducing services tends to compromise their ability to give disinterested advice. It is likely to shape their views of what kinds of activities are desirable.[57] And even if many individual doctors rise above the lure of incentives and provide neutral advice, patients will still have reasons to doubt their neutrality. This alone weakens the informed consent process. For although patients are ultimately responsible for deciding what medical care to accept, the process of making medical decisions involves communication, cooperation, and trust between patient and physician. If patients doubt the neutrality of their doctors, that process is impaired.

Physicians, like others, will always have private interests that may influence their judgment. But we can encourage institutions to temper self-interest, chan-nel it in socially desirable ways, and counter it.

The Problem with Hospital Incentives to Physicians

Hospitalized patients rely on physicians to act on their behalf more than other patients do. Usually the patients are weak or severely ill and lack the autonomy of patients living outside of hospitals. Ordinarily, they cannot switch physicians in mid-treatment. When hospitals pay physicians to promote the hospital's financial goals, this compromises physicians' loyalty to vulnerable patients.

Hospitals already enjoy an advantage over patients in competing for the loyalty of physicians. Patients consult doctors when they have a medical problem—just once in a while. Physicians have many patients, and each patient can augment a doctor's income by only a small amount compared to the total earned. The economic influence each patient exerts over a physician is small. And so, physi-cians have to divide their loyalty, or at least their time, between patients. But the relation between hospitals and physicians is entirely different. Most physicians have frequent, ongoing, and long-term relations with just a few hospitals.[58] Hospitals depend on physicians to admit patients, and many physicians, in turn, need hospital privileges to earn their livelihood. Physicians' clinical decisions affect hospital costs, hospital referrals, and other economic ties, which can, in turn, benefit physicians. Individual patients will come and go, but a doctor has to work with a small number of hospitals.

In short, even though there are growing tensions in their relations, hospitals and physicians increasingly depend on each other for employment and income and rely on each other's cooperation to make work manageable. Their relationship is one of economic symbiosis. Each party must work with, watch, court, and cater to the other. It is essential to both parties to promote good long-term relations with the other. How unlike the relations between physicians and their patients! Even though physicians are expected to be loyal to patients, hospitals have far greater leverage over physicians' decisions than do patients and far greater economic clout. These factors skew the relationship between hospitals, physicians, and patients in favor of common interests between hospitals and physicians—interests that can conflict with those of patients. As a result, hospitals and physicians often do not fully respect the rights of patients. The hospital has even been called "a human rights wasteland."[59] Hospital incentive plans did not create this structural imbalance between hospitals, physicians, and patients, but they are not neutral. They undermine physician loyalty to patients even further.

Are Physician Incentives Effective or Necessary?

Many HMO managers fear that without economic incentives for reducing the use of services, nothing will ensure that physicians use resources prudently.[60] They say that other approaches, such as administrative monitoring and penalties for overuse, are less effective.[61] They also discount the possibility that these incentives will encourage physicians to provide too few services. Peer review and quality assurance programs, they argue, would identify and deter underservice arising from other incentives that encourage overuse.[62]

If incentives to provide services cause physicians to use too many resources and to perform unnecessary procedures, would not incentives to reduce services result in too few services? If financial incentives do encourage physicians to reduce their services, will physicians reduce only unnecessary or wasteful services? Why should incentives have negative effects in one respect but not the other?

If peer review and quality assurance review programs can adequately control underservice, why can they not adequately control overuse? If administrative reviews of physicians' practices effectively identify and limit one kind of practice, then they should prove effective in the other. And if they are ineffective in one setting, why should we not suspect their efficacy in another?

No substantial evidence supports the claim that incentive plans are necessary to control use of services. The first HMOs did not use financial incentives to reduce the volume of services, and they significantly reduced hospitalization—with no discernible harm to patients.[63] Incentive plans did not even exist a few years ago. Other, more suitable methods for controlling unnecessary use of services exist; new ones can be developed.

Proponents of risk sharing acknowledge that strong incentives can produce negative effects, and they would prohibit such incentives. However, all risk-sharing and incentive plans compromise physician loyalty. There is no natural or easily identifiable threshold level for determining when incentives become too strong. Moreover, there are great obstacles to regulating risk-sharing and incentive plans based on the amount of risk borne. The danger of particular arrangements depends on the probability and extent of risk. Both are influenced by many factors—not by their broad structural features. So many different variations of risk-sharing plans exist that it would be impractical to evaluate each one, to distinguish the acceptable from the unacceptable, and harder still to monitor and regulate them—a quagmire of unknown dimensions.

Proponents also argue that the negative effects of incentives can be mitigated by spreading the total risk among a pool of physicians, limiting the risk assumed by any individual.[64] These measures could reduce the size of the incentive and prevent undue influence in clinical decision-making. Here, too, proponents of risk sharing want to have it both ways. They argue that if incentives are weak, no harm will be done. But even if weak, incentives will—they say—produce desirable changes in physician behavior. However, if incentives are strong enough to produce desirable changes, they could produce undesirable changes.[65]

Financial Incentives That Help Patients

Not all physician incentives are undesirable. Incentives rewarding behavior that promotes patients' interests should be encouraged. So should incentives that promote other desirable goals and do not compromise loyalty to patients. For example, HMOs and hospitals can use financial incentives to encourage physicians to provide high-quality care, devote extra hours of service, perform particularly hard or unpleasant work, produce high patient satisfaction, undertake research or publications, develop their skill and competence, or assume essential administrative duties.

HMOs and hospitals might also use incentives to encourage physicians to practice efficiently, that is, use the fewest resources needed to achieve a result. Many HMOs and hospitals claim they do just that. Their incentives, however, are usually designed only to reduce expenditures, which does not necessarily make a practice more efficient—it may reduce the benefits. Incentives to reduce the volume of services do not target waste. They discourage all services, not just inappropriate ones. To encourage efficient physician practices, HMOs should offer incentives directed to particular practices.

Effective incentive plans could build on existing peer review, often called "quality assurance" or "utilization review programs." Hospitals employ peer review organizations (PROs) to review patients' charts and evaluate the appropriateness of medical care. Often, third-party payers will deny payment for inappropriate medical procedures. HMOs use quality assurance programs to identify inappropriate underuse of medical care. Hospitals and HMOs could hire evaluators to review patients' charts and identify both inappropriate provision and denial of services. HMOs and third-party payers could then pay physicians bonuses if they made no, or very few, errors and impose penalties for overuse and underuse of services. Such incentives would discourage both skimping and waste, would reward physicians for providing good medical care, and would not undermine fidelity to patients. Reviewers could be independent experts unaffiliated with the hospital or HMO; the identity of the physicians evaluated would be kept confidential. At least two IPA HMOs, U.S. Healthcare and Ad-Med, have developed physician payment plans that include incentives both for reducing utilization and for promoting some measure of quality in care.[66] The plans attempt to counter incentives for quality with incentives for reducing services and are therefore preferable to incentives for reducing services alone. But neither program balances both incentives equally.

U.S. Healthcare has used several variations on its quality incentive formula. Initially, U.S. Healthcare paid primary care physicians by capitation. The payment plan included two main components: incentives for reducing services and incentives for so-called quality measures. The lower the volume of services each physician performed, the higher the capitation rate and the more frequently it was paid. The capitation rate was also adjusted upward or downward based on quality of care. Quality was measured by a review of medical records, results of patient satisfaction surveys, transfer rates out of physicians' offices, and what it called an assessment of physicians' "managed-care philosophy."

U.S. Healthcare reviewed medical records to determine whether physicians immunized infants, measured the blood pressure of high-risk individuals, and screened for high cholesterol. The patient survey asked about physician availability, waiting time, patient satisfaction with office personnel, and whether the physician appeared concerned with patients' welfare. Physicians received high or low scores on managed-care philosophy, depending on whether they used preventive care programs, participated in quality assurance advisory or membership committees, and helped patients receive high-quality care.

This program was headed in the right direction, but incentives were still skewed.[67] Physicians were not penalized for reducing services inappropriately, except for a few specified services included in the quality measures. There were too few of these measures, so inappropriate reduction of services was still rewarded. Incentives to reduce services overshadowed incentives to increase them. U.S. Healthcare's quality incentives encouraged only low-cost services, such as immunization, testing for cholesterol level, and blood pressure checks in high-risk groups. No direct financial incentive spurred the use of valuable but costly services. Moreover, many of the incentives for quality focused on patient satisfaction and participation in quality-review administrative work, which do not involve rewards for physicians providing services. Such incentives do not counteract conflicts of interest that discourage referrals to specialists and hospitals. They simply add incentives to provide patients with different low-cost services and keep them satisfied.

Measures of patient satisfaction and transfer rates out of a practice provide useful information to HMOs and can indicate quality problems. But they are also marketing tactics. They do not touch the most crucial aspects of medical care, and they do not encourage the provision of services most likely to be reduced by physician risk sharing. They do encourage physicians to play a role that sociologist Erving Goffman calls "cooling out the mark" (i.e., acting to reduce the patient's anger and frustration).[68] Physicians may please patients by reducing office waiting time and adopting a friendly, caring manner. They can help to prevent patients from choosing another provider due to frustration with the HMO, perhaps because of reduced services. Incentives to keep patients satisfied are generally desirable.[69] But when affirmed in conjunction with incentives to reduce services, they may help cover up, rather than eliminate, inappropriate reductions in medical care.

In 1992, U.S. Healthcare adopted a more complex compensation formula.[70] Multiple factors affect the payment doctors will receive, including quality measures. Still, each doctor's capitation rate can be adjusted upward by 5 percent if his or her patients' use of hospitals, specialists, and emergency rooms is low and downward by 2.5 percent if utilization exceeds targets. As with the previous formula, quality measures provide some check on utilization. But incentives still exist to use services frugally.

Incentives for Physicians to Allocate Scarce Resources

Using markets and administrative mechanisms, society limits the resources used for medical care. Budget constraints impinge on social goals. Increasingly, spending on medicine requires spending less on other desirable social goods, and beyond a certain point, further spending for medicine produces diminishing returns. Physicians are strategically situated to help society control medical expenditures because their clinical choices affect the allocation of resources. But resource allocation is at odds with physicians' traditional obligation: to act in the interests of their patients.

Physicians can play three distinct roles: (1) they can act as ideal fiduciaries, promoting their patients' interests without regard to those of other parties;[71] (2) they can act as neutral resource allocators, distributing resources to maximize social benefit or promote some principle of fairness; and (3) they can promote their own financial interests or those of third parties, such as HMOs or hospitals. Medical ethics adjures physicians to act as their patients' agents. But most physicians perform all three conflicting roles at different times.

As ideal fiduciaries, physicians have to promote the interests of their immediate patients even if the same resources could produce more good for still other patients. But physicians who treat a group of patients in triage or under severe budget constraints usually focus treatment on a few because very ill patients will die regardless of treatment, and patients with minor problems will survive and heal even if treatment is delayed or foregone. Doctors treat first those patients who would die without medical intervention. In triage, physicians' obligation to promote the best interests of each patient conflict with their obligation to care for all patients. Here, doctors must balance the interests of one patient against those of others.

Some countries control medical spending by imposing regional or hospital budgets that place physicians in a position similar to triage. Some Canadian provinces, for example, assign hospitals a budget for all patient care. To stay within the budget, hospitals set their own priorities on allocating funds. In this system, doctors have to consider the good of patients collectively. So, too, does this happen in Britain, where doctors have to make difficult decisions on how to use resources because the National Health Service has a limited budget.[72] Physicians working in staff model HMOs occupy a similar position. With limited resources, they must make difficult choices in caring for their patients. Too many resources donated to one kind of care or patient will leave less available to others or even threaten the solvency of the HMO.

Physicians caring for a group of patients under budgetary constraints cannot act as ideal fiduciaries; they are expected to adjudicate the allocation of resources. Even though this creates risks for patients, it also provides benefits. In theory, clinical choices and allocative choices are distinct; in practice, they merge. If physicians don't act as allocators, others will. This will constrain clinical choices and interfere with physician discretion. But since medicine constantly involves uncertainty, trade-offs, and conflicting goals, the art of doctoring requires discretion and subtlety of judgment.

To illustrate the risk to patients, consider a range of ways to pay physicians and the resource allocation roles they perform along a continuum from 1 to 6 (see Table 9–1). At one end (1), the physician is a nearly perfect agent for a single patient, acting solely on his or her behalf. At the other (6), the physician is an agent whose clinical decisions are highly self-interested. Between these extremes are several intermediate positions. Physicians can work for several patients (2). Here the interests of one patient may conflict with those of another, putting the doctor in the middle. For example, if a physician treating two patients must decide which he should admit to the one bed remaining in the intensive care unit, he is forced to choose between them, and the medical prognosis alone may not dictate an answer.

Table 9.1. Physician Payment Continuum.

PHYSICIAN PAYMENT CONTINUUM					
1	2	3	4	5	6
Salary paid to care for one patient	Salary paid to care for many patients	Salary paid to government. Physician administers budget for a group of patients.	Salary paid by providers or payers. Physician provides medical services to patients.	Physician paid by providers or payers, with financial incentives to reduce expenditures.	Physician paid a set fee per patient and bears the full risk of providing medical services.

Further along the continuum (3), the physician serves as an agent both for patients and for society. If a physician's budget covers the treatment of many patients, then society is, in effect, asking the physician to allocate resources. The physician must decide which medical care should be a priority and which must come second. Though acting on the behalf of patients, the physician is also an agent of society.

Next on the scale (4) is the salaried physician, paid by a hospital or a private firm to offer medical care to its patients or employees or remunerated by an insurance company to offer care to insured parties. In each instance, the physician is subject to pressure to limit medical interventions in order to protect the resources of the payer and has conflicts of interest.

In situation (5), the payer hires the doctor to provide services and offers incentives to reduce the use of resources. The physician is rewarded for limiting services.

At the end of the continuum (6), the physician is paid a set fee per patient to provide all the medical care that is necessary and is at full risk for the cost. Here, each time they make a clinical decision, physicians must balance their own interests against those of patients.

Some people say that if it is acceptable for physicians to help allocate resources, then encouraging them to do so with financial incentives is also acceptable. But the risks to patients are less onerous when physicians do not have a personal stake in the choices they make. Physicians practicing under budgetary constraints can act as disinterested judges of conflicting claims and promote the welfare of individual patients to the extent possible when the welfare of other patients is considered. The situation is different, though, when HMOs pay physicians to limit the use of resources. In that case, physicians are interested parties and watch their own purses. They are encouraged to use their own well-being as a criterion in making difficult medical allocation choices.[73] This tips the scales against patients. Doctors are more likely to limit medical care to increase their income.[74]

Is a Neutral Compensation Arrangement Possible?

One way to avoid perverse consequences is to pay physicians a salary. This form of payment would insulate doctors from direct financial incentives to provide more or fewer services; it would remove a major distorting influence in making clinical decisions. Paying a salary would probably eliminate the conflicts of interest in fee-for-service practice without creating the reverse conflict.[75]

However, employed physicians encounter both indirect and nonmonetary incentives to promote the interests of their employers. Employers can block salary increases or promotions. They can even dismiss physicians who perform too many medical procedures. No physician's salary is more secure than his or her employer's financial solvency, so salaried physicians have a reason to generate income for their employers.

It makes a difference who is employing the physicians. If the employer is a hospital or another provider, it may combine salary with other incentives to encourage patient admissions. If the employer is a large group practice, the incentive to refer services may depend on peer pressure. And when government agencies or other third-party payers employ physicians, they may discourage providing services. But in all of these situations, the absence of direct monetary rewards for providing or withholding service reduces the effect of the incentive.

Indirect and nonmonetary incentives arising from salaried employment can be distinguished from direct financial incentives for practical reasons. Indirect and nonmonetary incentives are ubiquitous. They often exert less effect than direct financial incentives. It would be difficult to identify them all or to gauge their seriousness, and it would therefore be exceedingly difficult, if not impossible, to control them or even to develop a policy in response.

The social significance of direct financial inducements is different. When we pay a physician to provide more or fewer services, we call forth self-interested behavior. We legitimize such motivations and actions and explicitly reward them. But physicians making clinical decisions ought to consider the interests of their patients and comply with appropriate standards of medical practice, not consult their own financial well-being.

Although physicians, like other people, are motivated by earning money, we should not encourage this motivation as a criterion for particular clinical choices. A combination of motives, drives, and desires prompts all persons to act as they do. It would be imprudent to try to suppress motives in order to promote desirable conduct. We need not worry about the complex range of motives of physicians or all the indirect incentives that influence them. But at least we can try to avoid encouraging self-interested action when it creates conflicts of interest.[76]

Are Existing Institutions and Regulations Adequate Protection?

Proponents of risk-sharing incentives claim that whatever drawbacks they may have are offset by existing institutions that provide a check. But as I show in a more extensive survey of existing policy, there is reason for great skepticism about the ability of current institutions to protect patients adequately.[77] Three main types of institutions are now used to counter incentives to undertreat: (1) peer review and quality assurance programs, (2) federal regulations, and (3) medical malpractice law.

Peer review and quality assurance programs sometimes help to deter underuse, but they have built-in limitations that make them insufficient safeguards to protect against incentives to underserve patients. They work best in identifying cases of clear abuse or violation of practice standards. They are less helpful when choices are subtle or when there is clinical uncertainty. In these situations, physicians will always need significant discretion because there is no medical consensus and reviewers will be unable to second-guess clinical judgments.

Federal regulations addressing incentives to undertreat patients are also only partial. Early on, the federal HMO act and regulations authorized and even encouraged HMOs to use physician risk-sharing plans. However, starting in 1992, the Medicare program received authority to regulate individual physician risk-sharing plans for certain HMOs. Still, the proposed regulations only aim to make sure that physicians do not bear a high level of financial risk (i.e. more than 20–30 percent of the doctor's salary, depending on circumstances) not to stop risk sharing.[78] Medicare regulations disallow hospital incentives modeled on the Paracelsus plan, which is akin to fee splitting. They prohibit hospitals from splitting with physicians the DRG payment they receive from Medicare, but not other inducements for reducing services.

Courts have not yet provided any check on risk-sharing practices and have not held physicians, HMOs, or hospitals accountable for conflicts of interest. Recently, some patients have challenged HMO risk-sharing arrangements through private lawsuits. They argue that these programs cause substandard care, that they are deceptive, and that they violate patients' rights as consumers in numerous other ways. So far, though, patients have lost these claims or settled out of court, or the cases are still pending. Although private lawsuits have the potential to be used as a remedy, it is unlikely they can serve this role well.[79]

The best protection for patients from physicians' conflicts of interest is to remove or reduce incentives that may prompt physicians to act in their own interests rather than those of their patients. There are, therefore, strong grounds to prohibit risk-sharing and other incentive plans altogether. If this is not politically acceptable, then the second best approach would be to limit the total amount of money physicians can gain or lose through risk sharing. The most practical way to do this would be to cap any physician's financial gain or loss at a small percentage of his or her baseline pay. This would provide a rule that would be easy to monitor, with effects easy to gauge. For example, a statute might restrict profit or loss under risk-sharing plans to 1–2 percent of baseline income or to a fixed dollar amount. Such a restriction would prevent providers from tempting physicians to change their behavior.[80] Although we cannot be sure that small financial incentives would not produce inappropriate conduct, strictly controlled risk sharing is preferable to risk sharing with stronger incentives.

Notes

1. This chapter draws on my analysis in chapters 5 and 6 of my book *Medicine, Money and Morals: Physicians' Conflicts of Interest* (1993). The book offers an extensive analysis of a wide range of physicians' financial conflicts of interest and proposed policy responses.
    A number of articles address incentives to increase services. *See:*
    Bruce Hillman *et al.*, Physicians' Utilization and Changes for Outpatient Diagnostic Imaging in a Medicare Population," 268 *JAMA* 2050–2054 (1992).
    Jean Mitchell and Jonathan Sunshine, Consequences of Physician Joint Ventures: The Case of Radiation Therapy Services, 327 *N. Engl. J. Med.* 1497–1501 (1992).
    Jean Mitchell and Elton Scott, Evidence of Complex Structure of Physician Joint Ventures, 9 *Yale J. Reg.* 489–520 (1992).
    Jean Mitchell and Elton Scott, Evidence on the Prevalence and Scope of Physician Joint Ventures, 268 *JAMA* 80–84 (1992).
    Jean Mitchell and Elton Scott, Physician Ownership of Physical Therapy Services: Effects on Charges, Utilization, Profits, and Service Characteristics, 268 *JAMA* 2055–2059 (1992).
    Marc Rodwin, The Organized American Medical Profession's Response to Financial Conflicts of Interest: 1890–1992, 70 *Milbank Q.* 703–741 (1992).
    Alex Swedlow *et al.*, Increased Cost and Rates of Use in the California Workers' Compensation System, 327 *N. Engl. J. Med.* 1502–1506 (1992).
    State of Florida Health Care Cost Containment Board and Department of Economics and Department of Finance, *Joint Ventures Among Health Care Providers in Florida* (1991).
    David Hemenway *et al.*, Physicians' Responses to Financial Incentives: Evidence from a For-Profit Ambulatory Care Center, 322 *N. Engl. J. Med.* 1059–1063 (1990).
    Bruce Hillman *et al.*, Frequency and Cost of Diagnostic Imaging in Office Practice—A Comparison of Self-Referring and Radiologist-Referring Physicians, 323 *N. Engl. J. Med.* 1604–1608 (1990).
    Alan Hillman *et al.*, How Do Financial Incentives Affect Physicians' Clinical Decisions and the Financial Performance of Health Maintenance Organizations?, 321 *N. Engl. J. Med.* 86–92 (1989).
    Marc Rodwin, Physicians' Conflicts of Interest: The Limitations of Disclosures, 321 *N. Engl. J. Med.* 1405–1408 (1989).
    Alan Hillman, Financial Incentives for Physicians in HMOs: Is There a Conflict of Interest?, 317 *N. Engl. J. Med.* 1743–1748 (1987).
    Blue Cross and Blue Shield of Michigan, Medical Affairs Division, *A Comparison of Laboratory Utilization and Payout to Ownership* (1984).
    Health Care Financing Administration, *Department of Health and Human Services, Region*

V Diagnostic Clinical Laboratory Services, Report No. 2-05-2004-11 (1983).

Michigan Department of Social Services, *Utilization of Medicaid Laboratory Services by Physicians with/without Ownership Interest in Clinical Laboratories* (1981).

A. W. Childs and E. D. Hunter, Non-Medical Factors Influencing Use of Diagnostic X-ray by Physicians, 10 *Med. Care* 323–35 (1972).

2. S. J. Reiser *et al., Ethics in Medicine: Historical Perspectives and Contemporary Concerns* (1977).

3. K. Kipnis, *Legal Ethics* (1986); P. D. Finn, *Fiduciary Obligations* (1977).

4. Incentives to reduce care also counter another distortion in medical markets, namely insurance, which removes financial barriers to access for insured people and thus eliminates any incentive they have to use resources frugally. A still more fundamental distortion is uncertainty, which makes patients depend on physicians and skews decisions. Kenneth Arrow, Uncertainty and the Welfare Economics of Medical Care, 53 *Am. E. R.* 941–973 (1963).

5. There is an exception: approximately 15 percent, or 37 million Americans, have no health insurance.

6. This is called a "prospective payment system" that pays hospitals using diagnosis related groups (DRGs). In fact, the system is more complex. If the cost of treatment greatly exceeds the DRG payment, Medicare will chip in and pay one-half of the extra cost. The payment is adjusted for hospital region, teaching status, and other criteria.

7. For a sample of views of proponents of such incentives, see the following articles:

Richard Egdahl and Cynthia Taft, Financial Incentives to Physicians, 315 *N. Engl. J. Med.* 59–61 (1986).

Mark Hall, Institutional Control of Physician Behavior: Legal Barriers to Health Care Cost Containment, 137 *U. Pa. L. R.* 431–536 (1988).

Mitchell Rabkin, Control of Health Care Costs: Targeting and Coordinating the Economic Incentives, 309 *N. Engl. J. Med.* 982–984 (1983).

8. For a summary of evidence of underuse of medical services and the effect on quality of care, *see Quality Problems and the Burdens of Harm: Evidence of Underuse in Medicare: A Strategy for Quality Assurance* (Kathleen Lohr, ed., 1990).

9. Alan Stone, Law's Influence on Medicine and Medical Ethics, 312 *N. Engl. J. Med.* 309–312 (1985).

10. "Health maintenance organization" is a legislative term used to describe prepaid group practices qualifying for certain federal benefits. In common usage, it often refers to prepaid group practice generally, and includes so-called competitive medical plans and many other similar arrangements.

11. *See*, Larry Brown, *Politics and Health Care Organization: HMOs As Federal Policy* (1983).

12. More recently, HMOs have developed three tiers. *See*, Alan Hillman *et al.*, Contractual Arrangements Between HMOs and Primary Care Physicians: Three Tiered HMOs and Risk Pools, 3 *Med. Care* 136–148 (1992).

13. Some analysts now suggest that differences in institutional structure are less significant than the different financial incentives and styles of management different HMOs use. *See*, Pete Welch *et al.*, Toward New Typologies for HMOs, 68 *Milbank Q.* 221–243 (1990).

14. There are numerous definitions of managed care. A few prominent ones are as follows.

"A coordinating and rationing strategy designed to make the unique role of the primary care provider the key to cost control." Deborah Freund and Robert Hurley, Managed Care in Medicaid: Selected Issues in Program Origins, Design, and Research, 8 *Annu. Rev. Public Health* 137–163 (1987).

"[A] health care plan that attempts to influence physician practice in contrast to traditional indemnity insurance that pays the health bills for services specified in the health benefit."

Richard Egdahl, *Managed Care in the U.S.*, Pew Seminar on Managed Care, Boston University Health Policy Institute, January 29, 1988.

"Management of resources used by physicians in the care of patients, driven by financial considerations." Michael Rabkin, Pew Seminar on Managed Care, Boston University Health Policy Institute, April 8, 1988.

15. Even in fee-for-service practice there is a variety of practice styles. *See* John Wennberg and A. Gittelshon, Small Area Variations in Health Care Delivery, 183 *Science* 1102–1108 (1973).

Nevertheless, fee-for-service encourages overuse of services. For a summary of evidence of overuse of medical services, *see* Institute of Medicine, Chap. 7 (1990).

16. Hillman, *supra* note 1.

17. I use the term "profitable" to cover both profit in for-profit HMOs and a "surplus" in non-profit HMOs.

18. Hillman, supra notes 12 and 13.

19. Marsha Gold and Ingrid Reeves, Preliminary Results of the GHAA-BC/BS Survey of Physician Incentives in Health Maintenance Organizations (HMOs), *Research Briefs* 1 (1987). Typically, bonuses are explicitly linked to the volume of services used. Sometimes, however, bonuses are based on HMO profits. Profit sharing provides the same incentives for physicians as bonuses based on the volume of services used. The main costs to an HMO are those of the medical services they provide.

20. Lewis Sullivan, Department of Health and Human Services, *Incentive Arrangements Offered by Health Maintenance Organizations and Competitive Medical Plans to Physicians* 2 (1988).

21. Gold, *supra* note 19.

22. For example, the California Primary Care Management Medicaid program gives physicians the option of bearing the risk for diagnostic tests, x-rays, and drugs. *See* Pete Welch et al., *Toward a Typology of HMOs Reflecting Financial Incentives to Physicians* (1989).

23. *See* Pete Welch, *Giving Physicians Incentives to Contain Costs Under Medicare: Lessons from Medicaid (The Urban Institute, Working Paper* 3872–01 (1989)).

24. Department of Health and Human Services, *Medicare: Physician Incentive Payments by Prepaid Health Plans Could Lower Quality of Care* (1988).

25. Stephen Moore, Cost Containment Through Risk-Sharing by Primary-Care Physicians, 300 *N. Engl. J. Med.* 1359–1362 (1979).

Stephen Moore *et al.*, Does the Primary-Care Gatekeeper Control the Costs of Health Care? Lessons From the SAFECO Experience, 309 *N. Engl. J. Med.* 1400–1404 (1983).

John Lavin, When Primary Doctors Run the Whole Show, 22 Dec. *Med. Economics* 25–42 (1980).

26. Based on Bluechoice documents in possession of author.

27. Primary care physicians can also receive income from providing services not covered in the capitation agreement on a fee-for-service basis and by sharing savings from their management of home care cases.

28. These figures assume a practice of 1,850 primary care patients.

29. Robert Berenson, Hidden Compromises in Paying Physicians, *Business and Health* 18–22 (July 1987).

30. Robert Berenson, Financial Confessions of a Sawbones: In a Doctor's Wallet, *The New Republic* 11-13 (May 18, 1977).

31. *Id.*

32. Gina Kolata, Being Thorough Can Be Costly-To the Doctor, *New York Times* § 4, at 6 (March 20, 1988).

33. Hillman, *supra* note 1.
34. Alan Hillman *et al.*, HMO Managers' Views on Financial Incentives and Quality, 10 *Health Affairs* 206–219 (1991).
35. Daniel Haney & Fred Bayles, *HMO Doctors Can Earn More For Doing Less*, Associated Press (November 19, 1991).
36. Michael Millenson, Health Care Debate Rages: Cost-Paring: Good Business or Bad Medicine?, *Chicago Tribune* §1, at 3-5 (June 14, 1987).
37. *Id.*
38. Some economists say that people are influenced most by marginal gains or losses from particular decisions. However, others say that money, like anything else, has decreasing marginal utility and will be less desirable as the supply increases. A growing literature suggests that physicians work to achieve a target income. If this is so, they will be less susceptible to incentives as they approach or exceed this target.

    For a discussion of the target income hypothesis, see the following articles: Jerry Cromwell and Janet Mitchell, Physician-Induced Demand for Surgery, 5 *J. Health Econ.* 293–313 (1986).

    Gail Wilensky and Louis Rossiter, The Relative Importance of Physician-Induced Demand in the Demand for Medical Care, 61 *Health and Society* 252–277 (1983).

    Uwe Reinhardt, The Theory of Physician-Induced Demand: Reflections After a Decade, 4 *J. Health Econ.* 87–93 (1985).

    Louis Rossiter and Gail Wilensky, A Reexamination of the Use of Physician Services: The Role of Physician-Induced Demand, 20 *Inquiry* 162–172 (1983).

    Frank Sloan and Roger Feldman, Competition Among Physicians, in *Competition in the Health Care Sector: Past, Present, and Future* (1978).

    Victor Fuchs, The Supply of Surgeons and the Demand for Operations, 13 *J. Human Resources* 35–56 (1978).
39. Hillman, *supra* note 12.
40. For a description of prospective payment using DRGs, see Bruce Vladeck, Medicare Hospital Payment by Diagnosis-Related Groups, 100 *Ann. Intern. Med.* 576–591 (1984).
41. Jeffrey Harris, The Internal Organization of the Hospital: Some Economic Implications, 8 *Bell J. Econ.* 467–482 (1977).
42. Mary Koska, Physician Practices Go Under the Microscope, *Hospitals* 32-37 (February 20, 1990).
43. William Tierney *et al.*, The Effect on Test Ordering of Informing Physicians of the Charges for Outpatient Diagnostic Tests, 322 *N. Engl. J. Med.* 1499–1504 (1990).
44. *See* the series of articles by Fred Bayles and Daniel Haney of the Associated Press entitled "Doctors for Sale." These articles deal with the carrots and sticks that hospitals use to get physicians to admit patients and practice in a manner that promotes hospitals' financial well-being. Released October 14, 1990: Hospitals Give Doctors Money, Freebies for Patients. Released October 15, 1990: Money for Patients: One Hospital's Story.
45. General Accounting Office, *Physician Incentives* (1988).
46. Paracelsus stopped its physician incentive plan following a 1985 investigation by the Department of Justice for Medicare fraud. Other hospitals with similar incentive plans have followed suit. Although the initial impetus for the Paracelsus investigation was the incentive plan, the Justice Department also investigated billing and other practices. As part of a settlement of all potential claims, Paracelsus agreed to pay $4.45 million in reimbursement, fines, and interest and to provide $100,000 in medical services to indigent persons living in Orange County. See the following sources: Department of Health and Human Services, Office of Inspector General, *Fact Sheet on the Paracelsus Investigation* (1988).

General Accounting Office, *Physician Incentives* (1988).

Kathryn A. Kreche, Abusing the Patient: Medicare Fraud and Abuse and Hospital-Physician Incentive Plans, 20 *Mich. J. L. Reform* 279–304 (1986).

The Paracelsus case was also instrumental in prompting Congress to pass legislation limiting risk sharing in HMOs. *See* 42 U.S.C. 1320a-7a(b).

47. Interstudy proposed the idea, and it has received considerable attention. However, it has rarely been used.

48. Glenn Richards, How Do Joint Ventures Affect Relations with Physicians?, 58 *Hospitals* 68–74 (1984).

49. *Id.*

50. James Dechene, Physician Incentive Programs: Are They Legal?, 4 *HealthSpan* 3–9 (1987).

51. Linda Perry, Physician Ownership May Give Hospitals a Shot in the Arm, *Modern Healthcare* 25-34 (June 30, 1989).

52. Often these arrangements involve a complicated series of ownership and leasing arrangements between the hospital and physicians.

53. For a review of recent developments and the legal issues, see Hall, *supra* note 7. See also Nathan Hershey, Applying Utilization Review Findings in Medical Staff Appointment and Reappointment Decisions, 1 *Quality Assurance and Utilization Review* 109–110 (1986).

54. Gerald Glandon & Michael Morrisey, Redefining the Hospital-Physician Relationship Under Prospective Payment, 23 *Inquiry* 166–175 (1986).

P.M. Ellwood, Jr., *When MDs Meet DRGs*, 57 Hospitals 62–66 (1983).

John Eller & Sanford Teplitzky, Considering Economic Factors in Hospital Privilege Decisions, 3 *HealthSpan* 11-14 (August/September).

For a study of one hospital's changed by-laws to account for physician costs, see Cantrell and Frick, Physician Efficiency and Reimbursement: A Case Study, *Hospital and Health Services Administration*, November/December at 43 (1986).

Economic Credentialing is Fine-For Tightrope Walkers, 15 *Hospital Peer Review* 49–51 (1990).

55. John Blum, Economic Credentialing: A New Twist in Hospital Physician Appraisal Processes, 12 *J. Legal Med.* 427–475 (1991).

Mary Koska, Hospital CEOs Divided on Use of Economic Credentialing, 65 *Hospitals* 42–48 (1991).

56. Hospitals frequently will maintain a referral service for patients who seek a physician for outpatient medical care. Some hospitals have excluded "high-cost" physicians from their referral programs (i.e., those who order a lot of tests and procedures), so that hospital revenues under Medicare's DRG reimbursement system are less than the costs of treating patients. Julie Franz, Clipping Doctors from Referral Program Spurs Them to Clip Costs, *14 Modern Healthcare* 116 (April 1984).

57. Theodore Schneyer, Informed Consent and the Danger of Bias in the Formation of Medical Disclosure Practices, 1976 *Wis. L. Rev.* 124–170 (1976).

58. The relationship between hospitals, physicians, and patients resembles that of courts, criminal defense lawyers, and clients. Marc Galanter says that criminal defense lawyers are "repeat players" that have a vested interest in the system which may compromise their loyalty to clients, who only interact with the justice system occasionally. Marc Galanter, Why the "Haves" Come Out Ahead: Speculations On The Limits of Legal Change, 9 *L. Soc. Rev.* 95–160 (1974).

59. George Annas, The Hospital: A Human Rights Wasteland, in his *Judging Medicine* 4-26 (1988).

60. However, more sober proponents acknowledge that not much is known about the effects of such incentive arrangements or about other crucial variables that affect the costs of caring for patients. *See, e.g.*, Physician Payment Review Commission, *Risk-Sharing Arrangements in Prepaid Health Plans, Annual Report to Congress* (1989).

61. The most common examples of such programs are Medicare's Professional Standards Review Program, private utilization review programs, and quality assurance programs. I discuss these in the section, "Are Existing Institutions and Regulations Adequate Protection?".

62. Sullivan, *supra* note 20.

63. The first HMOs were staff model HMOs that employed physicians on salary. They often reduced hospitalization by 30 percent. Harold Luft, *Health Maintenance Organizations: Dimensions of Performance* (1981).

64. *See, e.g.*, *Risk-Sharing Arrangements in Prepaid Health Plans*, chapter 15 (1987). The report's recommendations include the following:
    HCFA should require prepaid health plans to limit the total risk assumed by individual physicians or small groups through some form of reinsurance or "stop loss" provisions, and it should require them to rely primarily on incentives to groups of physicians rather than to individual physicians.
    See also the testimony of Karen Davis, Commissioner, Physician Payment Review Commission. *Fiscal Year 1990 Budget Issues Relating to Physician Incentive Payments by Prepaid Health Plans*, Hearings Before the Subcommittee on Health of the Committee on Ways and Means, House of Representatives, 101st Congress, 1st Session (Serial No. 101-30), April 25, 1989.

65. Some writers have commented on this problem. Dr. Stephen Moore acknowledges the need to reduce the risk physicians bear in order to prevent undue pressure on physicians when they have a few very ill patients. In such situations, doctors can do everything reasonably possble within the realm of accepted medical practice to eliminate waste yet still lose money. Here risk sharing can promote improper behavior. Yet Moore attributes the failure of the Safeco HMO to its providing incentives that were too weak. Moore, *supra* note 25.

66. U.S. Healthcare, a national HMO, and Ad-Med, a Florida-based HMO, have devised such programs. For a summary of the U.S. Healthcare program written by employees of U.S. Healthcare, see Neil Schlackman, Integrating Quality Assessment and Physician Incentive Payment, *Quality Review Bulletin* 234-237 (August 1989); Michael A. Stocker, Quality Assurance In An IPA, 3 *HMO Practice* 183–187 (1989).U.S. Healthcare has revised the incentive formula it uses three times and is likely to do so again in the future. For a discussion of the Ad-Med program by its medical director, see the chapter discussing age used in Peter Boland, *Making Managed Health Care Work* (1991).

67. The incentive payments are only part of the U.S. Healthcare quality assurance program. My criticisms are not directed to the whole program, only to the idea that incentives for their quality measures can appropriately counter incentives to reduce services.
    There is little public information about the effectiveness of the U.S. Healthcare program. U.S. Healthcare has published a brief description of the program (*see* note 66). It hired a consulting firm to evaluate the program and has released a four-page executive summary of the 100+-page report. The summary portrays the program very favorably. However, the report itself is not public. U.S. Healthcare acknowledges that the consultants also suggested a number of changes, including improvement of the review of medical records by using more comprehensive criteria, more objective measures, and better-trained reviewers. *See* Schlackman, *supra* note 66.

68. Erving Goffman, On Cooling the Mark Out, 15 *Psychiatry* 451–463 (1952).

69. One study found that patient satisfaction was correlated with quality of care. A. L. Stewart

et al., Functional Status and Well-Being of Patients With Chronic Conditions: Results From the Medical Outcomes Study, 262 *JAMA* 907–913 (1989).

70. *U.S. Healthcare's Quality Mission Statement* (1992), unpublished photocopy; telephone interview with Neil Schlackman, U.S. Healthcare, June 1992.

71. For a discussion of fiduciary obligations, see Chapter 14 in this volume at notes 119 to 124.

72. Thomas Halper, *The Misfortune of Others: End-Stage Renal Disease in the United Kingdom* (1989).

73. When physicians receive incentives to reduce services, they become what Dr. Geist calls "Self-serving denial-of-care agents for the benefit of 'buyer' of care seeking 'cost-control' of the 'health-care industry.'" Robert W. Geist, 291 *N. Engl. J. Med.* 1306, 1307 (1974).

74. Norman Daniels, Why Saying No to Patients in the United States is So Hard (Cost Containment, Justice, and Provider Autonomy), 314 *N. Engl. J. Med.* 1381–1383 (1986).

75. It might be argued that salaried practice does not make physicians neutral with respect to providing medical services because the risk of malpractice liability provides incentives for physicians to practice defensive medicine, *i.e.*, to perform minimally useful diagnostic tests merely to document the basis for their clinical decisions. Financial incentives to reduce diagnostic tests, it can be argued, are necessary to counter this tendency. However this approach to discouraging defensive medicine is roundabout and not particularly effective. A more direct approach would be for institutional providers to pay the cost of malpractice insurance.

76. For a thoughtful discussion of the undesirable consequences of using incentives to promote desirable behavior in another context, see, Steven Kelman, *What Price Incentives?: Economists And The Environment* (1981).

77. Rodwin, *supra* note 1 at chapters 5 and 6.

78. Requirements for Physician Incentive Plans in Prepaid Health Care Organizations. 5 *Federal Register* 59024–59041 (December 14, 1992).

79. For proposals advocating the use of private law suits as a remedy see, E. Haavi Morreim, Physician Investment and Self-Referral: A Philosophical Analysis of a Contentious Debate, 15 *Journal of Medicine and Philosophy* 425–448 (1990); E. Haavi Morreim, chapter 11 (this volume). But for further elaboration of why I believe private law suits are likely to be insufficient, see, Marc Rodwin, *Medicine, Money and Morals: Physicians' Conflicts of Interest* (1993) at chapter 6.

80. The average physician's salary in 1990 was $155,000. Suppose this was the baseline for a physician in an HMO with a risk-sharing plan that could increase or decrease his pay by 2 percent. Then the physician could increase or decrease his income by $3100. Thus, his income would be between $151,900 and $158,100. By sharing risk and making financially driven choices, he could affect his income by $6200.

10

Physician Rationing and Agency Cost Theory

Mark A. Hall

The Case For and Against Financial Incentives to Ration

This chapter examines *deflationary* conflicts of interest—those that encourage physicians to conserve resources—from the perspective of economic analysis known as "agency cost theory." It begins with the assumption, now widely accepted,[1] that the fundamental problem of public policy that must be resolved before this country can construct a respectable system for financing health care is how best to ration limited medical resources among competing beneficial uses, both within health care and among other societal needs. By rationing, I mean implicit or explicit denial of medical care that has some demonstrable benefit on the basis of its cost.[2]

There are fundamentally three different actors for making cost-sensitive treatment decisions: patients, physicians, and third parties.[3] Patients make their own rationing decisions when they pay for care out of pocket. However, most people have a strong desire not to think about money and be constrained by costs when they are facing the severe anxiety of serious illness, so they purchase insurance. If this insurance is to be comprehensive yet affordable, subscribers must appoint an agent for making cost/benefit trade-offs on their behalf. That agent might be the insurance company itself or some government review mechanism such as the courts, but there are strong reasons that subscribers might prefer having their physician make these decisions instead.[4]

Ethical and Legal Objections

Surprisingly, however, most ethicists[5] and physicians[6] who have written on the subject proclaim an absolute prohibition on physicians ever considering, to any degree, the costs of the treatment they recommend. In the words of Norman Levinsky, "physicians are required to do everything that they believe may benefit each patient without regard to costs or other societal considerations.... It is society, not the individual practitioner, that must make the decision to limit the availability of effective but expensive types of medical care."[7]

However, this view is an economic absurdity and is unsupported by any of the classic values underlying bioethical analysis—beneficence, autonomy, and justice.[8] Therefore, a divergent wing of less absolutist physicians and ethicists take a view that is more accommodating to physician rationing. They are willing to contemplate physicians incorporating economic costs into their clinical judgment in some manner, since they see this as superior to rationing by market forces or by insurer or governmental fiat.[9] Still, even this minority view imposes the constraint that physicians be strictly insulated from any personal stake in their economizing decisions. Physicians are allowed to mediate a conflict between the health care needs of one patient and those of a group, but they may not be financially rewarded for rationing. Thus, bedside rationing is permissible only if the savings go entirely to other patients within a closed financing system, as occurs in Great Britain, or in a nonprofit, group-model HMO that pays its physicians a straight salary.[10]

These views have strongly influenced public policy as expressed in Medicare legislation. In 1986, Congress enacted an absolute ban on hospitals making any payment, "directly or indirectly, to a physician as an inducement to reduce or limit services provided [to Medicare or Medicaid patients]."[11] Congress initially planned to extend this ban to HMOs but then realized this would fundamentally alter the entire industry. Instead, a 1990 law subjected Medicare HMOs to regulatory oversight of their physician incentive arrangements and prohibited "specific payment[s]...as an inducement to reduce or limit medically necessary services provided with respect to a specific individual."[12] States have not yet followed suit, but several have considered bills to require HMOs to disclose their financial incentive plans. Financial incentives are also proving controversial in litigation. In an increasing number of lawsuits, plaintiffs' lawyers are arguing that an HMO physician's decision to withhold treatment, such as a Pap smear or a biopsy to detect cancer, was inappropriately influenced by an undisclosed financial incentive plan.[13]

Elsewhere I have critiqued the absolutist position that would prohibit physician rationing in all its guises.[14] My purpose here is to address the more accommodating position that allows some bedside rationing but still prohibits inducing physicians to consider costs by sharing with them a portion of the savings. My essential position is that, recognizing that physician rationing in some form may be desired by some patients in some circumstances, the only issue becomes how best to motivate physicians to perform this task and to control for potential abuses. Considering the wide range of potential inducement and control mechanisms—ethical, legal sanction, government regulation, professional education, peer supervision, and so on—it is nonsensical to prohibit absolutely the one mechanism that has the greatest potential utility and ultimately is closest to the source of the problems we are trying to correct: financial motivation.

Influencing Physicians to Consider Costs

When I speak of physician rationing, I do not contemplate the crass and overt sacrifice of life or functional capacity that might occur if a doctor were to refuse treatment entirely to a deformed newborn infant or an aging diabetic. I mean declining marginally beneficial care, such as high-tech testing or expensive antibiotics, when the stakes are low and the confidence in the diagnosis or prognosis is already high. HMOs currently induce doctors to perform this function through various financial incentive arrangements described in more detail by Rodwin in the preceding chapter.[15] Two payment incentive arrangements are common for primary care physicians. First, HMOs pay them a fixed amount, either per annum (salary) or per enrollee (capitation), regardless of how much effort they devote to each patient's case. These base pay methods place primary care physicians at risk primarily only for their time. However, HMOs also use bonus and penalty devices to place them at *financial* risk for the costs of ordering expensive tests, specialist referral, and hospitalization services.[16]

HMOs have resorted to these explicit inducements because other mechanisms for instilling cost consciousness are notoriously futile if they are not coupled with reinforcing financial incentives.[17] Simply educating physicians or disseminating information about cost-effective practices has been a resounding failure.[18] For instance, consensus statements by prestigious National Institutes of Health panels have had little effect on changing erroneous physician practices.[19] Somewhat more success is achieved by intensive physician monitoring,[20] but the effect lasts only as long as the cumbersome and expensive process is continued and only as far as it reaches.[21] Therefore, direct monitoring is not cost effective.[22] More disturbing, peer review may only serve to cement in place existing bloated practice standards, since it tends to correct only extreme departures from the wide range of prevailing practice patterns.[23] In contrast, financial incentives generate an effective, pervasive, and ongoing influence on physicians' clinical judgment. Financial incentives are suited to counteracting the fee-for-service incentives that created inflated practice styles in the first place, and they fit the intuitive, judgmental thought processes that constitute actual clinical decision-making.[24]

Consenting to Conflicts of Interest

Nevertheless, incentives to consider the cost consequences of treatment decisions are subject to a serious ethical objection: By rewarding physicians for withholding admittedly beneficial care, they create an economic conflict of interest between the physician and the patient. As many medical ethicists have argued, while it may be permissible to ask doctors to save money on one patient in order to better treat others, it would defile physician rationing to allow them to keep the savings themselves. This is where virtually every medical ethicist draws the line on physician rationing.[25] It is difficult to understand why such a bright line can be maintained, however, since it is impossible to trace the path of potential savings this cleanly.[26] Money saved by salaried physicians even within a closed, nonprofit funding system may go to increased salaries next year or to corporate waste. Conversely, money saved under a for-profit HMO's physician incentive plan may ultimately benefit the patient by lowering the cost of insurance or allowing the provision of more comprehensive benefits.

But even if we adopt the simplistic tracing of savings that these ethicists propose, the absolutist prohibition of deflationary conflicts of interest cannot be maintained. The essence of the argument is based on patient autonomy. Properly informed insurance subscribers may rationally agree to place strategically structured incentives on their physicians in order to better induce them to act as both their medical treatment agents and their economic purchasing agents. Therefore, only undisclosed or extremely corrupting conflicts may be prohibited outright.

It is tempting to conclude, as Rodwin argues,[27] that *deflationary* conflicts are fundamentally worse because they pit the physician's personal interest against the patient's medical interest, whereas inflationary incentives encourage better medical care. But this categorical distinction is clearly an oversimplification. Fee-for-service reimbursement creates a highly conflicted incentive for physicians to provide unnecessary and harmful treatment, such as dangerous surgeries and medication, or simply to provide more care than a patient can afford copayments for. Deflationary incentives, on the other hand, can save the patient money or improve his or her health by making health insurance more affordable.

Some commentators argue that financial incentives are prohibited by the law of fiduciary obligation, observing that a patient's vulnerability and need for trust places the treatment relationship in this class of special legal protection. To the contrary, however, consenting to a reasonable financial conflict is fully consistent with most fiduciary positions. Fee–for–service payment, for instance, is not only considered legally appropriate, but many in the medical establishment consider it ethically mandatory. The array of payment methods used in other fiduciary settings, such as law, business agency, and trusteeship, confirms that fiduciary law does not mandate a particular fee arrangement. Fiduciaries of all types are paid by the hour, by the job, or by a percentage of the proceeds, whether or not this is contrary to the client's immediate interest. It is evident that any sufficiently clear, voluntary, and fair financial incentive can be consistent with most fiduciary positions. Thus, in each of the major categories of fiduciary status, beneficiaries may consent to at least some conflicts of interest.[28]

A fuller defense of waiving financial conflicts of interest under fiduciary principles would require a more exhaustive examination of this body of law, as well as a specification of how disclosure would be accomplished, tasks that I undertake elsewhere.[29] Here I wish to develop this line of defense by exploring a branch of economic analysis known as "agency cost theory." I will then apply these principles to the variety of rationing incentives commonly used by HMOs and explain how those incentives are presently regulated in order to demonstrate that both existing practice and regulation have remained within reasonable bounds.

Agency Cost Theory

The branch of economic analysis known as agency cost theory offers a more balanced perspective on conflict-of-interest problems than the moral absolutism sometimes generated by conventional medical ethics. Agency cost theory offers a generic framework for analyzing the ubiquitous problems that occur in all economic relationships that delegate influence or control over significant decisions.[30] This theory operates on a scale that integrates ethical, legal, and practical policy analysis, and it offers a perspective that is more appropriate for the role-based ethic that governs physicians. Agency cost theory recognizes that ethical and legal norms serve primarily instrumental goals that shape behavior in complex ways. Therefore, it avoids the categorical generalizations and unrealistic injunctions that can emanate from ethical analysis.

Agency cost theory is also superior to the fiduciary framework because it is more attuned to the complexities of conflicts that arise among groups of insured patients and across the multiple tiered relationships among physicians, patients, employers, and the insuring entity. Fiduciary law has developed in the one-dimensional setting of individual trustees administering funds for a single beneficiary. Agency cost theory, in contrast, has flourished in explaining how these basic fiduciary concepts should apply to the large, complex, and multi-tiered group relationships that characterize the interactions among corporations, shareholders, employees, and directors.

It might be objected that this economically oriented approach is suitable only for financial institutions and arrangements, not for health care. Granted that agency cost theory works well for widget salesmen and real estate agents, and perhaps even for lawyers, but, the objection goes, medicine is above crass concerns over transaction costs and economic efficiency. Unfortunately not. Health care, like any other service, must be paid for, and economic insights are helpful when we are examining how the commercial aspect—health insurance—should be structured. That the stakes are much greater than more material concerns does not subvert the agency cost perspective; whatever the stakes, whether health or money, it is important to recognize that unidirectional, cost-free moves are seldom possible. Enforcing the standard of care may produce defensive medicine; increasing the obligation to disclose risks may raise the patient's anxiety over complications. Larger stakes neither avoid nor resolve these tensions; they only heighten them, making it even more pressing to find the optimal balance between protection and discretion.

Summary Overview

Before exploring how agency cost theory applies to the particular problems that confront us, it is necessary to summarize its major tenets and analytical categories.[31] An *agent* is one who is authorized to act or decide on behalf of a *principal*. Agency relations are created because principals recognize that they are incapable of choosing or executing the correct course of action as successfully as are their designated agents, owing to some special expertise of the agent or some disability of the principal. However, any such delegation of authority creates an *agency risk* in that the agent's incentives and knowledge base never perfectly reflect those of the principal. Thus, every agency relationship entails two handicaps: (1) the agent may not fully understand the principal's objectives or (2) the agent may seize on opportunities to pursue his own benefit over the principal's, either by slacking in effort or by appropriating some of the value of the activity for himself. Agency relationships and these attendant risks permeate all aspects of economic, social, and political life. *Agency cost theory* categorizes and analyzes the various mechanisms that have been crafted for reducing this agency risk.

Earlier economic theory was deficient because it believed either that these imperfections did not exist or that they were unavoidable. Agency cost theory represents an important advance because it attempts to identify and analyze ways in which these agency risks can be minimized without unduly sacrificing the benefits that gave rise to the agency relationship in the first place. An *agency cost* is the cost (measured either by direct expenditure or by sacrifice in benefit) of either reducing or bearing these risks. Agency cost theory recognizes that there is no perfect set of agency incentives and structures: The extent to which these endemic risks can be reduced depends on the size of the risk and the costs imposed by the various techniques for its reduction.

The plethora of techniques for reducing agency risk can be lumped into two basic groups: *external monitoring* of the agent's performance and *internalizing incentives* for improving performance. Diminished effort, cheating, or other forms of poor performance can be detected either by the principal or by some other agent the principal retains for the purpose, as occurs, for instance, through quality assurance techniques in manufacturing. Alternatively, the agent's compensation can be structured in a manner to reward superior performance, as happens when sales agents are paid on commission. But each of these techniques involves a cost that compromises the benefit of the agency relationship. Monitoring is expensive and is never fail-safe. Incentives divert the profits that would otherwise go to the principal and may create a different set of counterproductive incentives, which themselves must be monitored.[32] The objective is to minimize the combination of losses that result from overprotecting and underprotecting. Overprotecting is costly and deters beneficial discretion; underprotecting allows opportunistic abuse to go uncorrected.[33]

A particular technique for agency risk reduction can be imposed through one or a combination of three mechanisms: (1) voluntary assumption by the agent, (2) individual contracting by the principal, or (3) legal imposition by society. "Bonding" is the term applied to the incentive that agents have to craft their own cost-reducing devices in order to make their services more attractive to principals. Bonding explains, for instance, the adoption of codes of ethics by professional groups in order to convince the public of their trustworthiness. The most common mechanism is *individual contracting*, which appears in numerous guises, such as hiring employees and agents and setting their range of authority or structuring compensation packages to reward or punish performance. Less obvious is the role society plays in reducing agency costs through *legal rules*. The principal such body of law is that relating to fiduciary responsibility, which shares precisely the same concerns about abuse of trust and dependency.[34] Thus, agency cost theorists observe that the law's imposition of fiduciary duties is a collective solution to a common set of problems that transcend a variety of agency relationships.[35]

Another branch of agency cost theory known as "relational contract" theory takes the agency cost analysis a step further by exploring the transaction costs involved in employing these various techniques and mechanisms. Relational contract theory explains that collective rules can be preferable to individually contracted rules because they reduce the time and effort involved in providing particularized specifications for complex and long-term relationships,[36] much as an arbitration agreement can refer to the uniform procedures specified by the American Arbitration Association. Fiduciary law offers just such an "off-the-rack" set of rules that apply generically to many agency relationships and to each instance of the governed relationships, without requiring the parties to consider and agree individually to a transaction-specific behavioral code. However, the parties to particular agency relationships may have a different view of what is best for them than the default rules the law offers. If the barriers to arriving at a superior set of specifications are not insurmountable (including adequate understanding and bargaining parity), then agency cost theory favors those restrictions that individuals negotiate over those the law imposes, so long as such arrangements do not harm anyone not a party to them.[37]

This analysis brings us to the point that is most critical to the present exposition: whether legal and ethical rules that address agency cost problems should be subject to individual exception. Agency cost theory answers "yes." "Because the fiduciary principle is a rule for completing incomplete bargains in a contractual structure, it makes little sense to say that 'fiduciary duties' trump *actual* contracts."[38] Indeed, the very reason fiduciary rules can afford to be so stringent and categorical is that individual beneficiaries concerned about the law's overprotective slant are often free to opt out. If the obligations were unalterable, they would have to be more centered and much more nuanced.[39]

Application to Physician Rationing

"In many respects, the physician–patient relation exemplifies the principal–agent relation almost perfectly;"[40] therefore, agency cost theory "offers powerful insights into the evolution and current organization of the health care industry."[41] Insured patients face a double-agency problem.[42] Patients appoint doctors as their medical treatment and spending agents because they lack the skill and training, and do not wish to bear the anxiety or risk, to make these decisions themselves.[43] But delegating this degree of discretion and authority[44] over such a critical matter creates serious problems in accurately pursuing patients' treatment interests—a *medical* agency problem. The full panoply of techniques and mechanisms just surveyed are employed to reduce these agency costs. Direct patient monitoring occurs via informed consent, which is an individual contracting mechanism. Incentives are used in the form of fee-for-service reimbursement to encourage optimal patient care. Bonding occurs through physicians' adherence to an ethical code, and malpractice and fiduciary laws apply collective norms for quality of care and patient loyalty.

However, the adoption of fee-for-service reimbursement to solve the *medical* agency problem creates a new *economic* agency problem of distorting physicians' spending decisions so that they fail to reflect what patients would have decided was cost effective were they willing and able to pay out of pocket.

Agency cost theory offers powerful insights into how this problem might be corrected. Physician rationing is a quintessential agency-cost solution. New forms of prospective payment, such as those embodied in HMOs, are intended to correct the abuse that results from giving physicians unconstrained authority over medical spending decisions under open-ended insurance.[45] The alternatives to physician rationing are much less acceptable. No rationing means that, for a number of people, no agency relationship will be formed at all, a situation that potentially characterizes over 35 million Americans who presently have no health insurance. For others, no rationing means that the treatment relationship will be less extensive because they can afford only reduced insurance coverage. Perhaps they will forego mental health or long–term care coverage, or perhaps they will have to pay such heavy deductibles and copayments that they will be covered only for catastrophic medical expenses. This blunt sacrifice of agency benefit is a more severe cost than the diminished autonomy or reduced medical benefit that comes from trimming marginally beneficial care more interstitially.

The next question becomes the appropriate rationing mechanism: physicians or outsiders? Third-party rationing exemplifies monitoring, while inducing physicians to ration exemplifies incentive-based control of agency costs. Agency cost theory tells us that there is no single best approach to reducing agency risk; each technique has its own strengths and weaknesses, so inevitably a mix will be crafted. Therefore, an absolute rule barring physician rationing would itself impose agency costs by foreclosing a possibly constructive solution to the deterioration of comprehensive insurance.

Categorical rule-based rationing, the primary alternative to internalizing rationing incentives at the bedside level, suffers from many troubling defects. In complex situations such as medical practice, categorical decision-making sacrifices accuracy and individuality.[46] Rule-based rationing also suffers from the biasing effects of interest group pressure on the political processes used to develop the rules. Moreover, rules alone are insufficient, since considerable areas of discretion will inevitably remain for physicians' judgment in the implementation and interpretation of the rules, discretion that can be channeled only with the use of internal incentives.

These concerns are amply borne out by Oregon's rationing of Medicaid services. Oregon has rank-ordered several hundred categories of treatment according to their expected benefits and has funded only that portion of the list that actuaries projected the state can afford with the amount the legislature appropriates.[47] Aaron and Schwartz aptly describe this as a "meat-ax" approach to rationing. All items above the funding line are covered, no matter how mild the condition is or how marginal the necessity is for the medical intervention.[48] "Patients with incapacitating lumbar disk disease are grouped with patients whose disease is barely symptomatic,"[49] and for breast cancer, "no distinction is made among different stages, cell types, or other factors likely to influence the choice of treatment and expected outcomes, nor are different treatments distinguished (*e.g.*, chemotherapy, radiation therapy, immunotherapy, or surgery)."[50] The effect of political bias is seen in the "distasteful and transparent coalition-building strategy" that targeted the rationing proposal only at the most politically and socially vulnerable components of the Medicaid population—indigent single mothers—leaving untouched the elderly and disabled, as well as the general population.[51] However, exactly the reverse was true for the groups Oregon consulted to construct the rankings: They were composed largely of health professionals and white, college–educated, upper–middle–class people.[52] Finally, the inevitability of reinforcing economizing incentives is demonstrated by the fact that Oregon intends to supplement its rationing list with a massive increase in the use of HMOs for its Medicaid population. The Office of Technology Assessment estimates that these prepayment incentives will be the primary source of any efficiency gains.[53]

Realizing that rules cannot be used to the complete exclusion of individualized, cost-sensitive decision-making, the third stage of agency cost analysis encounters the objection that physicians should not be induced to play a rationing role via financial incentives. Agency cost theory trivializes such an objection, when made in absolute terms, because it views financial incentives as merely one of a menu of motivational techniques, neither intrinsically optimal nor unvaryingly despicable. There is no greater intrinsic objection to rewarding a physician for economizing than there is to paying a lawyer a lump sum for handling a case or paying an architect a bonus for bringing a construction project in under budget. From an agency cost perspective, the only question is what techniques, in what combination, and at what strength work best. Agency cost theory takes seriously the objection that a financial conflict will erode the trust and confidence that are vital to the treatment relationship, but it allows a modulated and differentiated response depending on the actual strength and pervasiveness of this concern.

Finally, agency cost theory instructs us that fiduciary law's proscription of conflicts of interest is not absolute; this baseline rule merely sets a presumption that subscribers may choose to depart from in electing an alternative form of insurance. How stringently to set the baseline rule is influence by the transactional dynamics and burdens of opting out. Where bargaining positions are uneven and where only a single individual is affected, a strong presumption against conflicts is warranted. However, concerns about high-pressure bargaining are minimized where the rule affects the interests of a large group of beneficiaries. Moreover, the costs of contracting out of the rule increase with the size of the group. Providing detailed disclosure to each individual is costly, coordinating a group deliberation and decision is difficult, and obtaining unanimous agreement is impossible. Therefore, fiduciary law takes a more accommodating view of conflicted transactions in corporations than in trust administration.[54] Likewise, in this setting, where the interests at stake are represented by powerful employers, unions, or governmental representatives,[55] it is advantageous to set a default rule for physician rationing that more closely reflects the reasonable range of actual preferences among affected groups.

The Regulation and Practice of HMO Financial Incentive Plans

The more moderated approach of agency cost theory can be used to test the complex tableau of financial incentives presently in operation within HMOs and the manner in which federal law regulates them. When Congress first addressed HMO rationing incentives, as it did in 1990 for Medicare recipients, it recognized the impossibility of maintaining a sweeping prohibition.[56] The legislation bans only direct, patient specific incentives, leaving all others to the regulatory oversight of DHHS. Proposed regulations pending at the time of this writing establish certain categories of safe-harbor incentives and subject those that exceed these thresholds to more intensive oversight of patient care and patient satisfaction.[57] I will briefly summarize the major contours of each feature that shapes the strength of existing rationing incentives and how they are likely to be regulated. This survey will demonstrate that the HMO industry and the legal apparatus under Medicare have acted responsibly in setting the outer limits of financial motivation while leaving room for creative experimentation within those limits.

HMOs use three different forms of base pay—salary, fee-for-service, and capitation[58]—supplemented by a variety of bonus and penalty arrangements. One common technique is for the HMO to withhold a portion of a gatekeeping primary care physician's base pay until the end of an accounting period in order to place the physician at risk for excessive specialist referral or hospitalization costs that he orders. Another technique is to set the base payment rate lower to begin with and supplement it with a year-end bonus, based on productivity and efficiency measures.[59] As Rodwin describes,[60] various complex formulas are used to calculate these deficit-withhold and bonus-surplus amounts. The strength and effectiveness of these payment incentives vary according to five dimensions, each of which has multiple components:[61] (1) the types of services covered, (2) the practice setting and base reimbursement method, (3) the size of the incentive, (4) the incentive's immediacy, and (5) the presence of various counterbalancing monitoring mechanisms.

The Type of Services Covered

Cost-constraining financial inducements differ fundamentally according to whether they affect a doctor's time or his reimbursement. This distinction is captured in the difference between capitating primary care services and capitating referral and hospitalization services. Paying primary care physicians a set amount for each patient they are responsible for places primarily only their time at risk if the out-of-pocket expenses of referral services, hospitalization, prescriptions, and the like are paid for separately. Thus, like straight salary, primary care capitation imposes only mild financial disincentives to treat.[62] Therefore, the statute does not seek to regulate these compensation arrangements at all.[63]

The Practice Setting and Base Reimbursement Method

The impact of placing physicians at financial risk for the treatment costs they control depends next on the base payment method and the practice setting. Financial disincentives to treat are one tool used to neutralize the inflationary incentives that exist where physicians' base pay is fee-for-service.[64] They also are useful where direct monitoring techniques are infeasible. Thus, IPAs, where fee-for-service base pay is most common[65] and where monitoring is rendered more difficult by the dispersion of physicians in their individual offices, are most likely to place a portion of a physician's payment at risk by creating a withhold pool. However, physicians who practice in a group setting and who are paid a salary have fewer inflationary incentives and more monitoring devices, so that more targeted financial disincentives are unnecessary and possibly dangerous. Accordingly, withholds are uncommon in staff model HMOs.[66] Primary care capitation is a mixed bag. Its base incentive is more akin to salary, but it often applies in a nongroup setting. It also creates an inflationary incentive for excessive referrals to specialists. Accordingly, withholds are much more prevalent in primary care capitation plans than in salaried plans but somewhat less than in fee-for-service plans.[67]

The Size of the Incentive

The strength of a financial disincentive to treat also depends on its size in relation to the physician's base pay and on whether any stop-loss protection exists to limit the upper end of risk exposure. The trick is to find the golden mean. Too weak, and a financial incentive does not sufficiently constrain overutilization; too strong, and it may lead to substandard care or abusive practices. Either can lead to patient injury, but undertreatment is the more serious concern.

The little empirical work that has been done on the effect of deflationary financial incentives indicates that HMOs have erred on the side of weakness. The typical percentage withhold ranges from 10 to 30 percent of the physician's (or group's) base payment, with 20 percent being the most common amount.[68] This is within a range that is consistent with the bad debt amounts or negotiated discounts that physicians regularly accept for non-HMO patients. Therefore, these withhold levels are unlikely to be inordinately distracting and may arouse hardly any attention. One report of a failed HMO concluded that a 10 percent withhold "was too small an incentive to be taken seriously. Physicians considered the 10 percent risk a cost of doing business."[69] A comprehensive analysis of data from a large set of HMOs revealed that none of the more elaborate incentive arrangements presently in use had any discernible effect on the rate of hospitalization.[70] Accordingly, the proposed regulations under the federal statute set 15–25 percent as the safe-harbor threshold for "substantial financial risk" that triggers additional scrutiny and safeguards.[71]

At the other extreme, capitating *individual* physicians for the *entire* range of medical services is generally recognized as creating too great a risk.[72] This places the physician at risk not just for his own time but for 100 percent of the out-of-pocket costs of specialist referrals and hospitalization.[73] No such individual-physician, total-capitation arrangements are known to exist,[74] and they are likely to be prohibited by the proposed federal regulations.[75]

A third factor determining size is the presence of a stop-loss mechanism. Stop-losses can apply either at an individual patient level, capping the amount that a particular high-cost patient will be charged against the withhold pool, or at an aggregate level, capping the total dollar exposure. The competing concerns are that, absent a per-patient cap, physicians would have too great a tendency to withhold essential care from patients with catastrophic or chronic illnesses; however, setting such a cap too low will eliminate the economizing incentive from the very types of high-cost cases or high-utilizing physicians for which they are most needed. The federal statute requires some form of stop-loss whenever physicians are exposed to "substantial financial risk." The proposed regulations opted for a simple, aggregate stop-loss that is 5 percent higher than the substantial risk thresholds (which are 15 and 25 percent, depending on how frequently risk is assessed).[76]

The Incentive's Immediacy

The fourth critical dimension of financial incentive strength is the psychological immediacy of the incentive. There are at least four different factors other than raw percentage size that affect a given incentive's psychological impact on a physician's discrete mental decisions: the time horizon, the size of the physician group, the size of the patient pool, and whether the incentive is a bonus or a penalty. A penalty applied to each physician immediately after treating an individual patient is much more likely to get the physician's attention than a year-end bonus awarded to a large group of physicians treating a large pool of patients, even though the two amounts of money may be exactly the same. It is one thing to dock Dr. Jones' weekly paycheck $50 for ordering an expensive test for Mrs. Smith, and quite another to distribute a portion of the HMO's year-end profits to all doctors on a pro rata basis. The patient-specific penalty creates too great an incentive to deny necessary care, and the year-end group bonus is extremely unlikely to create anything more than a subliminal or background concern for the costs of treatment.

Accordingly, the federal statute prohibits "specific payment[s]...as an inducement to reduce or limit medically necessary services provided with respect to a *specific individual*,"[77] which is generally thought to place an absolute ban only on incentives directed immediately to particular patients, and only then if the incentives result in denying medically necessary care.[78] The paradigm Congress had in mind was a plan proposed by a for-profit hospital chain in California to reward physicians each month according to whether their patients were profitable under the Medicare program.[79] At the other extreme, the legislative history indicates that an incentive creates no substantial financial risk if it is applied to at least five physicians as a group or to a patient panel of 25, and is applied no less than semiannually.[80]

The time dimension of immediacy is reflected in the proposed regulations, which apply different substantial-risk thresholds of 25 and 15 percent, depending on whether risk is assessed annually or more frequently.[81] However, as with the other dimensions, there is no magic formula that strikes the perfect balance between excessive and insufficient impact.[82] Therefore, incentive plans that are worse than these levels are not banned, only subjected to plan-specific evaluation and the requirement of stop-loss protection.[83]

Counterbalancing Forces

Finally, incentive payments have a greater or lesser effect according to the existence of counterbalancing review and liability mechanisms. HMOs are the most closely monitored practice environment in existence as a consequence of state licensure, Medicare participation, and qualification for other federal benefits. In contrast with traditional solo office practice, HMOs are subject to grievance procedures, frequent subscriber satisfaction surveys, internal quality assurance and peer review processes, and external quality evaluations.[84] In addition, their physicians are subject to counterincentives in the form of professionally or expertly derived standards of appropriateness and their own internalized standard of professional ethics. Finally, patients are safeguarded from abusive decisions by the tort law penalties that result from malpractice and the market penalties that result from a bad reputation. This plethora of internal and external incentive and review mechanisms helps to keep treatment-denial incentives in check.

The Net Effect

Considering all of this, it is quite difficult without sophisticated empirical evidence, to determine the permissible range for any one factor or combination of factors. The best that can be done is to describe, for each factor in isolation, its direction and relative strength. But even this is unhelpful unless we know the ultimate effect on patient outcomes. The present state of empirical evidence provides no support for the blanket prohibition of HMO financial incentive plans that Rodwin and others urge. Virtually all studies of the aggregate quality of care in HMOs conclude that HMOs produce equal if not superior results to traditional reimbursement for most categories of patients,[85] and "evidence linking types of financial incentives to changes in quality of care is nonexistent."[86]

Even if such evidence existed, a simple prohibition would be impossible to justify since none of these factors operates in a one-dimensional field that allows us to maximize a single value. They each strike a balance between quality and cost, and they do so in a highly complex and interactive fashion that depends on the compound effects of all of the factors in simultaneous operation. As the DHHS concluded, "it is this ability to adjust factors to increase or mitigate the strengths of each different financial incentive that makes it impossible to classify, categorically, some factors as being too strong."[87]

In summary, although medical ethicists are virtually united in opposing financial rationing incentives, this is not where the ethical battle line should be drawn. The important issue is whether to allow physician rationing at all. If physicians are to be cost-conscious to any degree, as many ethicists agree they should be, then we have already allowed a conflicted interest in one form: that between the cost to the group versus the benefit to the individual. If we are willing to take this step despite the potential threat to patient trust, which we must be, then the exact manner of influencing physicians is of secondary importance—primarily a mechanical task of crafting the best strategic mix of incentives.

The ideal is for deflationary incentives to reinforce other mechanisms such as education, peer influence, and regulatory oversight that encourage physicians to adopt a more cost-effective practice style for the benefit of both their patients and themselves. The danger is that incentives will be so strong or arbitrary that physicians will be tempted to consciously sacrifice patient welfare for their own gain. There is certainly room for debate in striving for the correct balance between background reinforcement and conscious profiteering, but nothing of determinative importance inheres in the use of a financial motivation per se. In the words of one astute commentator, "Honest doctors do not knowingly and willingly place their own financial self-interest above the patient's best medical interests, and those who actively decide to cheat the system can easily find ways to do so, regardless of financial arrangements."[88]

Notes

1. *See generally* Symposium, The Law and Policy of Health Care Rationing: Models and Accountability, 140 *U. Pa. L. Rev.* 1505–1998 (1992). Those who still object to rationing are pursuing an underlying dispute over terminology or over the manner in which rationing is likely to occur.

2. Others prefer a more restricted use of the term. *See* Michael Regan, Health Care Rationing: What Does It Mean?," 319 *N. Engl. J. Med.* 1149–1451 (1988) (rationing is reserved for explicit, administrative decisions; it does not include ordinary price allocation); David Hadorn and Robert Brook, The Health Care Resource Allocation Debate: Defining Our Terms, 266 *JAMA* 33328 (1991) (advocating that rationing be reserved for unfair and discriminatory denial of services based on inability to pay). In some instances, this labeling dispute may simply be a rhetorical technique for allowing implicit rationing to occur by describing it in less inflammatory terms.

3. This analytical scheme, now standard in the literature, was first articulated by David Mechanic in *Future Issues in Health Care: Social Policy and the Rationing of Medical Services*, 19–21, 95–96 (1979) and in Rationing of Medical Care and the Preservation of Clinical Judgment, 11 *J. Fam. Prac.* 431–433 (1980).

4. For an analysis of insurers' role and a critique of the courts' role, see Mark Hall and Gerard Anderson, Health Insurers' Assessment of Medical Technology, 140 *U. Pa. L. Rev.* 1637 (1992).

5. *See, e.g.*, Robert Veatch, DRGs and the Ethical Reallocation of Resources, *16 Hastings Center Rep.* 32, 38 (June 1986) ("Asking physicians to be cost-conscious...[i]n effect would be ask[ing them] to remove the Hippocratic Oath from their waiting room walls and replace it with a sign that reads, `Warning all ye who enter here...but if benefits to you are marginal and costs are great, I will abandon you in order to protect society,'"); Edmund Pellegrino & David Thomasma, *For the Patient's Good: The Restoration of Beneficence in Health Care* 172, 173, 187 (1988) (gatekeeping is "ethically perilous," "morally unsound," and "moving in the direction of the code of the Soviet physician"); Tom Beauchamp and James Childress, *Principles of Biomedical Ethics* 213 (2d ed. 1983) ("Physicians are to do all they can for their patients without counting society's resources").

6. *See, e.g.*, Current Opinions of the Council on Ethical and Judicial Affairs of the American Medical Association 1986, p. 3, discussed in Edward Hirschfield, Should Third Party Payors of Health Care Services Disclose Cost Control Mechanisms to Patient Beneficiaries?, 14 *Seton Hall Leg. J.* 115, 130–131, 144–147 (1990) (physicians have "a duty to do all they [they] can for the benefit of [their] individual patients]"); Marcia Angell, Cost Containment and the Physician, 254 *JAMA* 1203, 1206-07 (1985) ("As individual physicians, we must do the very best we can for each patient,...spending whatever is necessary for effective medical care"); Erich Lowey, Cost Should Not Be a Factor in Medical Care, 302 *N. Engl. J. Med.* 697 (1990) (letter) (citing Nazi Germany in a vitriolic attack on cost/benefit analysis).

7. N. G. Levinsky, The Doctor's Master, 311 *N. Engl. J. Med.* 1573 (1984). The same view is shared by the few legal academics who have written on the subject. Barry Furrow, The Ethics of Cost-Containment: Bureaucratic Medicine and the Doctor as Patient-Advocate, 3 *Notre Dame J. L. Ethics and Pub. Pol.* 187 (1988); Maxwell Mehlman, Health Care Cost Containment and Medical Technology: A Critique of Waste Theory, 36 *Case West. Res. L. Rev.* 778 (1986).

8. For elaboration of this critique, see Mark Hall, *The Law, Ethics and Economics of Bedside Rationing* (unpublished).

9. Larry Churchill, *Rationing Health Care in America: Perceptions and Principles of Justice*, 106–112 (1984) (ethicist); Paul Menzel, *Strong Medicine: The Ethical Rationing of Health Care* 12–13 (1990) (ethicist); Howard Brody, Cost Containment as Professional Challenge, 8 *Theoretical Med.* 5–17 (1987) (ethicist); H. Gilbert Welch, Should the Health Care Forest Be Selectively Thinned by Physicians or Clear Cut by Payers?, 115 *Ann. Intern. Med.* 223–226 (1991) (physician); Christine Cassel, Doctors and Allocation Decisions: A New Role in the New Medicine, 10 *J. Health Politics, Policy and Law* 549, 550, 563 (1985) (physician).

10. The leading exponent of this compromise position is philosopher Norman Daniels. Norman Daniels, Why Saying No to Patients in the United States Is So Hard, 314 *N. Engl. J. Med.* 1380 (1986). *See also* Marc Rodwin, *Medicine, Money and Morals: Physicians' Conflicts of Interest in the United States* (1993), at chapter 6, which contains much of the same argument presented in his chapter in this volume; Christine Cassel, Doctors and Allocation Decisions: A New Role in the New Medicine, 10 *J. Health Politics, Policy and Law* 549 (1985).

11. 42 U.S.C. 1320a-7a(b). For a critique of this legislation, see Mark Hall, Institutional Control of Physician Behavior: Legal Barriers to Health Care Cost Containment, 137 *U. Pa. L. Rev.* 431, 499–504 (1988).

12. 42 U.S.C. §1395mm(i).

13. Harris Meyer, MD Incentives Suit Against HMO Dismissed; Issue Lingers, *American Medical News* 1 (January 12, 1990). So far, these allegations have not succeeded, either because the case was dismissed or settled prior to a decision on the merits *(see* Bush v. Dake, No. 86-25767, Mich. Cir. Ct., Saginaw County, April 27, 1989, summarized in 17 *Health Law Digest*, No. 8, at 16; Sweede v. CIGNA Health Plan of Delaware, C.A. No. 87C-SE-171-1-CV, Superior Court, New Castle County, Del., September 1988) or because the particular allegation was deemed deficient. *See* Pulvers v. Kaiser Foundation Health Plan, 99 Cal. App. 3d 565, 160 Cal. Rptr. 392, 394 (1979); Madsen v. Park Nicollet Medical Center, 419 N.W.2d 511, 515 (Minn. App. 1988); Teti v. U.S. Healthcare, Inc., C.A. No. 88-9808 (E.D. Pa.) (filed Dec. 27, 1988; dismissed Nov. 21, 1989). However, this area of common law remains very much unsettled.

14. Hall, *supra* note 8.

15. Marc Rodwin, Physician Conflicts of Interest in HMOs and Hospitals, Chapter 9 this volume.

16. For example, an HMO might withhold 20 percent of a physician's base pay until the end of the year to offset any excess beyond the budgeted amounts for these services attributable to that physician's patients, or the HMO might increase the base pay by distributing a portion of the savings that accrue for treating the physician's patients under budget, or both. These incentives can also be pooled among a group of physicians. For more detail, see *infra* text at notes 58 to 83.

17. *See generally* J.M. Eisenberg and S.V. Williams, Cost Containment and Changing Physicians' Practice Behavior, 246 *JAMA* 2195 (1981); S. A. Schroeder, Strategies for Reducing Medical Costs by Changing Physicians' Behavior. 3 *Int. J. Tech. Assess Health Care* 39 (1987).

18. *Id.*; D.E. Kanouse and J. Itzhak, When Does Information Change Practitioners' Behavior?, 4 *Int. J. Tech. Assess. Health Care* 33 (1988).

19. J. Kosecoff *et al.*, Effects of the National Institutes of Health Consensus Development Program on Physician Practice, 258 *JAMA* 2708 (1987) ("Practice failed to change even though the recommendations appeared to reflect the state of science and sound practice at the time and even though efforts to disseminate the recommendations were at least moderately successful at reaching an appropriate target audience of physicians"). *See also* J. Lomas et al., Do Practice Guidelines Guide Practice? The Effect of a Consensus Statement on the Practice of Physicians, 321 *N. Engl. J. Med.* 1306 (1989) ("We conclude that guidelines for practice may predispose physicians to consider changing their behavior, but that unless there are other

incentives or the removal of disincentives, guidelines may be unlikely to effect rapid change in actual practice").

20. Thomas Wickizer, John Wheeler, and Paul Feldstein, Does Utilization Review Reduce Unnecessary Hospital Care and Contain Costs?, 27 *Med. Care* 632 (1989); Howard Bailit and Cary Sennett, Utilization Management as a Cost-Containment Strategy, *Health Care Fin. R.*, 1991 Ann. Supp., at 87.

21. L. Goldman, Changing Physicians' Behavior: the Pot and the Kettle, 322 *N. Engl. J. Med.* 1524 (1990). In one dramatic example, an initial 30 percent decrease in the use of electro-cardiograms dissipated after nine months. Thereafter, test ordering rebounded to a rate of increase almost twice that of the control group. H. Sherman, Surveillance Effects on Community Physician Test Ordering, 22 *Med. Care* 80, 82 (1984).

22. One study reported a savings of $65 per patient, but at a cost of $62 per patient. J. Eisenberg, *Doctors' Decisions and the Cost of Medicare*, 116 (1986). Another found that physicians' compensatory behavior of increasing the use of unmonitored services erased entirely the net savings from monitoring. L.R. Myers and S.R. Schroeder, Physician Use of Services for the Hospitalized Patient: A Review, with Implications for Cost Containment, 59 *Milbank Mem. Fund Q.* 481, 501 (1981). *See also* Congressional Budget Office, *The Effect of PSROs on Health Care Costs: Current Findings and Future Evaluations* (1979) (finding similar mediocre results from the Medicare review mechanism).

23. Blumstein, The Role of PSROs in Hospital Cost Containment, in *Hospital Cost Containment: Selected Notes for Future Policy*, 461, 472–473 (M. Zubkoff, I. Raskin, and R. Hanft, eds., 1978) (peer review "seems to set current practice patterns as the minimum upon which to build"); CBO Report, *supra* note 22, at 42 ("peer review may alter utilization by patients of physicians whose standards are substantially different from the norm, but such review is unlikely to effect major changes in the standards of physicians as a group").
   Equally disturbing, peer review is highly inexact. A recent study of one Medicare Peer Review Organization's (PRO) quality review function found that it missed two-thirds of the cases with quality problems and that two-thirds of the cases it did identify had no quality problem. "Therefore, the PRO's final quality of care judgment...was only slightly better than random sampling at correctly identifying below standard care." Haya Rubin et al., Watching the Doctor-Watchers: How Well do Peer Review Organization Methods Detect Hospital Care Quality Problems?, 267 *JAMA* 2349 (1992).

24. *See generally Professional Judgment: A Reader in Clinical Decision-Making* (J. Dowie and A. Elstein, eds., 1988); Steven Schwartz and Timothy Griffin, *Medical Thinking: The Psychology of Medical Judgment and Decision Making* (1986); Symposium: The Structure of Clinical Knowledge, 14 *J. Med. and Philosophy* 103 (1989).

25. Note 10 *supra*. The leading exception is Haavi Morreim, but she seems to accept physician rationing more out of resignation, as a matter of practical necessity, than out of theoretical justification. *See Balancing Act: The New Medical Ethics of Medicine's New Economics*, 65–66 (1991) (conflicts of interest are now "inescapable for physicians"; "it is no longer plausible to demand that physicians literally always place patients' interests above their own").

26. E. Haavi Morreim, Fiscal Scarcity and the Inevitability of Bedside Budget Balancing, 149 *Arch. Intern. Med.* 1012, 1013 (1989).

27. *See supra* note 15.

28. *See Restatement of Agency* (1933), §390 comment a; *Restatement of the Law of Trusts* (Second) (1959) §170 comments a and t; Developments, Conflicts of Interest in the Legal Profession, 94 *Harv. L. R.* 1244, 1303–1304 (1981); Rev. Model Business Corporations Act, §8.61, .62, .63; L.S. Sealy, Some Principles of Fiduciary Obligation, 1963 *Camb. L. J.* 119, 136. The major counterexample is for government officials, to whom an absolute prohibition

applies. Marc Rodwin, Physicians' Conflicts of Interest: The Limits of Disclosure, 321 *N. Engl. J. Med.* 1405, 1407 (1989). However, this exception is justified by the absence of a specific beneficiary of the public trust capable of providing consent, other than the general electorate, which has expressed its views through the very law that prohibits conflicts.

29. Mark Hall, *Fiduciary Law: Patient Consent to Conflicts of Interest* (unpublished); Mark A. Hall, *Informed Consent to Rationing Decisions* (unpublished).

30. The only work so far to explore systematically the implications of agency cost theory for ethical problems in the treatment relationship is Allen Buchanan, Principal/Agent Theory and Decisionmaking in Health Care, 2 *Bioethics* 317–333 (1988). Much additional work needs to be done to develop Buchanan's introductory insights and to extend this framework to collective insurance arrangements.

31. This description is drawn from the following sources. The term "agency cost" was introduced in Michael Jensen and William Heckling, The Theory of the Firm: Managerial Behavior, Agency Costs, and Ownership Structure, 3 *J. Fin. Econ.* 305 (1976). Some of the more accessible general articulations are found in Joseph Stiglitz, Principal and Agent, in 3 *The New Palgrave* 966-72 (J. Eatwell, M. Milgate and P. Newman eds. 1987); Pratt & Zechhauser, "Principals and Agents: An Overview," in *Principals and Agents: The Structure of Business* (John Pratt and Richard Zeckhauser, eds. 1985) at 2; Kenneth Arrow, The Economics of Agency, in *id.* at 37. A very lucid introduction to the theory and how it applies generally to classic problems of medical ethics is found in Allen Buchanan, Principal/Agent Theory and Decisionmaking in Health Care, 2 *Bioethics* 317 (1988). *See also* J. Mirrlees, The Optimal Structure of Incentives and Authority within an Organization, 7 *Bell. J. Econ.* 105 (1976); S. Ross, The Economic Theory of Agency: The Principal's Problem, 63 *Am. Econ. Rev.* 134 (1973); J. Stiglitz, Incentives, Risk and Information: Notes Toward a Theory of Hierarchy, 6 *Bell J. Econ.* 552 (1975); Sanford Grossman and Oliver Hart, An Analysis of the Principal-Agent Problem, 51 *Econometrica* 7 (1983).

32. Thus, sales agents may be induced to offer their product to a reluctant buyer at far too steep a discount, one that would cause the principal a loss.

33. Anderson, *infra* note 35, at 761 ("The rules that exist sacrifice some fairness for efficiency and some efficiency for fairness. In criticizing or analyzing such rules, therefore, one must always keep in mind both the costs and the benefits").

34. Thus, it is wrong, as Buchanan does, to view fiduciary status as opposed to agency cost analysis. *Supra* note 30, at 322. Fiduciary rules help to solve agency cost problems. They are one instance of efficient agency risk reduction in action.

35. Much of the recent work in corporate law analyzes corporate fiduciary principles from an agency cost perspective. For a sampling, *see* Frank Easterbrook and Daniel Fischel, *The Economic Structure of Corporate Law* (1991); Frank Easterbrook and Daniel Fischel, Close Corporations and Agency Costs, 38 *Stan. L. Rev.* 271 (1986); Symposium, Contractual Freedom in Corporate Law, 89 *Colum. L. Rev.* 1395 (1989); Daniel Fischel, The Corporate Governance Movement, 35 *Vand. L. Rev.* 1259 (1982). For works that extend this perspective to fiduciary law generally, *see* Robert Cooter and Bradley Freedman, The Fiduciary Relationship: Its Economic Character and Legal Consequences, 66 *NYU L. Rev.* 1045 (1991); Kenneth Davis, Judicial Review of Fiduciary Decisionmaking—Some Theoretical Perspectives, 80 *Nw. U. L. Rev.* 1 (1985); Robert Clark, Contracts, Elites and Traditions in the Making of Corporate Law, 89 *Colum. L. Rev.* 1703 (1989); Alison Anderson, Conflicts of Interest: Efficiency, Fairness and Corporate Structure, 25 *UCLA L. Rev.* 738 (1978).

36. These are termed "relational contracts." Charles Goetz and Robert Scott, Principles of Relational Contracts, 67 *Va. L. Rev.* 1089 (1981); Macneil, Contracts: Adjustment of Long-

Term Economic Relations Under Classical, Neoclassical, and Relational Contract Law, 72 *Nw. U. L. Rev.* 854 (1978).

37. Clark, note 35 *supra*, at 1714–1715.
38. Easterbrook and Fischel, *supra* note 35, at 92.
39. Davis, *supra* note 35, at 47.
40. Arrow, *supra* note 31, at 49.
41. David Dranove and William White, Agency and the Organization of Health Care Delivery, 24 *Inquiry* 405, 413 (1987).
42. Health insurance also creates agency problems for the insurer, particularly when fee-for-service reimbursement is used and the standard for coverage is one of "medical necessity," which defers to professional medical judgment. For further elaboration from the insurer's perspective, see Hall and Anderson, *supra* note 4.
43. Gavin Mooney and Alistair McGuire, Economics and Medical Ethics in Health Care: An Economic Viewpoint, in *Medical Ethics and Economics in Health Care* (1988), at 16; Ake Blomquist, The Doctor as Double Agent: Information Asymmetry, Health Insurance and Medical Care, 10 *J. Health Econ.* 411 (1991); Robert Ohsfeldt, Contractual Arrangements, Financial Incentives, and Physician–Patient Relationships, in *Sociomedical Perspectives on Patient Care Relationship* (Jeffery Clair and Richard Allman, eds., 1993), chapter 6.
44. The delegation is so extensive that British health economist Alan Williams has noted the irony that the actual structure of a treatment encounter often appears more as if the doctor is the principal and the patient is the agent.
45. As Blomquist observes, however, the resulting incentive to undertreat raises yet a third agency cost problem. He maintains that the optimal solution is to adopt a liability rule that counters the HMOs' undertreatment incentive. *Supra* note 43.
46. Daniel Callahan, perhaps the leading advocate of rule-based rationing, acknowledges the inaccuracy and bluntness of rationing rules but revels in them nonetheless, indeed seemingly because of this very quality, as if some suffering were a necessary penitential ingredient in the public deliberative process that creates rationing rules to give the rules their requisite significance. *See* Daniel Callahan, Rationing Health Care: Will It Be Necessary? Can It Be Done Without Age or Disability Discrimination?, 5 *Issues in Law and Med.* 353, 364 (1989).
47. As most readers well know by now, this plan was initially rejected by the U.S. Department of Health and Human Services as discriminatory based on disability, but it was finally approved after certain revisions. *See, e.g.* Michael Astrue, Pseudoscience and the Law: The Case of the Oregon Medicaid Rationing Experiment, 9 *Issues In Law & Medicine* 375 (1994).
48. Schwartz and Aaron, The Achilles Heel of Health Care Rationing, *New York Times* A15 (July 9, 1990).
49. Robert Steinbrook and Bernard Lo, The Oregon Medicaid Demonstration Project—Will It Provide Adequate Medical Care?, 326 *N. Engl. J. Med.* 340, 342 (1992).
50. David Hadorn, Setting Health Care Priorities in Oregon: Cost-Effectiveness Meets the Rule of Rescue, 265 *JAMA* 2218, 2223 (1991). *See also* David Eddy, Oregon's Methods: Did Cost-effectiveness Analysis Fail?, 266 *JAMA* 2135, 2136 (1991) (diagnostic and procedure codes "cannot distinguish between a carotid artery bypass procedure done for a man with 90% occlusion and [angina] symptoms versus an asymptomatic man with 40% occlusion"); U.S. Office of Technology Assessment, Evaluation of the Oregon Medicaid Proposal 7 (1992) (even with 700 items, "the level of heterogeneity...means accepting that some patient with excellent expected outcomes with treatment must forego therapy, while other patients with patently worse treatment-specific prognoses receive it").
The rankings suffer from idiocy as well as ineffectiveness. The quality-of-life assessments used in public opinion surveys to assess the desirability of probable outcomes from each pro-

cedure were plagued by numerous absurdities. For instance, the disabling complication of "trouble speaking" was applied equally to conditions that range from a mild lisp to mutism, and "burn over large areas of the body" was ranked the same as an "upset stomach." Eddy at 2138; David Hadorn, The Oregon Priority-Setting Exercise: Quality of Life and Public Policy, 2 *Hastings Center Rep.* 11, 16 (supplement) (May/June 1991).

51. Lawrence Brown, The National Politics of Oregon's Rationing Plan, *Health Affairs* 28-35, (Summer 1991). *See also* Bruce Vladeck, Unhealthy Rations, *American Prospect* 101 (Summer 1991) .

52. Norman Daniels, Is the Oregon Rationing Plan Fair?, 265 *JAMA* 2232, 2234 (1991); Jack Nagel, Combining Deliberation and Fair Representation in Community Health Decisions, 140 *U. Penn. L. R.* 1965, 1976 (1992); Howard Leichter, Political Accountability in Health Care Rationing: In Search of a New Jerusalem, 140 *U. Penn. L. R.* 1939, 1961 (1992).

53. *Supra* note 50, at 19.

54. Davis, *supra* note 35, at 3.

55. It may be objected that these are the subscribers' enemies, not their friends, but they, after all, are the ones paying for the insurance benefit. Their level of generosity is dictated by labor market conditions and budget appropriations.

56. Omnibus Budget Reconciliation Act of 1990, sec. 4204, codified at 42 U.S.C. 1395mm(i). This statute rescinded for HMOs the total ban on hospital and HMO financial incentive plans that Congress initially applied to Medicare HMO patients in 1986. 42 U.S.C. 1320a-7(a(b). Inexplicably, though, the legislation left in place the ban on hospital financial incentive plans.

57. 57 Fed. Reg. 59024 (December 14, 1992), to be codified at 42 C.F.R. §417.479.

58. Capitation pays a set amount for each patient for whom the doctor is responsible, regardless of how much care each one requires.

59. For various case studies, typologies, and descriptions of the diverse array of HMO structures and payment methods, see W. Pete Welch, Alan Hillman, and Mark Pauly, Toward New Typologies for HMOs, 68 *Milbank Q.* 221 (1990); U.S. Department of Health and Human Services, *Incentive Arrangements Offered by Health Maintenance Organizations and Competitive Medical Plans to Physicians, Report to Congress* (1990); Physician Payment Review Commission, Risk-Sharing Arrangements in Prepaid Health Plans, in *Annual Report to Congress* 275 (1989); Alan Hillman, W. Pete Welch, and Mark Pauly, Contractual Arrangements Between HMOs and Primary Care Physicians: Three-tiered HMOs and Risk Pools, 30 *Med. Care* 136 (1992).

60. *See* note 15 *supra*.

61. Readers may notice a superficial similarity between this categorization scheme and Rodwin's description in Chapter 9 in this volume. However, our schemas were developed independently and have important differences.

62. Primary care services are associated with the costs of office management, equipment, and materials, but these enjoy sufficient economies of scale that the major disincentive to treat is the inconvenience of a heavy patient load. However, financial disincentives do exist when primary care capitation extends to the costs of outpatient testing and ancillary care services, as is often the case. *See* Alan Hillman, Mark Pauly, Keith Kerman, and Caroline Martinek, HMO Mangers' Views on Financial Incentives and Quality, 10 *Health Affairs* 207, 211 (Winter 1990).

63. It applies only where "the plan places a physician...at substantial financial risk for services *not provided by the physician*." 42 U.S.C. §1395mm(i). *See* 57 Fed. Reg. 59029 (December 14, 1992).

64. Lawrence Casalino, Balancing Incentives: How Should Physicians Be Reimbursed?, 267 *JAMA* 403 (1992) (advocating a combination of fee-for-service and capitation payments).

65. Over half of IPAs provide fee-for-service reimbursement, whereas fewer than 10 percent of other HMO models employ this method. Stated otherwise, of the HMO models using fee-for-service payment, 75 percent are IPAs. Alan Hillman, Financial Incentives for Physicians in HMOs: Is There a Conflict of Interest?, 317 *N. Engl. J. Med.* 1743, 1745 (1987).

66. In a universal survey of all HMOs existing in 1986 (but with a response rate of only 51 percent), Hillman found that whereas two-thirds of all HMOs withhold a portion of payments from primary care physicians, only 21 percent of plans with salaried physicians do so. Alan Hillman, *supra* note 66.

67. Hillman found that 82 percent of fee-for-service plans use withholding, as do 67 percent of capitation plans, compared to only 21 percent of salaried plans. *Id.*

68. Group Health Association of America, Preliminary Results of the GHAA-BC/BS Survey of Physician Incentives in Health Maintenance Organizations, November 1987, in Vol. II of *DHHS Report*, at 5; Hillman, *supra* note 66; Hillman et al., *supra* note 62. The very few cases of withholds as high as 50 percent are unique situations where the HMO was in such dire financial distress that the doctors most likely had little expectation that the withhold would be returned in any event. Therefore, their extreme was unlikely to affect the physicians' behavior very greatly. *DHHS Report, supra* note 59, at V-38.

69. Stephen Moore and Diane Martin, Does the Primary-Care Gatekeeper Control the Costs of Health Care? Lessons from the SAFECO Experience, 309 *N. Engl. J. Med.* 1400, 1402 (1983). It is remarkable to compare this autopsy of the HMO's collapse with the glowing reports of its initial success reported in an earlier article in the same journal. Stephen Moore, Cost Containment Through Risk-Sharing by Primary-Care Physicians, 300 *N. Engl. J. Med.* 1359 (1979).

70. Alan Hillman, Mark Pauly, and Joseph Kerstein, How do Financial Incentives Affect Physicians' Clinical Decisions and the Financial Performance of Health Maintenance Organizations?, 321 *N. Engl. J. Med.* 86, 91 (1989). The study found that only the method of base payment—salary or capitation—had a significant effect on hospitalization. Withhold funds did have some effect on the use of outpatient services, however.

71. 57 Fed. Reg. 59027 (December 14, 1992), to be codified at 42 C.F.R. § 417.479(d). The higher versus lower percentage applies according to whether the physician (or group's) risk is calculated annually or more often. The additional scrutiny comes in the form of requiring patient satisfaction surveys. The additional safeguards come in the form of imposing a stop-loss level of 5 percent higher than the threshold level.

72. I stress individual because, as discussed next, if total capitation payments are made to a sufficiently large group, then the disincentive to treat is much more attenuated and depends much more heavily on how the profits and losses are distributed within the group than on the capitation payment itself.

73. Observe that this percentage figure is not comparable with the 10–30 percent figure just cited since that compares the out-of-pocket risk against the base physician payment amount, not against the total costs of treatment. To make such a comparison, we would need to know how to allocate the total HMO premium between primary care and other services. Using an arbitrary 50/50 allocation, the relevant risk percentage here would be 50 percent of the physician's base pay; alternatively, the at-risk range previously mentioned could be converted to 20–60 percent of total treatment costs.

74. *DHHS Report, supra* note 59, at V-40.

75. 57 Fed. Reg. 59029 (December 14, 1992), to be codified at 42 C.F.R. § 417.479(e), (f).

76. 57 Fed. Reg. 59032 (December 14, 1992), to be codified at 42 C.F.R. §417.479(g).

77. 42 U.S.C. 1395mm(i).

78. *See* Proposed Rule, 57 Fed. Reg. 59033 (December 14, 1992), to be codified at 42 C.F.R. §417.479 (c).

79. U.S. General Accounting Office, *Physician Incentive Payments by Hospitals Could Lead to Abuse* 14 (July 1986). Observe, however, that if the timing were changed from monthly to semiannually, this incentive arrangement would be quite acceptable, considering the factors previously discussed, which have a diluting or mitigating effect. It is a (a) small percentage (b) bonus (c) set against a background of fee-for-service practice (d) in a single institution, and (e) it would be aggregated over a large number of patients and a significant length of time.

80. House Report No. 101-899, Committee on Ways and Means, October 18, 1990. This report also suggests that payments greater than 10 percent of total compensation from the plan are suspect, but this recommendation is not likely to be followed by DHHS in its regulations. *See* text at notes 68–71 *supra*.

81. 57 Fed. Reg. 59027 (December 14, 1992), to be codified at 42 C.F.R. §417.479(d).

82. Taking physician group size, for instance, too large of a group will induce free-rider behavior in which no doctor sees it in his interest to economize, since he will receive only a tiny fraction of the savings produced by his own treatment decisions. *DHHS Report, supra* note 59, at V-12.

83. 42 U.S.C. §1395mm(i)(8)(A)(ii); 57 *Federal Register* 59032 (December 14, 1992), to be codified at 42 C.F.R. §417.479(g).

84. *See generally DHHS Report, supra* note 59, at chapter IV (summarizing the multiple sources of state and federal law).

85. *See generally* F.C. Cunningham and J.W. Williamson, How Does the Quality of Care in HMOs Compare to That in Other Settings? An Analytic Review: 1958–1979, 1 *Group Health J.* 4 (1980) (in a review of studies of HMO quality, found HMOs superior and the rest found them equivalent); J. Bates and M. J. Conners, Assessing Process of Care under Capitated and Fee-for-Service Medicare, *Health Care Financing Review*, 1987 Ann. Supp., at 57 (reviewing the literature and concluding that the quality of care in HMOs is at least equal to that of fee-for-service); Ellwood and Paul, But What About Quality?, Health Affairs 135 (Spring 1986) (same). The notable exception is for sick poor patients. One study found that they fared somewhat worse in HMOs under some, but not all, measures of health status. J. Ware, R. Brook, W. Rogers, E. Keeler, A. Davies, C. Sherbourne, G. Goldberg, P. Camp and J. Newhouse, Comparison of Health Outcomes at a Health Maintenance Organization with Those of Fee-for-Service Care, 120 *Lancet* 1017 (1986).

86. HHS Report, *supra* note 59, at V-8.

87. *Id.* at V-20.

88. Alan Hillman, Health Maintenance Organizations, Financial Incentives, and Physicians' Judgments, 112 *Ann. Intern. Med.* 891, 892 (1990).

This work was supported by a grant from the Robert Wood Johnson Foundation. The analysis and conclusions are entirely my own. However, I benefitted greatly from the insightful comments and critique I received from Allan Buchanan and Marc Rodwin.

11

Conflicts of Interest for
Physician Entrepreneurs

E. Haavi Morreim

One of the more controversial ethical issues of medicine's new economics concerns physicians who refer patients to facilities in which they are investors. A number of physicians made such investments, particularly in the late 1980s and early 1990s, and news reports have cited a growing list of alleged abuses.[1] In 1989, the Office of the Inspector General (OIG) of the Department of Health and Human Services (DHHS) found that 12 percent of physicians who treat Medicare patients referred them to laboratories or other facilities in which they have a financial interest. These physicians' patients received about 45 percent more clinical laboratory services and 13 percent more physiological testing services than other Medicare patients.[2]

By 1991, the Florida Health Care Cost Containment Board reported that at least 40 percent of physicians in Florida had invested in ancillary facilities, and more than 90 percent of the state's diagnostic imaging facilities were owned partly or wholly by physicians.[3] The Florida study alleged widespread problems of overutilization, overpricing, reduced access, and poorer quality of care, particularly in clinical laboratories, diagnostic imaging, physical therapy, and rehabilitation centers.[4]

More recently, a study by the General Accounting Office (GAO) found that physicians with imaging equipment in their offices or practices ordered magnetic resonance imaging (MRI) scans, computerized tomography (CT) scans, ultrasound, echocardiography, and other sophisticated imaging tests two to five times more often than physicians who referred their patients outside their practices for these studies.[5]

In September 1991, a DHHS departmental appeals board ruled that the Hanlester Network of clinical laboratories, which received most of its business from referring investor-physicians, may have received illegal remuneration in return for referrals. Though the Network did not literally base dividends on the number of referrals, it energetically reminded its physician partners that the success of the venture depended on their referrals, rewarded high-volume referring physicians with invitations to buy a larger share of the business, and pressured those sending insufficient business to increase referrals or sell back their interest.[6]

Concerns over the conflicts of interest and alleged abuses associated with self-referral have led to new rounds of government restrictions.[7] In 1989 Congress amended the Social Security Act to prohibit physicians from referring Medicare patients to clinical laboratories in which they have a financial interest.[8] Though the prohibition did not encompass other facilities, such as diagnostic imaging centers, the law did require entities providing Medicare-covered services to supply the government with information concerning their ownership, including the identities of physician investors and the occasions on which they referred their own patients to that entity.[9]

That law was considerably broadened in 1993. It now covers inpatient and outpatient hospital services, radiology and other diagnostic services, radiation therapy, durable medical equipment, physical and occupational therapy, parenteral and enteral nutrition equipment and supplies, prosthetics and orthotics, home health care services, and outpatient prescription drugs. Various exemptions are included in the law, such as for certain in-office equipment and services.[10] Through a separate bill, these restrictions applicable to Medicare were also extended to Medicaid.

In July, 1991, the OIG published its long-awaited safe-harbor guidelines.[11] Required by the Medicare and Medicaid Patient and Program Protection Act of 1987,[12] these guidelines outline more precisely what sorts of activities will not be subject to prosecution as kickbacks or other financial abuses. In general, they specify that no more than 40 percent of an enterprise's investors can be physicians in a position to refer patients to the business, and no more than 40 percent of revenues can come from referrals by investor physicians.

States, too, are enacting legislation. Whereas some states have long restricted self-referral and other conflicts of interest,[13] others have added new legislation. In their 1992 legislative sessions, Florida, New York, New Jersey, Illinois, and Missouri all enacted bans on self-referral, some applying to virtually all self-referral and others affecting only certain areas, such as diagnostic imaging, physical therapy, and the like.[14] Other legislatures have enacted or considered a range of similar measures.[15]

Professional organizations are also scrutinizing investment arrangements more closely. In December 1991, the American Medical Association (AMA) altered its previously permissive stance on self-referral, declaring it to be unethical except where there is a genuine need for the facility and no alternative financing is available.[16] After internal dissension caused it to reverse its stand in June 1992, the organization again reaffirmed its opposition in December 1992.[17] The AMA states that it will actively investigate physicians who fail to comply.[18] While such organizations have no official enforcement power, any decisions to revoke physicians' memberships must be reported to state medical boards, which, in turn, report the information to the National Practitioner Data Bank.[19] Since hospitals must consult the data bank in their credentialing decisions, information in it can affect physicians' staff privileges and thereby their livelihoods.

A number of commentators, believing there are no other ways to control this threat to patients' welfare and the nation's health budget, propose close government regulation or an outright ban on physician self-referral.[20] However, I oppose that approach. First, it is *undesirable* to prohibit or unduly restrict physician investment because, in the process, one can discourage useful arrangements that can serve patients and the health care system. Indeed, virtually the entire debate thus far has misconstrued the issue. Once we understand that the real question concerns not physicians' prerogatives to self-refer but rather patients' right to choose their own providers, the idea of global restriction becomes untenable.

Second, it is *unnecessary* to prohibit or unduly restrict physician investment legislatively, because the law already contains a variety of powerful tools by which to suppress and penalize abusive self-referral. These include such common law doctrines as informed consent, fiduciary duty, and bad faith breach of contract, as well as antitrust laws governing appropriate conduct of entrepreneurs in the marketplace.

Prohibition: Undesirable

We can justify physician investments the same way we justify any form of entrepreneurship. A free market enhances people's freedom to choose the products and services that they deem best, and it promotes important information. Where consumers don't buy a product, manufacturers can learn what is undesirable in that product and improve it. Reciprocally, buyers who are free to try a variety of products can discover sooner which ones best meet their needs.[21] Vigorous competition in health care can foster creativity, with new products and services, greater efficiency, better quality of care, and the host of benefits we hope for in a free marketplace.

The Federal Trade Commission has noted a number of potential advantages in physician investment: Quality of care can improve when the physician has an economic interest to ensure that his[22] facility is of high quality; physicians, who are most familiar with their patients' needs, can best identify community health care needs and provide an important pool of equity capital to finance worthwhile projects; and vigorous competition can enhance efficiency.[23] To gain those advantages, investors must be permitted a measure of freedom to enjoy the rewards of a successful effort. "Unless the builders of better mousetraps are rewarded and the builders of inferior mousetraps are not, better mousetraps will not be built."[24]

Thus, if local physicians believe that existing mammography units charge patients too much or are insensitive to their needs, thereby discouraging important preventive care, they may establish their own facility with a lower price and better service. If a group of physicians believe that the local for-profit laboratory has inadequately trained staff or emphasizes productivity at the price of accuracy, they can establish a superior alternative.[25] If restrictive legislation deters physicians from making such useful investments, health care can be harmed.

A second problem is posed by the fact that existing and proposed prohibitions on self-referral apply only to free-standing units, not to in-office facilities. This is true, for instance, of Medicare's ban on self-referral to clinical laboratories.[26] And yet it is difficult to justify this differential treatment. The potential benefits of in-office testing services are substantial, just as they are for free-standing units. Quicker test results mean that the patient can save time, avert inconvenience, and even sometimes shorten an illness.

However, the danger of abuse in the office is at least as great as it is in free-standing units. Aside from the possibility of poor-quality service—a danger that spawned federal regulation of in-office laboratories[27]—there are the familiar hazards of overutilization and overcharging.[28] In a 1990 survey of in-office radiological testing, Hillman and colleagues discovered that for several common procedures, physicians who had their own equipment ordered four times as many studies, and ran costs up to seven times higher, than physicians who referred their patients to a radiologist.[29] More recent studies confirm similar findings.[30] Additionally, the prospect of easy money from a captive audience could inspire some physicians to acquire excessive amounts of in-office equipment.

Legislators' exclusive focus on free-standing facilities does not merely neglect the serious problems posed by in-office facilities. It reopens the door to the entire array of self-referral abuses, merely transposed to a different setting. So long as prohibitions apply to free-standing but not to in-house facilities, a determined physician-investor can often escape restriction altogether. With the aid of a good carpenter, he can establish an examination room at the independent facility and hold office hours there periodically, thereby transforming the formerly free-standing facility into an office-based one. Or he and his coinvestors can acquire a new building that houses both physician offices and the referral facility, as for instance when an orthopedic group joins with its physical therapy unit under one roof. Such maneuvers could shield many self-referral arrangements.

Thus, a fully effective ban might have to prohibit physicians from owning any but the most rudimentary examination equipment. And yet that sort of proscription could easily harm patient care by increasing the inconvenience and delay in securing important tests and treatments. As a result, it is difficult to justify prohibiting or heavily restricting physicians' referring their patients to free-standing facilities without similarly restricting office-based facilities. If we are reluctant to refuse patients the advantages of in-office laboratories and x-rays, then we are hard pressed to justify refusing them whatever advantages they might enjoy by using their physicians' free-standing facilities.

Finally, there is a far more fundamental problem. Few people would deny that physicians should be free to spend their money as they wish, including investing in health care facilities. Rather, the debate is over whether physicians should be permitted to refer their own patients there. Self-referral, not mere investment, creates the conflicts of interest and potential for abuse. And yet, the way in which the issue is usually framed—whether the physician should be permitted to self-refer, or whether he should be required to send the patient elsewhere—misconstrues the real problem. It assumes a morally anachronistic picture of the physician–patient relationship in which the physician "refers" the patient. That is, he simply chooses, unilaterally, where the patient will receive ancillary care.[31] If the patient objects or expresses a particular preference, the physician may agree to an alternative but, on this traditional picture, the physician ordinarily presumes to make the choice.

A few decades ago, much of the medical community held this same presumption with respect to virtually any therapeutic decision. The Hippocratic tradition encouraged physicians not to involve patients in decision-making or even to inform them truthfully about their condition.[32] Contemporary medical and legal doctrine has long since rejected such paternalism in favor of an informed consent in which the physician describes all reasonable therapeutic options so that the patient can choose among them, based on his own values and goals.[33]

This patient participation often includes the decision on whether to seek care from additional providers, yet curiously, it seems not to include the choice of which person or institution will provide that service. There is a historical explanation. Up to the past decade or so, virtually all the costliest, most sophisticated technologies were located in hospitals, partly because hospitals were the obvious financiers of such projects and partly because insurers generally paid for such interventions only if they were performed in a hospital. Since physicians usually had staff privileges at only one or two hospitals, the decision to use such a technology automatically dictated the facility at which the procedure would be performed.

As health care costs continued to rise, however, payers began to favor out-patient over inpatient care, creating a vigorous market for free-standing diag-nostic and therapeutic facilities.[34] As a broad variety of options now exists, it is difficult to justify this odd vestige of history and paternalism. When the physician refers the patient to a particular diagnostic center or physical therapy agency, he is unilaterally deciding where the patient will spend his money and in whom the patient will put his trust. This practice is an anachronism. The choice of ancillary facilities or consultant specialists can involve values every bit as important and personal as the choice of medical treatments—matters such as price, quality, convenience, and courtesy—and the patient is entitled to decide where and on whom he will spend his own money.

Therefore, the important question is not whether the physician should be permitted to refer a patient to his own facility—defined here as the physician's presuming to send the patient directly to his own facility without discussing alternatives or empowering the patient to make the final choice. Clearly, the answer is no. Self-referral, intrinsically a preemption of patient choice, is wrong. Rather, the question is whether the patient should be permitted to choose to use his own providers, including a facility in which his physician has a finan-cial interest. To ban self-referral is, in essence, to forbid the patient to make that choice. It is nearly as restrictive as, and potentially no less harmful than, self-referral itself. Whereas a physician's self-referral dictates where the patient will spend his money and receive his care, a government prohibition dictates to the patient, just as rigidly, where he can *not* choose to go and where he will *not* spend his money. Either way the patient loses. His choices are preempted, whether by his physician or by his government.

Suppose, for example, that a group of physicians has invested to bring out-patient cardiac catheterization facilities into their locality. Suppose further that although inpatient cardiac catheterization is safe and effective, the outpatient alternative is more comfortable for patients, requires less time away from work, and costs less.[35] Prohibiting self-referral would mean not only that the physician-owners of this facility cannot presume to send their patients there, but also that their patients cannot choose to go there, even if they are fully advised of the alternatives and of their own physician's financial interests. Or suppose, in like manner, that two home nursing agencies serve an area, one with a very good reputation and moderate prices, the other mediocre at best, with higher prices. If it happens that a patient's own physician is an investor in the former (a facility perhaps created because the latter was inadequate), then again, a prohibition on self-referral would mean not just that the physician cannot automatically direct his patients to his own agency, but also that the patient himself is forbidden to choose what he believes to be better care at lower cost.

Once it is clear that the real ethical issues concern patient choice, the next question concerns how to address abusive conduct by physicians. The mere fact that a physician is an investor in a facility his patient uses does not mean that any wrong has occurred. Nevertheless, given the enormous sums of money to be made in the market for ancillary health care, the potential for patient abuse is serious. As we will see, a variety of legal devices is already in place for penalizing abusive physician investors.

Prohibition: Unnecessary

Three levels of abuse in self-referral can be distinguished. At the most basic level, even a benevolently motivated self-referral fails to honor the patient's right to make informed decisions. Second, in more serious cases the physician begins to make judgment calls in his own favor. The indications for further diagnostic workup may be equivocal, for example, and the physician may give the benefit of the doubt to himself as he proposes that the further testing be done and then refers the patient to his own diagnostic facility. Third, the physician may commit blatant abuse, such as by sending patients for interventions that they clearly do not need or to a facility of clearly inferior quality.

Failure of Informed Consent

As defined above, all self-referral is at least somewhat abusive. The physician preempts the patient's preferences in favor of his own. Even where the physician self-refers from the belief that his own facility is truly the best for the patient, or where he intends to waive the patient's fees and thereby erase any financial gain for himself, he still bypasses the patient's judgment. We do not permit such paternalism for treatment decisions, and we should not accept it for referral choices. In medical malpractice law there is already a strong tradition requiring physicians to secure informed consent for treatment choices. Such informed consent should now apply to economic factors, so that the patient can consider the costs of proposed treatments, the merits of various providers, and the physician's conflicts of interest.[36]

This requirement for information is not satisfied if the physician simply tells the patient that he is an investor in the facility, as required in many states' disclosure laws.[37] The patient may be utterly puzzled as to why the physician is dropping this little fact into the conversation, or he may think that the physician is designating the referral site as an extension of his office. Or he might see the disclosure as an advertisement of its quality: "my doctor wouldn't have bought it if it weren't the best in town."

Nor is the information requirement satisfied if, after recommending his own facility, the physician provides a list of alternatives and promises not to be vindictive if the patient chooses one of them.[38] Real disclosure requires that the physician provide the patient with the factual basis on which to make an intelligent decision. Important differences exist among referral options. One facility may be close to the patient's home or workplace; another may have more convenient hours; one may be less expensive; another may be a "preferred provider" favored by the patient's insurance carrier; another may have different equipment, with its advantages and disadvantages. It is already well recognized that in choosing among therapies, a patient needs to know more than just the name of each therapy. He needs to know the risks and benefits, and to have some idea of what it would be like to actually experience each option. Comparable information is needed for choosing among ancillary providers.[39]

In addition to the law of informed consent, patients may be protected by various states' consumer protection laws. Some commentators argue that unnecessary testing, disclosure of medical and economic information, and a variety of other issues are covered by laws such as deceptive trade practices acts.[40] Such remedies vary from state to state.

Breach of Fiduciary Duty

At a second level of abuse, self-referral can begin in subtle ways to favor the physician's interests over the patient's. Much of medicine requires judgment calls in which competing answers can be justified. The conclusion that an MRI scan is medically indicated, for example, requires a judgment that the scan is likely to reveal information that will be useful in treating the patient, and that the improvement in the patient's care is likely to be worth the cost and risk. In many instances there is no "gold standard" for making such judgments, and good physicians can differ. Where a physician has an investment in an imaging facility, he can easily find himself casting the benefit of the doubt toward intervention.

Even where the physician's recommendation falls within an acceptable standard of care, therefore, he may still violate his fiduciary duty obligating him to hold his patient's interests paramount, even above his own.[41] Fiduciaries generally are expected to refrain from engaging in conflicts of interest and, where they cannot, they must disclose the problem to the beneficiary and permit the latter to decide how the situation will be managed. Where the physician subtly shifts his standards of medical judgment in ways that benefit his own interests, and where he keeps his conflict of interest hidden, he violates this duty.

The case of *Moore v. Regents of the University of California* applies both informed consent and fiduciary law to physicians' economic conflicts of interest.[42] When Dr. David Golde treated John Moore for hairy cell leukemia, he verified, after removing Moore's spleen, his prior scientific hunch that Moore's cells might be capable of producing a medically useful and potentially lucrative cell line for treatment of other patients. On a number of occasions over the next seven years, Golde required Moore to return to UCLA from his home in Seattle to provide samples of blood, blood serum, skin, sperm, and bone marrow aspirate. These samples were in fact used to advance Golde's research, but Golde told Moore that such visits were necessary to his health and could be performed only by himself or his associates.[43] Much of the cost, including travel costs, was at Moore's expense.[44]

The California Supreme Court denied Moore's claim to a property interest in the cell line and its profits but ruled that he did have a cause of action against Golde. That cause "can properly be characterized either as the breach of a fiduciary duty to disclose facts material to the patient's consent or, alternatively, as the performance of medical procedures without first having obtained the patient's informed consent."[45] Although consent questions typically arise regarding medical rather than financial matters,

> "the concept of informed consent...is broad enough to encompass the latter....The possibility that an interest extraneous to the patient's health has affected the physician's judgment is something that a reasonable patient would want to know in deciding whether to consent to a proposed course of treatment. It is material to the patient's decision and, thus, a prerequisite to informed consent."[46]

Therefore, the court reasoned:

> These principles lead to the following conclusions: (1) a physician must disclose personal interests unrelated to the patient's health, whether research or economic, that may affect the physician's professional judgment; and (2) a physician's failure to disclose such interests may give rise to a cause of action for performing medical procedures without informed consent or breach of fiduciary duty....Accordingly, we hold that a physician who is seeking a patient's consent for a medical procedure must, in order to satisfy his fiduciary duty and to obtain the patient's informed consent, disclose personal interests unrelated to the patient's health, whether research or economic, that may affect his medical judgment.[47]

While the *Moore* case focused on conflicts of interest in research, it encompasses the conflicts embedded in self-referral. Indeed, the court based a significant portion of its reasoning on a California statute requiring physicians to disclose in writing any investment interest in health care facilities to which they may refer their patients.[48]

Fraud, Kickbacks, Negligence, and Bad Faith

At a third level, the most serious abuse occurs when a physician flagrantly exploits his patients for personal gain. He commits fraud, collects a kickback, refers patients for clearly unnecessary or poor-quality care, or care at unreasonably high prices, solely to enrich himself.

Powerful legal tools already exist to combat such abuse. As noted above, the federal government pursues kickbacks and other financial abuses of tax funds through the Medicare and Medicaid Patient and Program Protection Act of 1987[49] and through the OIG's safe harbor guidelines.[50] Of 1258 cases investigated up to the early 1990s, over 800 were deemed worthy of pursuit and, of these, some 600 resulted in some form of settlement or penalty.[51]

Patients who have been injured by abusive self-referral may also have potent civil recourse. If a physician refers the patient to a facility that he knows or should know to be poor in quality and the patient is harmed, the patient may have a cause of action not only against the facility but also against the physician who sent him there.[52] When the physician is an investor, juries are unlikely to believe that the physician was unaware of his own facility's quality.

In some instances, an aggrieved patient may also be able to sue under a doctrine called "bad faith breach of contract." Although this approach has not been applied to self-referral, the theory is plausible and consistent with case law. And because such suits are generally lodged in tort rather than contract, they afford a prevailing plaintiff more than just economic damages for the extra cost of an unnecessary or high-priced intervention. They could also support recovery for emotional distress, attorneys' fees, and, in particularly egregious cases, costly punitive damages.[53]

Ordinarily, those who enter into a contract are free to set terms as they wish, including the manner in which they will address a breach of that contract. Commonly, such breaches are redressed by requiring the offending party to place the other in the position he would have enjoyed had the contract been fulfilled.[54] Thus, a contractor bidding to build a home or bridge might agree to complete the structure by a certain deadline or to pay a fine for every day over deadline until the project is complete. If he makes neither the deadline nor the late payments, a court can force him to make good.

Some contracts, however, differ from ordinary commercial agreements in that the parties do not bargain with equal power. One party is dependent on the other for an important service, while the latter writes the terms of their agreement and may even hold the power to determine how the agreement will be fulfilled. While the law requires all who enter into a contract to meet their obligations in good faith, those who fail in cases like these may be subject to added damages through the doctrine of bad faith breach of contract, or "bad faith."[55]

Courts have not established clear criteria to define bad faith cases, but several common elements have emerged: (1) the weaker party's purpose in entering the contract is not personal gain, but to protect himself or to secure some other essential service; (2) one of the parties enjoys a superior bargaining position that enables it largely to dictate the terms of the contract; (3) the weaker party must place his trust in the stronger, thus creating a fiduciary relationship; and (4) the stronger party acts to deprive the weaker one of that to which he is entitled under the contract.[56]

Health insurers refusing to pay a subscriber's claim for medical and hospital costs, for instance, have sometimes been found to breach good faith requirements. These rulings suggest no reason to confine the doctrine to insurance companies. "[B]oth the tort of bad faith failure to exercise due care in discharge of a contractual duty and the granting of damages for mental anguish caused by a willful and wanton breach of contract are grounded in basic common law, and not solely in the area of insurance law."[57] "'Bad faith, then, is not simply bad judgment or negligence. It imports a dishonest purpose and means a breach of known duty, i.e., good faith and fair dealing, through some motive or self-interest or ill-will.'"[58]

While bad faith doctrine has not hitherto been applied to physicians or to abusive self-referral, such a move could satisfy all four elements identified above. (1) The physician–patient relationship generally begins with a contract in which the patient's aim is not financial gain but personal security and health. (2) The physician, far more knowledgeable and powerful than the vulnerable, often ill patient, is usually able to secure the patient's agreement to whatever plan of action he recommends.[59] Indeed, courts have been quick to call contracts between health care providers and patients adhesory.[60] (3) Thus, the patient must trust in the physician to be knowledgeable, competent, and motivated by the patient's best interests, thereby creating a fiduciary relationship.[61] (4) Finally, where a physician uses this superior power to his own advantage by self-referring the patient for needless, poor-quality, or excessively priced care, he has deprived the patient of the central benefit of their contractually created fiduciary relationship: medical care designed to promote the patient's interests, even above the physician's.[62] He has actively disregarded the patient's rights, whether the right to adequate-quality care, informed consent, or fiduciary disclosure of conflicts of interest.

Bad faith doctrine in this context should be restricted, as elsewhere, to the most egregious abuses. The physician who refers the patient to his own facility in the sincere belief that it offers better service at lower cost has wronged the patient by preempting informed choice. But he has acted in good faith, even if erroneously. In contrast, the physician who sets up a "mill," running large numbers of patients through for tests and treatments at high cost with little or no medical justification, acts in bad faith. If courts do accept this extension of bad faith doctrine, patients victimized by such abusive self-referral could collect extensive damages from physicians and, in the process, deter other physicians from similar conduct.

Patients and society as a whole can be harmed on yet another level by self-referral. To self-refer is to dictate which product or provider the patient will choose and where the patient will spend his money. The physician thereby harms the free enterprise system and the consumers who rely on it to enact their personal values in the marketplace. Arguably, this injury constitutes an antitrust violation.

Antitrust: Basic Law and Values

One of the clearest statements of the purpose of antitrust law comes from the U.S. Supreme Court in *Times-Picayune v. United States*: "Basic to the faith that a free economy best promotes the public weal is that goods must stand the cold test of competition; that the public, acting through the market's impersonal judgment, shall allocate the Nation's resources and thus direct the course its economic development will take."[63] Antitrust law aims to protect consumer welfare by fostering free enterprise and vigorous competition, thereby maximizing the nation's welfare.[64]

Antitrust law in the United States began with the Sherman Act of 1890, enacted in response to the monopolies, trusts, and widespread price fixing of the nineteenth century. Its two main provisions were, in Section 1, to prohibit all conspiracies, contracts, and combinations to restrain trade among the states and, in Section 2, to prohibit monopolization, as well as conspiracies and attempts to monopolize in interstate trade.[65] The Sherman Act was supplemented in 1914 by the Clayton Act and the Federal Trade Commission (FTC) Act. These two laws tried not only to specify more precisely what activities are violations of antitrust law, but also to establish the government's regulatory authority to prohibit actions that, while not yet fully violations of the Sherman Act, were likely over time to lessen competition or restrain trade.[66]

For a 100 years, then, most commerce has been subject to antitrust scrutiny by the Justice Department and the FTC. However, not until 1975 did medicine, law, and other learned professions come explicitly within its ambit.[67] Since then, physicians have faced antitrust scrutiny in a variety of areas, particularly price fixing, boycotts of alternative providers such as chiropractors, restraints on innovative forms of health care delivery such as HMOs, restraints on advertising, and peer review.[68] The list is not yet closed, however. As argued below, self-referral can potentially offend antitrust law in several ways. We begin by looking at the restraints of trade prohibited by Section 1 of the Sherman Act and related laws, and then consider monopoly practices proscribed in Section 2 of this act and elsewhere.[69]

Section 1: Restraints of Trade

Together, Sherman Section 1, the Clayton Act, and the FTC Act forbid a wide range of practices that can harm competition. Note, they do not mean to protect individual competitors.[70] Indeed, one sure result of a free market is that some competitors will be losers: If Smith buys his car from Jones, then he does not buy it from Baker. Rather, these laws aim to preserve fairness of competition, thereby promoting freedom for buyers and sellers and, with it, the diversity of goods and services that can best meet our needs with quality and efficiency.[71]

Many of the most common antitrust offenses concern groups of people conspiring to corner large segments of a market. Later, we will examine such offenses as monopolization and boycott. However, competition can be offended on a much smaller scale. Individual physician entrepreneurs who thwart the market via self-referral can be guilty of tying arrangements.

Tying Arrangements

Tying arrangements were first specifically outlawed in the Clayton Act, Section 3.[72] They are also encompassed by Sherman Section 1 and by Section 5 of the FTC Act, which gives the FTC broad authority to intervene where actions either constitute unfair competition or will likely lead to violations of the Sherman or Clayton acts.[73]

In a typical tie-in, a seller with substantial market power over one product (the *tying* product) requires its buyers to purchase a second product (the *tied* product) as a condition for buying the first. Many of the first tying cases arose in patent law, where a firm with a legitimate monopoly on one product, such as a patented salt processing machine, required the buyer also to buy a second, separate and distinct product—all of its salt—from that company.[74]

Over time, the legal and economic criteria for tie-ins have varied. The seller need not have a literal monopoly over the tying product. "Appreciable market power,"[75] a "special ability,"[76] an advantage not shared by competitors,[77] or even the uniqueness or special desirability of the tying product[78] can also suffice to describe the seller's influence over the first product. In some instances, the sheer inequality of bargaining power between buyer and seller has sufficed because such inequality, like market power, can induce the buyer to accept the second product whether or not he wants it.[79] In a recent decision, the Supreme Court held that a significant cost or other impediment associated with switching to another seller can endow that seller with the necessary power over the buyer in the aftermarket for the tied product.[80] In whatever form, this initial power enables that seller to exercise leverage over the buyer[81] to induce him to buy a product or patronize a seller he might not otherwise want.[82] If a not insubstantial volume of competition in the second market thereby is significantly foreclosed or unreasonably restrained,[83] the arrangement may constitute an illegal tie-in.

Two other requirements are also important. First, the two products must be distinct from each other.[84] There is nothing wrong with selling shoes with shoelaces as one product, or even with pairing flour and sugar in a special sale at a grocery store.[85] The tying prohibition aims not to forbid such useful arrangements but rather to ensure that those who have significant market power in one area do not use that power to hinder competition in another area. Second, as with all antitrust law, the violation must affect, or be "in the flow of," interstate commerce, unless the activity is scrutinized under the antitrust law of a particular state.[86]

Tying arrangements are condemned for a number of reasons. They can foreclose the market to competitors, who may find it too costly to compete in both product lines.[87] They preclude competition between products on the basis of their merits,[88] thereby potentially insulating inferior products.[89] And they preclude consumers from exercising their own judgment about which products they really want to buy and from whom.[90] Tie-ins have traditionally been regarded by courts as so pernicious, and so utterly devoid of any possible justification, that they are held illegal per se—that is, they are declared illegal without any need to examine the seller's intentions or even to look for actual harm to competition.[91]

Although courts have not yet applied the antitrust tie-in doctrine to self-referral, arguably they can and should. Let us consider in turn the five elements outlined above: (1) the first (tying) product has market power or other special desirability, (2) which the seller uses as leverage to force the consumer to purchase the tied product, (3) which is distinct from the first product, (4) adversely affecting competition in the second market (5) on an interstate level.

Market Power or Other Special Desirability. An individual physician cannot be said to possess market power, except perhaps in a rural area. And yet he does have considerable power because he offers something unique or specially desirable.[92] The patient needs medical care, sometimes to save his very life, and cannot gain access to the most potent tests and treatments without the prescription of a physician, who alone is legally licensed to diagnose and treat illness. The physician possesses vastly greater knowledge and power relative to the ill, vulnerable patient and thereby enjoys a position of influence over the patient.[93]

In this sense, physicians have the kind of power at which antitrust law aims, even more perfectly than the most powerful monopoly. In ordinary business, the firm's power over the consumer is indirect: It influences his decisions by producing something he wants and perhaps by being the only firm to do so. It controls supply and advertises vigorously because it cannot manipulate demand directly.

In medicine, unlike virtually any other enterprise, the physician has direct power over the consumer. That is, the physician actually controls the "demand" side of the economic equation.[94] In many cases, once a disease requires that something be done, the physician can literally dictate purchase decisions to the patient-consumer. Although the doctrine of informed consent requires physicians to involve patients in decisions, patients often do not challenge medical recommendations.[95] Such extraordinary power was noted by a California appellate court in upholding that state's law forbidding physicians to own pharmacies:

> The doctor dictates what brand the patient is to buy...orders the amount of drugs and prescribes the quantity to be consumed. In other words, the patient is a captive consumer. There is no other profession or business where a member thereof can dictate to a consumer what brand he must buy, what amount he must buy, and how fast he must consume it and how much he must pay with the further condition to the consumer that any failure to fully comply must be at the risk of his own health. If the doctor interferes with the patient's free choice as to where he purchases his prescribed medicine, the patient then becomes a totally captive consumer and the doctor has a complete monopoly.[96]

Leverage to Force the Consumer to Purchase the Tied Product. In ordinary business transactions, consumers are expected to seek information on their own about the various products they might buy. Medicine is different. A major reason patients seek medical advice is to learn about their options for diagnosing and treating whatever is wrong. Indeed, the law of informed consent says that the physician cannot proceed with significant interventions unless he has not only explained the nature and risks of what he proposes to do but has also described the reasonable alternatives. Thus, it is the physician's job to provide the patient with options.[97]

Where the physician engages in self-referral, he withholds information and choice from the patient. He directs the patient to his own facility, and the patient knows neither that the physician is an investor nor that there are alternatives. In this sense, he forces[98] the patient to use his facility: By offering no options, he leaves the patient no choice. Further, it is not reasonable to expect the patient to secure such information on his own. The specialized nature of health needs and medical knowledge usually means that the physician is best, if not solely, equipped to determine which facilities will meet the patient's particular needs. Even when the physician offers an alternative after recommending his own facility, he still exercises leverage over the patient. In this fiduciary relationship of influence, his recommendation carries weight that an ordinary commercial suggestion or advertisement does not.[99]

Nor is it reasonable to expect the patient to switch to a different physician in order to get further information about medical options and facilities, or to secure a physician who is not tied to a particular ancillary provider. Once a patient has developed a relationship with one physician, it becomes very difficult to change to another. A switch could require the patient to repeat embarrassing personal intimacies and costly or risky examinations, and the concomitant delays could be medically risky, if not catastrophic. Thus, once he has chosen a particular physician, the patient may essentially be "locked in" to that provider as his source of information as well as treatment.[100]

Admittedly, such leverage does not constitute the coercive, explicit agreement usually found in tie-in cases. However, arm-twisting coercion is not actually required.[101] Where the physician steers the patient to his own facility, he uses a concealed coercion that is in effect no different from a seller's requiring a buyer to sign an explicit agreement to purchase a tied product. By steering the dependent patient to his own facility, the physician implicitly requires that "if you receive my medical care, you will patronize my ancillary facility." Reciprocally, if the physician empowers the patient with information and permits the latter to make a real choice, he does not exert the leverage implicit in tie-ins.

Distinctness of Tying and Tied Products. Some kinds of intervention, such as a physical examination, are part of any medical visit and cannot be considered a tie-in. The kinds of intervention for which a physician might choose to make a special, optional investment in free-standing or in-office equipment, however, are usually easily separable from the physician's basic personal care. Arguably, the appropriate criterion is whether the patient could accept or reject the proposed intervention, or purchase it elsewhere, while still remaining in the care of that physician. Thus, one might decline an MRI scan and still be Dr. Jones's patient; one can agree to the scan but go to an imaging center other than Dr. Jones's and still be Dr. Jones's patient.

This approach essentially follows existing tie-in doctrine: Generally, two products are separate if consumers might wish to purchase them separately.[102] The question is whether there is or could be a demand[103] to buy them separately in two distinct markets.[104] If the patient's illness permits the leisure to discuss and actually use an alternative provider, then arguably the secondary, referred intervention can be regarded as a separate product.

Adverse Effect on Competition in the Second Market. Where physicians direct patients to their own facilities, competition is inevitably hurt. Consumers—the patients—are precluded from making choices at all, let alone those based on the merits of the competitors. They may unwittingly be forced into facilities that are of poorer quality, higher priced, less convenient, or less courteous. At the same time, prospective competitors may be unable to enter the market, and existing competitors may be forced quickly out of business.[105]

Interstate Level. Under current case law, many instances of self-referral will satisfy the interstate requirement.[106] In *Summit Health v. Pinhas*, an ophthalmologist lost his staff privileges at a Los Angeles hospital. The Supreme Court found that interstate commerce was sufficiently affected to permit antitrust review. The hospital serves, and receives revenues—including federal Medicare dollars—from many out-of-state patients. Further, peer review proceedings can affect a physician's ability to work, not just in one state but throughout the nation.[107] The same is true in most cases of self-referral. The physician may have many out-of-state patients; their bills may be paid by insurers from other states; the equipment in the facility to which he refers them may have been manufactured in another state; other partners in the venture may be from out of state; the affected competitors may have patients or equipment from other states.[108]

To avoid antitrust problems, the physician must provide thorough disclosure. It is not sufficient simply to recommend his own facility and then add the name of an alternative—leaving the burden on the patient to challenge that recommendation if he wants the alternative. Rather, the physician must provide all the information that may be material to the reasonable patient's decision—for example, prices, hours of operation, scheduling availability, and proximity to home.

Because the physician is a fiduciary, he has the duty to be affirmatively forthcoming with such information. Moreover, in conflicts of interest such as referral to an investment facility, the physician bears the burden of proving that he did meet this obligation.[109] That is, if the patient subsequently accuses the physician of self-referral, the physician must prove that he provided all the essential information and opportunity for choice. In fact, that burden should be fairly easy to satisfy if, for example, the physician has some standardized information sheets comparing the features of alternative facilities. He or his office staff can then discuss various options and answer questions. Such a conversation should not only identify which facility the physician owns, but should also include an honest explanation that such ownership represents a conflict of interest and should help the patient to choose whichever option best suits his particular circumstances. The physician would also be wise to enter a note in the patient's chart that the options were discussed, which one the patient chose, and why.

Other Anticompetitive Acts

Also relevant are exclusionary practices known as "boycotts" and "exclusive dealing." Here entrepreneurs attempt to exclude rivals via agreements with buyers rather than by earning buyers' business through better products and lower prices.[110] In exclusive dealing, the seller does not rely on his market power to coerce the buyer to purchase a second product. Rather, he secures the latter's agreement not to deal in the goods of a competitor.[111] As with tying, one uses one's economic power as a leverage to affect one's competitors.

As with tie-ins, we must deviate somewhat from existing case law to find a fit between exclusive dealing and self-referral. And yet, as with tie-ins, we need not go far. Here, too, the physician uses the leverage inherent in the relationship to induce the patient not to patronize the competitors of his investment facility. The basic situation is the same, although it is described with different language. In making a case for exclusive dealing, we would not say that the physician covertly coerces the patient by declining to identify any choices, as we would under the tying doctrine; rather, we would say that he secures the patient's "agreement," since usually the patient does, in some sense, agree to go to the referral facility.[112]

In boycotts, a group of competitors conspire to not to deal with a supplier, customer, or other competitor.[113] These concerted refusals to deal can be used to gain market power at the expense of competitors or to enforce an agreement such as price fixing among the group's members.[114] Boycotts are generally considered per se offenses of antitrust law,[115] though it is possible for courts to handle boycott-like activities more gently.[116]

Self-referral could constitute a group boycott. If the physicians as joint venturers in a free-standing facility agree that they will not refer their patients to competing facilities, they can hinder those competitors from their normal access to patients' business.[117] Such actions might also, under certain conditions, amount to a conspiracy or an attempt to monopolize.[118]

Monopolization

Consider the following hypothetical scenario.[119] Suppose that nearly every urologist in a town of 1 million people enters into a joint venture for the purchase of a new lithotripter, a device used to crush kidney stones with ultrasound. Although there is already a five-year-old lithotripter in the area, the new one allows patients to be treated with less pain, reducing the need for anesthesia and obviating the need for the patient to spend two to three days in the hospital. It is also mobile for greater patient convenience. However, some studies show that patients treated with the newer model may be more likely to require retreatment due to inadequate breakup of stones.

The new unit costs nearly $2 million and is jointly owned by the urologists and its out-of-state manufacturer. Although it is cheaper to operate, its charges of $7100, not counting the physician's fee, are about twice the going rate in some areas of the country, though allegedly comparable with the rates of other regions. The price is also higher than that of the older unit for which the charge is $6000 to $6500, including the inpatient stay. According to a private memorandum from the partner company that built the new unit, a conservative estimate is that its investors could profit by about $4 million over the next eight years, paying individual physicians approximately $50,000 a year.

For many patients, insurance does not cover the higher costs of the newer machine. Medicare will pay only $4628, and many insurers with preferred provider agreements will pay only 70 percent of their $5000 maximum reimbursement at a nonpreferred facility. Because those patients receive only $3500, they are left to pay the remaining $3600 out of pocket, plus their share of the $2000 physician's fee. Some patients report that their urologist did not inform them of his financial interest in the new lithotripter, or of its costs, or of the alternatives. After the new lithotripter arrives, urologists stop referring their patients to the older model, which is owned by six medical centers and thirty urologists. Within a few months, it closes for lack of business. Most patients now have no alternative, except for a few slots at a unit in the local veteran's hospital and one older unit owned by some physicians who are also partners in the new group.[120]

Antitrust law does not prohibit monopolies.[121] There are natural monopolies, such as where a town is only large enough to support one newspaper. Some monopolies are granted by government (*e.g.*, utilities companies) or patent law, and some firms create monopolies through sheer energy, creativity, and efficiency. Rather, the Sherman Act is interested in those who make monopoly—the ability to fix prices or exclude competition from the market—their goal.[122] Sherman Act offenses range from conspiracy, to attempt, to actual monopolization. Conspiracy to monopolize requires concerted action among conspirators with an intent to monopolize, plus some overt act that furthers their plan. An attempt requires a dangerous probability of success. A charge of monopolization requires that the defendant actually have monopoly power and that there be "'willful acquisition or maintenance of that power as distinguished from growth or development as a consequence of a superior product, business acumen, or historic accident.'"[123] Such power is used "'to foreclose competition, to gain a competitive advantage, or to destroy a competitor.'"[124]

Two further conditions must be met. As in every federal antitrust case, interstate commerce must be affected. Additionally, one must specify the relevant market in terms of both product and geography. That is, to have a monopoly over product X, one must define what X is and distinguish it from products that only resemble X. And one must specify over what territory this monopoly ranges, whether the entire nation or just a town.[125]

Under these definitions, one finds several possible antitrust violations in the above scenario. If the investing urologists agreed that none of them would use the old unit once the new one was installed, a conspiracy would exist. Indeed, one would not even need to prove that the partners had a written or even an explicit oral agreement.[126] In this case, the fact that only urologists were permitted to invest in the facility[127] might constitute further evidence of conspiracy with an intent to monopolize.

Once the physicians begin consistently to refer their patients to the new lithotripter, and to refrain from offering them any information or choice, their conduct may constitute an overt act in furtherance of the conspiracy—conspiracy to monopolize.

Their systematic self-referral may additionally provide the "dangerous probability" element necessary to establish attempted monopolization. Given physicians' influence over patients, self-referral virtually guarantees that most, if not all, patients will go where they are sent. Competing facilities can advertise to solicit patients, of course, but for highly specialized medical services like lithotripsy, advertising to the general public is not likely to be cost-effective. Most people will never need these services, and the patient who does is unlikely to know, until he consults his physician, which facilities in town actually fit his needs.

Finally, the prompt demise of the older facility seems to yield an actual or virtual monopoly. Nearly every urologist in town joined the venture, thus ensuring that if all or most of them self-referred to their new facility, it would quickly enjoy a monopoly. The urologists thus began with the physician's usual control over demand, as they could determine whether, when, and where a patient would receive lithotripsy. Even a patient who sought a second opinion could only receive one from another partner in the venture. Through their collective numbers, the physicians added a second level of power. Once the chief competitor was defunct, they also controlled the supply by possessing the only widely available unit in town. The two remaining facilities in town, including the one at the veterans' hospital, were of limited availability.

Here, however, we must consider the "relevant market," both product and geographic. As in the case of tying arrangements, the buyer's perspective generally determines the issue. If two products are sufficiently close that the buyer would be willing to substitute one for the other, then they are the "same" for purposes of antitrust analysis.[128] Patients who were forced to pay an extra $3600 out of pocket for the new facility might argue that both were the same product because they both were lithotripters designed to serve the same purpose. The urologists, however, might argue that their unit is medically different and that the older one went out of business because it was an inferior product. As antitrust is applied to medicine, such definitional questions will require some difficult lines to be drawn among myriad advancing technologies. Some new equipment constitutes the "same product" with a few improvements over previous models, while other changes represent an entirely new product.

The relevant geographic market can be defined more easily as a reasonable travel distance for patients. If the nearest similar facilities are over 100 miles away then, particularly for city dwellers who normally find all necessary medical resources within the metropolitan area, 100 miles would be an unreasonable distance. Further, any attempt to receive lithotripsy in another city would also require the patient to enlist another physician and thereby, quite possibly, to repeat some or all of the medical evaluation that led the first physician to prescribe the lithotripsy treatment. The patient might have to pay for duplicate testing, take more time away from work, and endure extra discomfort. The burdens of traveling to another area thus would be extensive and, arguably, unreasonable.[129]

The lithotripter scenario can also satisfy the interstate requirement. The manufacturer, who is also a major partner, is from another state;[130] patients who use the facility may be from other states; many of their insurers are based in other states.

Just as with tie-ins and other anticompetitive acts, the problem is not that the patient uses a facility in which his physician is an investor. Rather, the real issue is the covert coercion implicit in self-referral. Consumer judgment is bypassed entirely as the physician exploits the patient's ignorance and dependency. Once again, physician investors could easily avoid antitrust problems by providing full disclosure and fully free choice for their patients. Some patients might gladly pay a higher lithotripsy fee in exchange for less pain, no hospitalization, and greater convenience. Others will prefer to save several thousand dollars out of pocket and to reduce the chance of needing retreatment. If one facility runs out of business with such full disclosure and free choice, then that is the action of the marketplace. Monopoly gained through superior performance does not offend antitrust law.

Enforcement

Admittedly, no cases have arisen that specifically pursue self-referral on antitrust grounds. The federal government, however, was, as of 1992, actively investigating a number of cases.[131] In addition, two recent court cases come are of interest: *Key Enterprises v. Venice Hospital*, and *Advanced Health-Care Serv. v. Radford Com. Hospital*.[132]

Prior to entering a joint venture with a durable medical equipment (DME) supplier, Venice Hospital had not recommended any particular DME supplier to patients about to be discharged or permitted any DME representatives even to speak with patients. Such arrangements were made through independent home health nurses. After purchasing a half interest in a DME firm, however, the hospital began to insist that these nurses recommend this firm in preference to any competitor as a condition of their continued access to patients prior to discharge. The hospital also permitted its own DME representative, clad in a white lab coat, to visit patients directly, and instituted a variety of other changes that made it difficult for competing firms to secure patients' business. Prior to the joint venture, the largest competing DME supplier had 73 percent of the business in that market; within a few months afterward, the hospital's firm received 85 percent of the hospital's business and 61 percent of the overall market. One firm had already gone out of business, and the demise of another appeared imminent.[133]

The Eleventh Circuit Court of Appeal held that the hospital had violated antitrust laws on several counts. The hospital was guilty of anticompetitive acts, as it channeled patients' choices. Admittedly, a patient could choose any DME vendor.

> However, a patient's freedom to choose under these circumstances may be illusory. The evidence presented in this case shows that patients rarely have a preference for a DME vendor. The patients know very little about the equipment or the companies that rent the equipment. Thus, they are very susceptible to rec-ommendations made by anyone who appears to be knowledgeable on the subject. It therefore becomes very easy to channel patient choice by limiting the patient's exposure to the competition.[134]

To let its own representative speak with patients and to require the nurses to rec-ommend its vendor thus "was a 'decision by a monopolist to make an important change in the character of the market.'"[135] The hospital restricted competition unnecessarily, without any justification in terms of efficiency, quality, price, con-venience, or other benefit to patients.[136]

The court also held that although the case did not strictly fit the requirements for a tying case (contrary to the ruling of the district court), it did constitute reciprocal dealing—a variant of exclusive dealing.[137] It further found that the hospital was guilty of both Section 2 conspiracy and an attempt to monopolize. Its policies attempted to exclude competitors by unduly influencing the nurses to recommend its DME vendor. Given that the hospital had 80 percent of the patient admissions in its area,[138] its near-monopoly market power also ensured that this conspiracy to monopolize the DME market had a "dangerous probability" of success.[139] Alternatively stated, the hospital had engaged in monopoly leveraging. It used its power in one market to gain power in the second market by other than competitive means.[140]

The other case, *Advanced Health-Care Serv. v. Radford Com. Hospital*, likewise featured hospitals owning DME enterprises and exploiting their advantage over patients to secure an edge over competing DME ventures. Here, too, the court found that competitors of hospitals' DME ventures had antitrust causes of action, including conspiracy and an attempt to monopolize, anticompetitive activity, mis-use of essential facilities, exclusive dealing, and unreasonable restraint of trade.[141]

In general, antitrust law is enforced on several fronts. Sherman Act violations are enforced solely by the Antitrust Division (AD) of the Justice Department. They can be prosecuted as felonies, though that remedy is usually reserved for more serious offenses such as price fixing and other per se offenses.[142] Alternatively, the AD can use civil remedies such as consent decrees in which antitrust violators agree, for instance, to cease and desist from their activities.[143]

The AD and the FTC both enforce the Clayton Act, using formal hearings or informal measures such as consent decrees.[144] And the FTC alone pursues the unfair methods of competition and other anticompetitive behaviors proscribed under the FTC Act. These investigations are intended to "'stop in their incipiency acts and practices which, when full blown, would violate' the Sherman and Clayton Acts."[145]

Private citizens may hold the strongest enforcement tools.[146] Section 4 of the Clayton Act permits citizens who are injured by antitrust violations to collect treble damages, plus litigation costs including reasonable attorneys' fees.[147] The injury must, of course, be measurable, and it must be demonstrably caused by the anticompetitive behavior.[148]

Two groups are potentially injured by self-referral: competing facilities and patients. Suits by competing businesses will likely be the more potent source of enforcement against physicians' self-referral, because such businesses can quickly suffer large monetary damages that, when trebled, amount to large sums of money. For instance, radiologists who allege that their diagnostic imaging businesses have been harmed by self-referring physicians' competing facilities[149] may be especially interested in filing such a suit.

Patients, too, can be compensated for their losses. In *Key Enterprises* the court noted that, as home health nurses recommended Venice Hospital's DME vendor, and as its DME representative visited patients in the hospital,

> the channeling of patient choice is sufficient to show injury to consumers. The antitrust laws do not require the consumer to suffer some form of monetary damage before a defendant's anticompetitive conduct is actionable...("Coercive activity that prevents its victims from making free choices between market alternatives is inherently destructive of competitive conditions and may be condemned even without proof if its actual market effect.")[150]

Another case is particularly pertinent. In *Blue Shield of Virginia v. McCready*,[151] the plaintiff, Carol McCready, challenged her insurer's policy of refusing to pay for psychologists' services unless the treatment was supervised and billed through a psychiatrist. McCready, who had secured a psychologist's services directly, alleged that Blue Shield's refusal to reimburse her constituted a conspiracy to boycott psychologists. The Supreme Court ruled that she had standing under the Clayton Act to seek treble damages and attorneys' fees. As the Court noted, the plaintiff

> alleges that Blue Shield sought to induce its subscribers into selecting psychiatrists over psychologists for the psychotherapeutic services they required, and that the heart of its scheme was the offer of a Hobson's choice to its subscribers. Those subscribers were compelled to choose between visiting a psychologist and

forfeiting reimbursement, or receiving reimbursement by forgoing treatment by the practitioner of their choice. In the latter case, the antitrust injury would have been borne in the first instance by the competitors of the conspirators, and inevitably—though indirectly—by the customers of the competitors in the form of suppressed competition in the psychotherapy market; in the former case, as it happened, the injury was borne directly by the customers of the competitors.... Although McCready was not a competitor of the conspirators, the injury she suffered was inextricably intertwined with the injury the conspirators sought to inflict on psychologists and the psychotherapy market.[152]

The Court's reasoning in *McCready* can plausibly be extended to patients of physicians engaging in self-referral. Suppose, for example, that patients of self-referring urologists object to paying several thousand dollars more out of pocket for visiting the newer, costlier lithotripter than they would have paid had they been able to choose the older, cheaper, PPO-approved facility. If 1,000 patients are awarded $3000, trebled, the losing urologists would pay $9 million, plus litigation costs and attorneys' fees. Because such suits would not be brought under negligence or malpractice law, all damages and costs would be paid not by the physicians' malpractice insurers but out of their own pockets.

The prospect of such payouts surely represents a formidable deterrent to abusive self-referral. If we also add the prospect of damages in suits for breach of fiduciary duty, breach of informed consent, kickbacks, and bad faith breach of contract, as discussed in Section III, it is difficult to imagine that physicians would not quickly transform their self-referral habits into careful conversations to help patients make their own referral choices.

If this deterrence is so powerful, then we do not need legislation that would ban or substantially limit physicians' freedom to invest in potentially useful ancillary facilities, or that would forbid patients to choose where they wish to spend their money and receive their treatment. Existing legal remedies, well used, are potent enough to deter abusive self-referral while permitting the entrepreneurial freedom that can foster creative new ways to meet formidable problems in delivering and distributing health care.

More important, such an approach instates the patient not as a commodity whose needs and funds are to be exploited for others' benefit but as a consumer with economic power.[153] Many thoughtful observers have suggested that one of the most important reasons why health care costs continue to escalate is that patients do not function as consumers. Where products and services are chosen by physicians, received by patients, and paid for by insurers, the connection between cost and value is lost. Neither really asks whether the value of something is worth its cost.[154]

Adequate health care reform, on this view, will require that patients have far more choice and responsibility for their health care.[155] Admittedly, health care will probably never have all the elements of a fully functioning free market.[156] Nevertheless, greater involvement of patients—buyers—in health care decisions carries an important opportunity to contain costs while fairly allocating limited resources.[157] And if that is to be the case, enforcement of antitrust and common law protections for patients as consumers will be an essential tool, far superior to legislative prohibitions that strip patients of options in the health care market.

ACKNOWLEDGMENT: The author acknowledges with gratitude the very helpful comments provided on earlier drafts of this chapter by Clark Havighurst, J.D., Lance Stell, Ph.D, Lawrence Pivnick, J.D., Roy Spece, J.D., and Fidel Davila, M.D.

Notes

1. B. McCormick, Fraud-Busters Grapple with "Epidemic" of Abuse, *American Medical News* 4, 5 (December 9, 1991).
2. R.P. Kusserow, *Financial Arrangements Between Physicians and Health Care Businesses: Report to Congress.* Pub. OA1-12-88-01410 (1989).
3. B. McCormick, AMA Council Takes New Look at Ethics of Self-Referral, *American Medical News* 1, 44 (September 16, 1991).
4. State of Florida Health Care Cost Containment Board, *Joint Ventures Among Health Care Providers in Florida*, vol. II (1991); J. M. Mitchell and E. Scott, Physician Ownership of Physical Therapy Services: Effects on Charges, Utilization, Profits and Quality, 268 *JAMA* 2055 (1992).
5. U.S. General Accounting Office, *Medicare Diagnostic Imaging Rates*, GAO/HEHS-94-129R.
6. Inspector General v. Hanlester Network et al., Decision No. 1275, 9/18/91; B. McCormick, Physician Self-Referral: The Noose Tightens After Ruling on Labs, *American Medical News* 1, 60, 61 (October 7, 1991).
   On remand, the administrative law judge ruled that the network should be excluded from participating in Medicare for two years, and excluded permanently the three labs that comprised the network. Inspector General v. Hanlester Network et al., Docket No. C-448, Decision No. CR181. DHHS Departmental Appeals Board, Civil Remedies Division, 3/10/92; T. S. Crane, The Problem of Physician Self-Referral Under the Medicare and Medicaid Antikickback Statute: The Hanlester Network Case and the Safe Harbor Regulation, 268 *JAMA* 85, 91 (1992).
7. These are in addition to previous laws proscribing kickbacks, referral payments, and other abuses. For further discussion, see E. H. Morreim, Physician Investment and Self-Referral: Philosophical Analysis of a Contentious Debate, 15 *Med. Philosophy* 425, 427–428 (1990); J. K. Iglehart, The Debate Over Physician Ownership of Health Care Facilities, 321 *N. Engl. J Med.* 198 (1989); T. N. McDowell, Physician Self-Referral Arrangements: Legitimate Business or Unethical "Entrepreneurialism", 15 *Am. J. Law Med.* 61, 71–73 (1989); D. A. Hyman and J. V. Williamson, Fraud and Abuse: Regulatory Alternatives in a "Competitive" Health Care Era, 19 *Loyola U. L. J.* 1133, 1196 (1988).

8. Omnibus Budget Reconciliation Act of 1989, 42 USC §§ 1395nn, 1395q; *see also* 56 (145) Fed. Reg. 35957 (July 29, 1991); N. B. Caesar, The Feds Are Looking Harder at Your Medical Investments, 68(19) *Med. Econ.* 78 (1991).

9. Omnibus Budget Reconciliation Act of 1989, Section 6204, PL 101-239, section 1877; Caesar, *supra* note 8, at 80. Federal regulations implementing this act were issued on March 11, 1992. Medicare Program, *Physician Ownership of, and Referrals to, Health Care Entities that Furnish Clinical Laboratory Services,* 57(48) Fed. Reg. 8588 (1992).

10. Omnibus Budget Reconciliation Act of 1993, 42 U.S.C. § 1395nn.

11. Medicare and State Health Care Programs: Fraud and Abuse; OIG Anti-kickback Provisions, 56 (145) Fed. Reg. 35952 (July 29, 1991); J. K. Iglehart, Efforts to Address the Problem of Physician Self-Referral, 325 *N. Engl. J. Med.* 1820 (1991).

12. 42 U.S.C. § 1320a-7(b)(7).

13. Mich. Comp. Laws Ann §400.604; Calif. Business and Professions Code §654.2; R. P. Kusserow, *supra* note 2, at 5–6.

14. Florida Chapter Law No. 92-178; N.J. Stat. Ann §45:9–22.5 (West 1992); New York Chapter No. 803, Laws of 1992; Mo. Rev. Stat. § 334.252 91992), Mo. Rev. Stat. § 334.253 (1992); Illinois Public Act 87-1207. B. McCormick, Self-Referral Restrictions Hit New York, *American Medical News* 3, 47 (August 24/31 1992).

15. Mark Rodwin, *Medicine, Money, and Morals: Physicians' Conflicts of Interest* 117 (1993).

16. Council on Ethical and Judicial Affairs, Conflicts of Interest: Physician Ownership of Medical Facilities, 267 *JAMA* 2366, 2368 (1992).

17. AMA Reaffirms Rule on Facility Referrals with Financial Links, *Wall Street Journal* B-6 (December 9, 1992).

18. J. Hamilton, AMA Checks Ethics of Doctors' Venture, *Memphis Commercial Appeal* A-1, A-15 (September 25, 1991). Signifying the controversial nature of self-referral, the AMA's own House of Delegates voted just six months later to repudiate the Council on Ethical and Judicial Affairs' (CEJA) restrictive stance. Despite the disagreement of the larger body, the CEJA opinion would stand as official AMA policy. *See* T. M. Burton, Physicians Who Own Labs May Refer Patients to Them for Tests, *Wall Street Journal* B-6 (June 24, 1992). The House of Delegates finally approved the restriction in any event. *See, e.g.,* AMA Rules Against Self-Referrals, *Chicago Tribune* N20 (December 1992).

19. F. Mullan, R. M. Politzer, C. T. Lewis, S. Bastacky, J. Rodak, and R. G. Harmon, The National Practitioner Data Bank: Report from the First Year, 268 *JAMA* 73, 79 (1992); J. R. Bierig and R. M. Portman, The Health Care Quality Improvement Act of 1986, 32 *St. Louis L. J.* 977, 996, 1014, (1988); B. McCormick, AMA Council Takes New Look at Ethics of Self-Referral, *American Medical News* 1, 44 (September 16, 1991).

20. R. M. Green, Medical Joint-Venturing: An Ethical Perspective, 20 *Hastings Cent Rep.* 22, 26 (1990); Rodwin, *supra* note 15; M. A. Rodwin, Physicians' Conflicts of Interest: The Limitations of Disclosure, 321 *N. Engl. J. Med.* 1405, 1408 (1989).

21. W. D. Slawson, A Stronger, Simpler Tie-In Doctrine, 25 *Antitrust Bull.* 671, 678–679 (1980).

22. Throughout this chapter I will observe the somewhat old-fashioned but still correct custom of using the masculine pronoun in its gender-neutral form to stand as the singular indefinite pronoun. To substitute plural pronouns such as "they" and "their" where the singular is required is grammatically incorrect; consistently using the feminine pronoun instead of the masculine is no less "biased"; and alternating between the two seems awkward and contrived. Therefore, although the masculine form is used, no gender bias is intended.

23. McDowell, *supra* note 7; Hyman and Williamson, *supra* note 7; M. Mitka, Hospitals Look to Joint Ventures for Capital, *American Medical News* 9, 13 (January 28, 1991).

24. Slawson, *supra* note 21.

25. Similarly, if a local hospital is unable or unwilling to maintain or upgrade its technology, local physicians can fill in the need. E. Neuman, Medical Ventures Born out of Need of Profit?, 8(23) *Insight on the News* 12, 16, 38–39 (1992).

26. Omnibus Budget Reconciliation Act of 1989, Section 6204, PL 101-239, section 1877; L. Jones, Forms Ask for Lab Ownership Data, *American Medical News* 3, 14 (August 26, 1991).

27. Clinical Laboratory Improvement Amendments of 1988, Public Law 100-578. *See also* DHHS, Medicare, Medicaid, and Clinical Laboratories Improvement Programs: Laboratories Regulations, 57 (40) Fed. Reg. 7002 (January 28, 1991).

28. C. Stevens, Why "Safe Harbors" Leave Doctors in Danger, 68(22) *Med. Econ.* 155, 156–157 (1991).

29. B. J. Hillman, C. A. Joseph, M. R. Mabry, J. H. Sunshine, S. D. Kennedy, and M. Noether, Frequency and Costs of Diagnostic Imaging in Office Practice—A Comparison of Self-Referring and Radiologist-Referring Physicians, 323 *N. Engl. J. Med.* 1604, 1608 (1990).

30. B. J. Hillman, G. T. Olson, P. E. Griffith, J. H. Sunshine, C. A. Joseph, S. D. Kennedy, W. R. Nelson, and L. B. Bernhardt, Physicians' Utilization and Charges for Outpatient Diagnostic Imaging in a Medicare Population, 268 *JAMA* 2050, 2054 (1992).

31. Note, for example, the AMA's policy on this issue: "Patients should be given a list of effective alternative facilities if any such facilities become reasonably available" (Council on Ethical and Judicial Affairs, Conflicts of Interest: Physician Ownership of Medical Facilities, 267 *JAMA* 2366, 2368 (1992)). Note that this policy does not suggest that all physicians should routinely offer the patient an array of referral choices. It only expects this of the investor-physician. Note also that the other facilities are described not as one of two options offered on an equal footing but as alternatives to the physician's first choice recommendation (namely, his own facility). This entire recommendation, then, buys into the traditional, anachronistic picture in which the physician is entitled to decide where the patient will receive ancillary care.

32. Howard Brody, *The Healer's Power* 120ff (1992); D. Oken, What to Tell Cancer Patients: A Study of Medical Attitudes, 175 *JAMA* 86, 94 (1961).

33. Salgo v. Leland Stanford Jr. University Bd. of Trust, 317 P.2d 170 (Cal. 1957); Natanson v. Kline, 354 P.2d 670 (Kan. 1960); Cobbs v. Grant, 502 P.2d 1 (Cal. 1972); and Canterbury v. Spence, 464 F.2d 772 (D.C. 1972)

34. R. P. Kusserow, *supra* note 20.

35. J. Hamilton, Homey Lab Offers Catheterization, *Memphis Commercial Appeal* C-3 (February 16, 1992).

36. E. H. Morreim, Economic Disclosure and Economic Advocacy: New Duties in the Ethical Standard of Care, 12 *J. Legal Med.* 275, 329 (1991); E. H. Morreim, Conflicts of Interest: Profits and Problems in Physical Referral, 262 *JAMA* 390, 394 (1989); Moore v. Regents of the Univ. of Cal., 793 P.2d 479, 483 (Cal. 1990).

37. Rodwin, *supra* note 20; Kusserow, *supra* note 2.

38. This essentially is what is required in the AMA guidelines. Council on Ethical and Judicial Affairs, *supra* note 31.

39. Hence, good disclosure is hardly satisfied in the rather simplistic scenarios offered by Katz in Chapter 12 of this volume. To tell the patient that he can use a facility the physician owns or go to another one does not begin to convey useful information, either about the conflict of interest or about the nature of the choices available. Neither does posting a sign in the waiting room.

Katz is quite right that the physician needs to ensure that the disclosure does not give the patient the awkward choice of either using a facility he does not want or impugning the physician's integrity. Katz's concerns can be met, however, with a bit more creative effort. The physician can indicate that he has an ownership interest and that, because this creates a conflict of interest, it is especially important that the choice be made according to the factors that are important to the patient. He can then ask the patient, for instance, whether it is important that the proposed diagnostic test be done someplace close to home, or whether it is particularly important that the test not interfere with his work schedule. For many patients, the decisive question will be which facility his insurer regards as preferred, so that the patient's out-of-pocket costs will be least. In many cases, it may be useful for someone other than the physician to provide such information. Patients may be more willing to share their questions and concerns with office staff than with the physician, whose time they do not want to burden, any more than they want to impugn his integrity.

40. R. M. Alderman, The Business of Medicine-Health Care Providers, Physicians, and the Deceptive Trade Practices Act, 26 *Houston L.Rev.* 109, 145 (1989); R. Craswell, Tying Requirements in Competitive Markets: The Consumer Protection Issues, 62 *Boston U. L.Rev.* 661, 700 (1982).

41. M. J. Mehlman, Fiduciary Contracting: Limitations on Bargaining Between Patients and Health Care Providers, 51 *U. Pitt. L.Rev.* 365, 417 (1990); E. H. Morreim, Conflicts of Interest: Profits and Problems in Physician Referral, 262 *JAMA* 390, 394 (1989); Morreim, *supra* note 36.

42. Moore v. Regents of the Univ. of Cal., 793 P.2d 479 (Cal. 1990).

43. *Id.* at 481.

44. H. R. Bergman, Case Comment: Moore v. Regents of the University of California, 18 *Am. J. Law Med.* 127, 145 (1992).

45. Moore *supra* note 42, at 483.

46. *Id.* at 483–484.

47. *Id.* at 483–485.

48. *Id.* at 484.

49. 42 U.S.C. § 1320a-7(b)(7).

50. Medicare and State Health Care Programs: Fraud and Abuse; OIG Anti-kickback Provisions, 59 (145) Fed. Reg. 35952 (July 29, 1991); Hanlester case.

51. McCormick, *supra* note 6. Some of these cases include United States v. Bay State Ambulance and Hosp. Rental Serv., 874 F.2d 20 (1st Cir. 1989); United States v. Greber, 760 F.2d 68 (3rd Cir. 1985); United States v. Kats, 871 F.2d 105 (9th Cir. 1989); United States v. Lipkis, 770 F.2d 1447 (9th Cir. 1985); and United States v. Ruttenberg, 625 F.2d 173 (7th Cir. 1980).

52. J. H. King, *The Law of Medical Malpractice* 216 (2d ed., 1986); Batty v. Arizona State Dental Board, 112 P.2d 870 (Ariz. 1941).

53. F. B. Stern, Bad Faith Suits: Are They Applicable to Health Maintenance Organizations?, 85 *W. Va. L. Rev.* 911, 928 (1983); T. A. Diamond, The Tort of Bad Faith Breach of Contract When, If at All, Should It Be Expected Beyond Insurance Transactions?, 64 *Marquette L.Rev.* 425, 454 (1981); G. O. Kornblum, The Current State of Bad Faith and Punitive Damage Litigation in the U.S., 23 *Tort and Insurance L.J.* 812, 841 (1988).

54. G. D. Schaber and C.D. Rohwer, *Contracts* (1984).

55. In one bad faith case, for example, an on-the-job injury left a man, Fletcher, completely disabled. His disability insurance company denied, delayed, and limited benefits with stalling tactics and bureaucratic maneuvers. Fletcher and his family suffered substantial financial distress, falling behind on house payments, experiencing a cut-off of utilities, removing a daughter from school for a period of time to care for Fletcher so that his wife could work part-time, and being forced to seek donations from family and friends to cover basic expenses.

Fletcher v. Western National Life Insurance Co., 89 Cal. Rptr. 78 (Cal. App. 1970). Although this concept emerged first in insurance law, it has since extended to other areas, such as employment law. For more detailed discussion of bad faith doctrine, see P. M. Callahan, Some Thoughts on the Avoidance of Extra-Contractual Damages in California Insurance Litigation, 14 *Western State L.Rev.* 72, 172 (1986); J. Hubble, Survey: Good Faith and Fair Dealing: An Analysis of Recent Cases, 48 *Montana L.Rev.* 193, 211 (1987); S. B. Katz, The California Tort of Bad Faith Breach, the Dissent in Seaman's v. Standard Oil, and the Role of Punitive Damages in Contract Doctrine, 60 *So. Cal. L.Rev.* 509, 537 (1987); Kornblum, *supra* note 53; C. M. Louderback and T. W. Jurika, Standards for Limiting the Tort of Bad Faith Breach of Contract, 16 *U.S.F. L.Rev.* 187, 227 (1982); Diamond, *supra* note 53; Stern, *supra* note 53.

56. Louderback and Jurika, *supra* note 55.

57. Rederscheid v. Comprecare, Inc., 667 P.2d 766, 767 (Colo. App. 1983).

58. Aetna Life Ins. Co. v. Lavoie, 470 So. 2d 1060, 1066 (Ala. 1984) (citing Gulf Atlantic Life Insurance Co. v. Barnes, 405 So.2d 916, 924 (Ala. 1981)). *See also* Hughes v. Blue Cross of Northern Calif., 245 Cal. Rptr. 273 (Cal. App. 1 Dist. 1988); Mordecai v. Blue Cross-Blue Shield of Ala., 474 So.2d 95 (Ala. 1985); Linthicum v. Nationwide Life Ins. Co., 723 P.2d 675 (Ariz. 1986); Taylor v. Prudential Ins. Co. of America, 775 F.2d 1457 (11th Cir. 1985).

59. Key Enterprises of Delaware, Inc. v. Venice Hosp., 919 F.2d 1550, 1557 (11 Cir. 1990).

60. Tunkl v. Regents of University of California, 383 P.2d 411 (Cal. 1963); Emory University v. Porubiansky, 282 S.E. 2d 903 (Ga. 1981).

61. Lockett v. Goodill, 430 P.2d 589 (Wash. 1967); Batty v. Arizona State Dental Board, 112 P.2d 870 (Ariz. 1941); Berkey v. Anderson, 82 Cal. Rptr. 67 (Cal. App 2 Dist. 1969); Moore v. Regents of the University of California, 793 P.2d 479 (Cal. 1990).

62. Morreim, *supra* note 7.

63. *Times-Picayune* v. United States, 345 U.S. 594, 605 (1953).

64. Ernest Gellhorn, *Antitrust Law and Economics* 1 (3d ed., 1986).

65. 15 U.S.C.A. §§ 1–7; Gellhorn, *supra* note 64, at 21–22; E. W. Kintner, *An Antitrust Primer* (2d ed., 1973); B. M. Peters and W. C. Maneval, Medical Staff Credentialing: A Prescription for Reducing Antitrust Liability, 19 *Law, Med. Health Care* 120, 122 (1991).

66. Gellhorn, *supra* note 64, at 30–31; E. W. Kintner, *supra* note 65, at 21–23, 50, 115–116.

67. Goldfarb v. Virginia State Bar, 421 U.S. 773 (1975).

68. M. Rose and R. F. Leibenluft, Antitrust Implications of Medical Technology Assessment, 314 *N. Engl. J. Med.* 1490, 1493 (1986); L. B. Costilo, Antitrust Enforcement in Health Care: Ten Years After the AMA Suit, 313 *N. Engl. J. Med.* 901, 904 (1985); Clark Havighurst, Professional Peer Review and the Antitrust Laws, 36 *Case Western Res. L.R.* 1117, 1137 (1986); Barry Furrow, Sandra Johnson, Timothy Jost, Robert Schwartz, *Health Law: Cases, Materials and Problems* 785 (2d ed., 1991; Wilk v. American Medical Assn, 895 F.2d 352 (7th Cir. 1990), cert. denied 111 S. Ct. 513 (1990); Patrick v. Burget, 108 S. Ct. 1658 (1988); Arizona v. Maricopa County Medical Society, 457 U.S. 332 (1982); F.T.C. v. Indiana Federation of Dentists, 106 S.Ct. 2009 (1986); American Medical Association v. United States, 317 U.S. 519 (1943); United States v. American Soc. of Anesthesiologists, 473 F.Supp. 147 (S.D.N.Y. 1979); B. McCormick, No Criminal Charges for Allergists, *American Medical News* 1, 37 (August 5, 1991); P. McGinn, Justice Dept. Insists Ariz. Dentists Are Guilty of Antitrust, *American Medical News* 1, 25 (May 23, 1991).

69. The antitrust analysis presented below draws on that presented by Haavi Morreim, *Blessed Be the Tie that Binds? Antitrust Perils of Physician Self-Referral*, 14 *J. Legal Med.* 359 (1993).

70. Key Enterprises of Delaware, Inc. v. Venice Hospital, 919 F.2d 1550, 1560 (11th Cir. 1990); Clark Havighurst, Professional Peer Review and the Antitrust Laws, 36 *Case Western Res. L.Rev.* 1117, 1122 (1986); E. Gellhorn, *Antitrust Law and Economics 8* (3d edition, 1986); C.C. Havighurst, Doctors and Hospitals: An Antitrust Perspective on Traditional Relationships, 1984 *Duke L. J.* 1071, 1142 (1984).

71. W.D. Slawson, A Stronger, Simpler Tie-In Doctrine, 25 *The Antitrust Bull.* 671, 678-79 (1980); A. Goldman, Ethical Issues in Advertising, in *Just Business: New Introductory Essays in Business Ethics* 235 (T. Regan ed., 1984).

72. Section 3 of the Clayton Act, 38 Stat. 730 (1914) as amended, 15 U.S.C.A. § 14 (1973).

73. Kintner, *supra* note 65, at 115, 116.

74. International Salt Co. v. United States, 332 U.S. 392 (1947).

75. Clark Havighurst, Doctors and Hospitals: An Antitrust Perspective on Traditional Relationships, 1984 *Duke L.J.* 1071, 1237, 1242; Slawson, *supra* note 21.

76. Jefferson Parish Hospital Dist. No. 2 v. Hyde, 466 U.S. 2, 13 (1984).

77. Spartan Grain & Mill Co. v. Ayers, 735 F.2d 1284 1288 (11th Cir. 1984).

78. U.S. v. Loew's, Inc., 371 U.S. 38, 45 (1962); T.A. Baker, The Supreme Court and the Per Se Tying Rule: Cutting the Gordian Knot, 66 *Va. L. Rev.* 1235, 1241 (1980); Kinter, *supra* note 65, at 52.

79. Atlantic Rfg. Co. v. FTC, 381 U.S. 357, 368 (1965); Baker, *supra* note 98, at 1304; Craswell, *supra* note 40; Kintner, *supra* note 65, at 52.

80. In the Eastman Kodak case, Kodak attempted to dominate the market for parts and service for its copiers and micrographic equipment. The Court noted that once a firm has bought such a costly piece of equipment, it becomes very difficult to switch to another brand even if one does not want to buy parts and service from that same marketer. In that sense, the existence of "significant information and switching costs" renders the buyer "locked in" to the seller. Eastman Kodak Co. v. Image Technical Services, Inc., 112 S.Ct. 2072, 2085, 2087 (1992).

81. Northern Pacific Railway v. U.S., 356 U.S. 1, 6 (1958); *Times–Picayune* v. United States, 345 U.S. 594, 608, 611 (1953); Key Enterprises of Delaware, Inc. v. Venice Hospital, 919 F.2d 1550, 1561 (11th Cir. 1990); Gellhorn, *supra* note 64, at 314; W. S. Bowman, Jr., Tying Arrangements and the Leverage Problem, 67 *Yale L.J.* 19, 29 (1957); Baker, *supra* note 78, at 1238, 1316; L. Kaplow, Extension of Monopoly Power through Leverage, 85 *Columb. L. Rev.* 515, 515 (1985).

82. Jefferson Parish Hospital Dist. No. 2 v. Hyde, 466 U.S. 2, 3, 12 (1984); Eastman Kodak Co. v. Image Technical Services, Inc., 112 S.Ct. 2080 (1992). Note, Havighurst argues that this criterion is overbroad: Havighurst, *supra* note 70.

83. *Times-Picayune* v. United States, 345 U.S. 594, 608 (1953); Gellhorn, *supra* note 64, at 320; Jefferson Parish Hospital Dist. No. 2 v. Hyde, 466 U.S. 2, 17 (1984); Bob Maxfield, Inc. v. American Motors Corp., 637 F.2d 1033, 1036 (5th Cir. 1981), cert. denied 102 S. Ct. 315 (1981); Spartan Grain & Mill Co. v. Ayers, 735 F.2d 1284, 1288 (11th Cir. 1984); Slawson, *supra* note 21; Kintner, *supra* note 65, at 56.

84. Jefferson Parish Hospital Dist. No. 2 v. Hyde, 466 U.S. 2, 21, 39 (1984); Bob Maxfield, Inc. v. American Motors Corp., 637 F.2d 1033, 1037 (5th Cir. 1981), cert. denied 102 S.Ct. 315 (1981).

85. Bowman, *supra* note 81.

86. Gellhorn, *supra* note 64, at 38.

87. Baker, *supra* note 78; *Times-Picayune* v. United States, 345 U.S. 594, 605 (1953).

88. *Times-Picayune* v. United States, 345 U.S. 594, 605 (1953); Jefferson Parish Hospital Dist. No. 2 v. Hyde, 466 U.S. 2, 12 (1984); Baker, *supra* note 78; Kintner, *supra* note 65, at 47.

89. Jefferson Parish Hospital Dist. No. 2 v. Hyde, 466 U.S. 2, 14 (1984).
90. Assoc. Gen. Contractors of Cal. v. Cal. St. Council, 103 S.Ct. 897, 903 (1983); Jefferson Parish Hospital Dist. No. 2 v. Hyde, 466 U.S. 2, 12 (1984); Craswell, *supra* note 79; B. M. Peters and W. C. Maneval, Medical Staff Credentialing: A Prescription for Reducing Antitrust Liability, 19 *Law, Med. & Health Care* 120, 123 (1991).
91. Jefferson Parish Hospital Dist. No. 2 v. Hyde, 466 U.S. 2, 9 (1984); Craswell, *supra* note 40; M. Rose and R. F. Leibenluft, Antitrust Implications of Medical Technology Assessment, 314 *N. Engl. J. Med.* 1490, 1491 (1986); Gellhorn, *supra* note 64, at 248; Kintner, *supra* note 65, at 20.
92. U.S. v. Loew's, Inc., 371 U.S. 38, 45 (1962); Baker, *supra* note 78; Kintner, *supra* note 65, at 56.
93. Baker, *supra* note 78; Craswell, *supra* note 90; Kintner, *supra* note 65, at 52.
94. G. B. Shaw, *The Doctor's Dilemma* 7 (1911).
95. F. H. Miller, Secondary Income from Recommended Treatment: Should Fiduciary Principles Constrain Physician Behavior?, in *The New Health Care for Profit* 153, 159 (B. H. Gray ed., 1983).
96. Magan Medical Cl. v. California State Bd. of Med. Exam., 57 Cal. Rptr. 256, 263 (Cal. App. 2 Dist. 1967).
97. The Supreme Court has recognized that where consumers face significant information and switching costs, competition can be adversely affected. Eastman Kodak Co. v. Image Technical Services, Inc., 112 S.Ct. 2072, 2085, 2087 (1992). In medical care, the patient relies on the physician to provide information about medical options and their associated risks and benefits. Indeed, such reliance is the fundamental way in which patients address the otherwise prohibitive task of acquiring medical information on their own.
98. Jefferson Parish Hospital Dist., No. 2 v. Hyde, 466 U.S. 2, 3, 12 (1984); Faulkner Advertising Assoc. v. Nissan Motor Corp., 905 F.2d 769 (4th Cir. 1990).
99. Miller, *supra* note 95; Mehlman, *supra* note 41.
100. Eastman Kodak Co. v. Image Technical Services, Inc., 112 S.Ct. 2072, 2087 (1992).
101. "It is clear that such coercive conduct is sufficient to run afoul of the Sherman Act; however, it is equally clear that '[r]eciprocal trading may ensue not from bludgeoning or coercion but from more subtle arrangements.'" Key Enterprises of Delaware, Inc. v. Venice Hosp, 919 F.2d 1550, 1561 (11 Cir. 1990)(citing FTC v. Consolidated Foods Corp., 85 S.Ct. 1229, 1222 (1965)).
102. Jefferson Parish Hospital Dist., No. 2 v. Hyde, 466 U.S. 2, 37 (O'Connor, et al dissent) (1984); and Eastman Kodak Co. v. Image Technical Services, Inc., 112 S.Ct. 2072, 2080 (1992).
103. In cases where no second market currently exists enabling buyers to express their preference for separating the two, we cannot say that there "is" a demand for the separation. However, we can still ask whether there could reasonably be enough consumer interest to create such a second market.
104. Jefferson Parish Hospital Dist., No. 2 v. Hyde, 466 U.S. 2, 19, 21 (1984); *Times-Picayune* v. United States, 345 U.S. 594 (1953); Faulkner Advertising Assoc. v. Nissan Motor Corp., 905 F.2d 769, 774 (4th Cir. 1990).
105. M. Waldholz and W. Bogidanich, Doctor-Owned Labs Earn Lavish Profits in a Captive Market, *Wall Street Journal* A-1, A-6 (March 1, 1989); E. Neuman, Medical Ventures Born Out of Need or Profit?, 8(23) *Insight on the News* 12-16, 38,39 (1992); J. Brice, Radiologists Often on Losing Side in Fight for Outpatient Imaging, 11(6) *Diagnost Imag* 83, 87 (1989); J. Hamilton, David Fares Well Among Goliaths, *Memphis Commercial Appeal* C-3 (April 21,

1991); J. Hamilton, Doctors' Kidney-Stone Crusher Zaps Insurers, Patients $7,100, *Memphis Commercial Appeal* A-1, A-14 (June 2, 1991); J. Hamilton, Kidney Machine Attracts Attention, *Memphis Commercial Appeal* C-3 (June 9, 1991).

106. It is possible that future courts will apply more strictly the requirement of interstate commerce. In Summit Health Ltd. v. Pinhas, 111 S. Ct. 1842, 1899 (1991), Justice Scalia commented in his dissent, joined by Justices O'Connor, Kennedy, and Souter: "Federal courts are an attractive forum, and the treble damages of the Clayton Act an attractive remedy. We have today made them available for routine business torts, needlessly destroying a sensible statutory allocation of federal–state responsibility and contributing to the trivialization of the federal courts."

107. Summit Health Ltd. v. Pinhas, 111 S. Ct. 1842 (1991); Lorain Journal Co. v. United States, 72 S.Ct. 181 (1951).

108. Thus far, it looks eminently plausible to consider self-referral to be a possible tie-in. A potential objection needs to be addressed, however. Many scholars have argued that tie-ins should not be deemed per se illegal, as they currently are. They suggest that many tying arrangements can benefit consumers by offering better quality, lower price, or higher efficiency in production. Tie-ins, therefore, ought to be analyzed according to the rule of reason, by which the defendant can justify his conduct if he can demonstrate that, on balance, it promotes more than hinders competition. Jefferson Parish Hospital Dist. No. 2 v. Hyde, 466 U.S. 2 (1984), concurring opinion of O'Connor et al, at 32–44; Baker, *supra* note 81; Slawson, *supra* note 21; Craswell, *supra* note 40; Gellhorn, *supra* note 64, at 42, 195; R.H. Bork, *The Antitrust Paradox* 365-381 (1978). Note that the Supreme Court has expressly rejected this reasoning. *See* Eastman Kodak Co. v. Image Technical Services, Inc., 112 S.Ct. 2072 (1992) and Jefferson Parish Hospital Dist. No. 2 v. Hyde, 466 U.S. 2 (1984).

This dispute is important in antitrust law, and there is probably much merit in these commentators' view. Fortunately, we need not settle the dispute here. Even if self-referral were judged to be a flagrant tying arrangement, and tie-ins continued to be per se violations, the physician can escape the entire problem quite easily. He needs only to inform the patient about referral options and empower the patient to make the choice. As noted above, there is nothing wrong with a patient's patronizing his physician's ancillary facility. Competition is offended only if the patient is covertly coerced to go there.

109. Morreim, *supra* note 36; Mehlman, *supra* note 41; Cobbs v. Grant, 502 P.2d 1 (Cal. 1972).

110. Gellhorn, *supra* note 64, at 281.

111. *Id.* at 328.

112. Further, some commentators might prefer an exclusive dealing approach in that courts address it under the rule of reason rather than as a per se offense. *See* Jefferson Parish Hospital Dist. No. 2 v. Hyde, 466 U.S. 2 (1984), O'Connor conc. opinion, at 44; Bob Maxfield, Inc. v. American Motors Corp., 637 F.2d 1033 (5th Cir. 1981), cert. denied 102 S.Ct. 315 (1981)); Kintner, *supra* note 65, at 53-54, 58. To the extent that courts may hamper commerce with overzealous antitrust adjudication, the rule-of-reason approach may make the exclusive dealing doctrine somewhat more attractive. *See* Havighurst, *supra* note 70, at 1151. As argued above, however, a physician can easily escape these antitrust allegations. He needs only to empower the patient with information to make the referral choice.

113. Peters and Maneval, *supra* note 90.

114. Gellhorn, *supra* note 64, at 212–213; F.T.C. v. Indiana Federation of Dentists, 106 S.Ct. 2009 (1986).

115. Gellhorn, *supra* note 64; Leibenluft, *supra* note 91.

116. F.T.C. v. Indiana Federation of Dentists, 106 S.Ct. 2009 (1986).

117. *See, e.g.*, Key Enterprises of Delaware, Inc. v. Venice Hosp, 919 F.2d 1550 (11 Cir. 1990); Advanced Health-Care Serv. v. Radford Com. Hosp., 910 F.2d 139 (4th Cir. 1990).

118. Some commentators propose that self-referral can constitute price-fixing or predatory pricing. *See, e.g.,* J. Hamilton, Kidney Machine Attracts Attention, *supra* note 105. However, it is unlikely that self-referral offends these antitrust rules. Even if a number of physicians invest in a facility, such as a diagnostic center, and even if that center has just one price list, this does not constitute price fixing. It is simply the price offered by one center. Even if this center happens to be the only one in the town, and even if it caused the only competing center to go out of business, there is still no price fixing. The center is a single business entity, and it is entitled to charge a particular price.

Nor, in a health care context, is there likely to be predatory pricing. In predatory pricing, a large firm sells its goods at extraordinarily low prices in order to drive competitors out of business so that, thereafter, it can charge as much as it pleases. In health care such price competition is rare, if not impossible. The prevailing reimbursement system, in which an insurer either pays "usual, customary and reasonable" charges or uses a set fee schedule, does not lend itself to the under-cutting prominent in predatory pricing. These incentives, somewhat perversely, actually encourage all providers to price their services as highly as possible. Therefore leverage that physicians use is not rock-bottom prices but rather their direct influence over consumer choices.

119. All features of this story have been described in newspaper reports but, because of the possibility of factual error, it is offered as hypothetical.

120. Hamilton, David Fares Well Among Goliaths, *supra* note 105; Hamilton, Doctors' Kidney-Stone Crusher Zaps Insurers, Patients $7,100, *supra* note 105; Hamilton, Kidney Machine Attracts Attention, *supra* note 105; J. Hamilton, Local Venture Won't Follow New Guidelines, *Memphis Commercial Appeal* C-3 (August 18, 1991); J. Hamilton, Memo Sees Fortune from Crusher of Kidney Stones, *Memphis Commercial Appeal* C-3 (August 25, 1991); J. Hamilton, Urologists Expected to Reject Device Tied to Fee Cut, *Memphis Commercial Appeal* C-3 (September 8, 1991); J. Hamilton, AMA Checks Ethics of Doctors' Venture, *Memphis Commercial Appeal* A-1, A-15 (September 25, 1991); J. Hamilton, Testimony Slated on Lithotripter, *Memphis Commercial Appeal* B-1 (October 9, 1991); J. Hamilton, Mid-South Urologists Drive Treatment Cost Up, Panel Told, *Memphis Commercial Appeal* A-7 (October 18, 1991); J. Hamilton, Legislators Quiz Doctors' Lock on Kidney Therapy, *Memphis Commercial Appeal* A-1, A-15 (November 19, 1991). Subsequent to these initial events, the urologist-investors took various measures to accommodate public concern about the arrangement, including offering discounts on fees to specified groups.

121. Monopoly is commonly defined as the power to set price and exclude competition. *See* Aspen Skiing Co. v. Aspen Highlands Skiing Corp., 105 S.Ct. 2847, 2854 (1985); Key Enterprises of Delaware, Inc. v. Venice Hospital, 919 F.2d 1550, 1568 (11th Cir. 1990); Havighurst, *supra* note 68; United States v. Loew's Inc., 371 U.S. 38, 44 (1962).

122. 105 S. Ct. 2847, 2854 (1985); Key Enterprises of Delaware, Inc. v. Venice Hospital, 919 F.2d 1550, 1568 (11th Cir. 1990); Kintner, *supra* note 65, at 101, 104; E. Gellhorn, *Antitrust Law and Economics* 121, 135 (3d ed. 1986); Slawson, *supra* note 21; Peters and Maneval, *supra* note 90.

123. Eastman Kodak Co. v. Image Technical Services, Inc., 112 S.Ct. 2072 (1992), citing United States v. Grinnell Corp., 384 U.S. 563, 570, 571 (1966); Lorain Journal Co. v. United States, 72 S.Ct. 181, 186 (1951); Peters and Maneval, *supra* note 90.

124. Eastman Kodak Co. v. Image Technical Services, Inc., 112 S.Ct. 2072, 2090 (1992), citing United States v. Griffith, 334 U.S. 100, 107 (1948).

125. Kintner, *supra* note 65, at 102-103.

126. "It is elementary law that direct evidence is not necessary to establish the existence of a conspiracy. As long ago as 1914 the Supreme Court held that the existence of a conspiracy viola-

tive of the Sherman Act may be inferred from the actions of the persons charged. In fact, the more sophisticated the businessman, the less likely the possibility that there will exist direct evidence of illegal combination; for example, a written agreement to fix prices. As the preceding cases indicate, agreement may be express or implied. The 'gentlemen's agreement' is a familiar term in antitrust law. Such an agreement, or the unwritten understanding, or the unspoken understanding, or even a 'knowing wink,' if designed and used to restrain competition, is just as vulnerable as a signed and sealed written contract to restrain trade." Kintner, *supra* note 65, at 28.

127. Hamilton, AMA Checks Ethics of Doctors' Venture, *supra* note 120.
128. Brown Shoe Co. v. United States, 370 U.S. 294, 325 (1962).
129. As noted in the Eastman Kodak case, significant costs of switching to another seller can render a buyer effectively locked in to a particular seller. Eastman Kodak Co. v. Image Technical Services, Inc., 112 S.Ct. 2072, 2087 (1992).
130. Hamilton, Memo Sees Fortune from Crusher of Kidney Stones, *supra* note 120.
131. K. J. Arquit (Director, Bureau of Competition, Federal Trade Commission), A New Concern in Health Care Antitrust Enforcement: Acquisition and Exercise of Market Power by Physician Ancillary Joint Ventures (prepared remarks delivered to National Health Lawyers Association, Washington, D.C., January 30, 1992).
132. Key Enterprises of Delaware, Inc. v. Venice Hospital, 919 F.2d 1550 (11th Cir. 1990); Advanced Health-Care Serv. v. Radford Com. Hosp., 910 F.2d 139 (4th Cir. 1990).
133. Key Enterprises of Delaware, Inc. v. Venice Hospital, 919 F.2d 1550, 1566 (11th Cir. 1990).
134. *Id.* at 1557.
135. *Id.* at 1558.
136. *Id.*
137. Reciprocal dealing is very similar to tying, except that both parties face each other as both buyer and seller: a buyer with substantial market power agrees to buy something from a second party, but only on the condition that the latter will purchase some specified product from the former. The first buyer uses its greater power as leverage to secure the agreement. In this case, the hospital permitted home health nurses continued access to the hospital, which they needed for their livelihood, but required them to agree to recommend the hospital's DME vendor. *Supra* note 133, at 1561.
138. *Id.* at 1552.
139. *Id.* at 1565.
140. *Id.* at 1566. Although the Eleventh Circuit Court of Appeals later granted a petition to rehear the case en banc, an out-of-court settlement by the litigating parties rendered the request for rehearing moot and prompted the court to term its decision to rehear the substantive antitrust issues "improvident." At that point, the case was returned to the panel with instructions to dismiss the appeal, vacate the district court's judgment, and remand to the district court with instructions to dismiss.
141. Advanced Health-Care Serv. v. Radford Com. Hosp., 910 F.2d 139 (4th Cir. 1990). On remand, the district court found that the hospital's DME business was not actually guilty of antitrust violations. However, its finding was based on the plaintiff's lack of factual evidence to substantiate its claims. The substantive legal principles articulated by the circuit court remain in force. Advanced Health-Care Services v. Giles Mem'l. Hosp., 846 F.Supp. 488 (W.D. Va. 1994).
142. Kintner, *supra* note 65, at 30, 136.
143. *Id.* at 131-138.
144. *Id.* at 24, 131-148.

145. *Id.* at 23, 148. Some commentators regard self-referral as a form of kickback. So far, kick-backs have not been treated as antitrust violations, but kickbacks and referral payments are proscribed as felonies under the 1977 Medicare/Medicaid Anti-Fraud and Abuse Amendments. The 1987 Medicare and Medicaid Patient and Program Protection Act permitted the Department of Health and Human Services (DHHS) to exclude offenders from federal insurance programs or to fine them. The 1989 "Stark" law forbidding self-referral to clinical laboratories is strictly civil, sanctioned by denials of payment, program exclusion, and/or civil money penalties. *See* Omnibus Budget Reconciliation Act of 1989, Section 6204, PL 101-239, section 1877; Medicare and State Health Care Programs: Fraud and Abuse; OIG Anti-kickback Provisions. 56 (145) Fed. Reg. 35952–35984, 35957 (July 29, 1991).

146. Richard Posner, Exclusionary Practices and the Antitrust Laws, 41 *Chicago L. Rev.* 506, 534 (1974); Kintner, *supra* note 65, at 150.

147. 15 U.S.C.A. §§ 12–27.

148. Kintner, *supra* note 65, at 152; Grand Light & Supply Co., Inc. v. Honeywell, Inc., 771 F.2d 672, 681 (2d Cir. 1985).

149. M. Waldholz and W. Bogidanich, Doctor-Owned Labs Earn Lavish Profits in a Captive Market, *Wall Street Journal* A-1, A-6 (March 1, 1989); J. Brice, Radiologists Often on Losing Side in Fight for Outpatient Imaging, 11(6) *Diagnost. Imag.* 83, 87 (1989).

150. Key Enterprises of Delaware, Inc. v. Venice Hospital, 919 F.2d 1550, 1559 (11th Cir. 1990).

151. Blue Shield of Virginia v. McCready, 102 S.Ct. 2540 (1982).

152. *Id.* at 2550-2551.

153. When the patient lacks the capacity to make his own health care decisions, a surrogate decision maker is normally identified to act on the patient's behalf.

154. D. M. Eddy, What Do We Do About Costs?, 264 *JAMA* 1161, 1170 (1990).

155. S. M. Butler and E.F. Haislmaier, *Critical Issues: A National Health System for America* (1989); S. J. Reiser, Consumer Competence and the Reform of American Health Care, 267 *JAMA* 1511, 1515 (1992).

156. T. R. Marmor, R. Boyer and J. Greenberg, Medical Care and Procompetitive Reform, 34 *Vand. L.Rev.* 1003, 1008 (1981).

157. R. E. Moffit, Surprise! A Government Health Plan That Works, *Wall Street Journal* A-14 (April 2, 1992); Clark Havighurst, Practice Guidelines for Medical Care: The Policy Rationale, 34 *St. Louis University L.J.* 777, 819 (1990); P. E. Kalb, Controlling Health Care Costs by Controlling Technology: A Private Contractual Approach, 99 *Yale L. J.* 1109, 1126 (1990).

12

Informed Consent to Medical Entrepreneurialism

Jay Katz

This chapter explores one question: Can informed consent protect physicians and patients from the adverse consequences of patient referral to facilities in which physicians have a financial interest? Thus, my focus is on informed consent as a safeguard against the impact of physicians' increasing entrepreneurial activities on the physician–patient relationship. Put most generally, the concerns raised over such practices are these: that patients will be exposed to unnecessary or unduly expensive tests and procedures and, therefore, can no longer trust that their physicians will place their interests before interests in financial gain. I shall leave largely unconsidered wider societal concerns that the newly discovered opportunities for economic gain, beyond fee-for-service, will significantly increase health care expenditures by excessive resort to laboratory tests and other procedures.

I shall say more about the legal doctrine of informed consent later on. For now, let me call attention to the often overlooked fact that this doctrine is a hybrid concept, with "informed" denoting physicians' disclosure obligations and "consent" patients' explicit or implicit agreement to a medical intervention. What constitutes consent has remained ill defined in law; what constitutes adequate disclosure has also not been specified in law and surely not in medical practice.

In a previous article and in Chapter 11, E. Haavi Morreim has emphasized physicians' new disclosure obligations and has suggested that informed consent be expanded to include "economic [disclosures], so that the patient can consider costs of the proposed treatments, merits of various providers, and even his physicians' potential conflict of interest."[1] Morreim's faith in the doctrine of informed consent would have greater merit if two issues did not haunt its meaningful implementation.

First, the nature and quality of the dialogue between physicians and patients continue to be so unsatisfactory that the authoritarian nature of their interaction has remained essentially unchanged. Proponents of disclosure of financial interests as a mechanism of control have left unconsidered whether physicians in *customary* practice make meaningful disclosures and, therefore, whether a consent can be obtained in the situations under consideration here that amounts to more than voluntary submission.

Second, the practice of medicine in the current climate of medical knowledge gives physicians wide discretion to justify the ordering of many tests and procedures. Therefore, economic gain, even with the best contrary intentions, can readily infiltrate decisions to do more rather than less. This dilemma is inherent in the ubiquitous uncertainties[2] that accompany the practice of contemporary medicine and about which patients are customarily told little, if anything. For informed consent to remedy any concerns about the impact of entrepreneurialism on the physician–patient relationship would require an unambiguous legal doctrine and a professional commitment to disclosure; both still elude us. The call for legislative restrictions on ownership of diagnostic and other facilities is an understandable response to these problems.

In what follows, I shall first discuss the two major proposals that have been advanced to resolve the concerns over economic conflicts of interest: total prohibition of such arrangements or disclosure of such practices to patients. I shall then explore whether the doctrine of informed consent in the current climate of physician–patient decision-making can assure patients of a meaningful choice. In the final section, I shall argue that disclosure of financial interests can only undermine physician–patient trust, for such disclosures leave patients only with two choices: to acquiesce to the referral or, by refusing to do so, to impugn their physicians' professional and moral integrity. A few hypothetical scenarios will illustrate the impossibility of physicians and patients arriving at a mutually satisfactory resolution of the dilemmas posed by economic conflicts of interest.

Prohibition or Disclosure?

Arnold Relman, the distinguished former editor of *The New England Journal of Medicine*, was among the first to alert the medical profession and the public to the emergence of a huge new industry—the "medical–industrial complex," as he called it—that supplies health care services for profit.[3] He called attention to the increasing financial interests of physicians in all "health care businesses. . . proprietary hospitals, nursing homes, dialysis units," and so on, and included among them "diagnostic laboratories."[4] Relman was critical of the American Medical Association's (AMA) Judicial Council's opinion that "[i]t is not in itself unethical for a physician to own a for-profit hospital [and laboratories], or an interest therein, provided that the physician does not make unethical use of that ownership."[5]

In his path-breaking 1980 article, Relman seemed most concerned about the impact of such financial interests on "public trust" and the "[great] potential for mischief."[6] He argued that "physicians should derive no financial benefit from the health-care market except from their own professional services."[7] He never wavered in this belief, but he was resigned that "[t]he new medical–industrial complex is now a fact of American life."[8] Therefore, he only called for further study "to ensure that the medical-industrial complex serves the interests of patients first and of its stockholders second."[9]

The Institute of Medicine (IOM), in its 1986 report on the *For-Profit Enterprise in Health Care*, addressed "physicians' investments in facilities to which referrals are made."[10] It recommended, echoing Relman, that "[i]t should be regarded as unethical and unacceptable for physicians to have ownership interest in health care facilities to which they make referrals or receive payments for making referrals."[11] Like Relman, however, the IOM had little confidence that such an ethical stance would prevail. Thus, it recommended that "[i]n the absence of prohibition of such arrangements which reward physicians for writing prescriptions, making referrals, and ordering tests, it is essential that *disclosure standards* be developed to make certain that patients, referring physicians, and third-party payers are aware that the conflict of interest exists so that they *can respond appropriately*."[12] The terms "disclosure" and "appropriate response" were left undefined.

The IOM, in accord with Relman, was upset about physicians' loss of "moral authority to speak on health matters" as a consequence of such economic arrangements, particularly today when the public has become concerned about rising health care costs. The IOM probably believed that disclosure to affected parties would ameliorate the problem, but without giving the matter careful consideration. The AMA's House of Delegates shared this belief, when it recommended in 1984 that "[t]he physician has an affirmative ethical obligation to disclose to the patient or referring colleagues his or her ownership interest in the facility or therapy prior to utilization."[13] When in 1991 the House of Delegates first accepted its Council of Ethical and Judicial Affairs' opinion that "physicians should generally not engage in self-referral," it reversed its vote six months later.[14] Soon thereafter the Delegates did another about-face.[15]

None of the proposals for disclosure makes clear whether, after physicians' acknowledgment of financial interest, it then becomes patients' obligation to raise questions or whether their acquiescence to such an arrangement constitutes consent. Since physicians are accustomed to having their recommendations accepted without question in their ordinary diagnostic and therapeutic encounters with patients, it is likely that the AMA's and IOM's recommendations for disclosure will only be viewed as a formalistic requirement to apprise patients of physicians' financial interests, which only "difficult" patients will question. If more needs to be discussed when economic matters are in issue, it deserves articulation, particularly since the medical profession, including the AMA, is still so dubious about the extent to which physicians can and should go in inviting patients to make decisions jointly with them. After all, physicians still all too commonly assert that they would neither recommend diagnostic tests nor send patients to their own laboratories unless doing so were in patients' best interests.

Consent and Informed Consent in Medical Practice

Proposals for disclosure of financial conflicts of interest, as I have already suggested, have addressed neither the extent of information to be disclosed nor the nature and quality of consent that should be obtained. The IOM recommendations merely ask for disclosures to which patients "can respond appropriately." Morreim is more specific. In her 1991 article on financial conflicts of interests, she asks that the doctrine of informed consent, which mandates that patients "receive the information necessary to make their own medical decision," be extended to include "economic information."[16] In her view, the dangers posed by the "new economics of care" are adequately safeguarded by the legal doctrine, which bases "physician's disclosure duties not on what physicians generally disclose, but upon the *material* facts the patient will need in order to intelligently chart [his or her own] destiny with dignity."[17] According to Morreim, the "material economic information" that must be provided includes "such matters as . . . the conflicts of interest that *limit [physicians'] loyalty* to the patient's interests, and [their] *economically prompted deviations* from the medical standard of care."[18] While she identifies an important issue, her solution is more problematic, for the question remains: Can patients, or indeed physicians, cope with the revelation that loyalty to the patient may no longer be the polestar of their interaction? I shall return to this question later; for now, I suggest that

Morreim overstates the case for either the informed consent process to ensure protection of patients' interests "to chart [their] own destiny" or for the safeguards provided by the "material facts" standard of care.[19]

Informed consent, in both *current* medical practice and legal theory, is no safeguard for controlling the abuses of self-referral. As I have already suggested, in the context of medical practice, informed consent has not substantially affected physicians' conviction that they must retain the authority to decide what is best for their patients. And the legal doctrine of informed consent, which has generally been narrowly construed to require only disclosure of the risk of any recommended therapeutic intervention, does not significantly enhance shared decision-making between physicians and patients. Both of these contentions require brief elaboration.

From the perspective of practice, physicians continue to believe that diagnostic and therapeutic decisions are theirs to make. As stated by the influential sociologist Talcott Parsons:

> [The physician's] competence and specific judgments and measures cannot be competently judged by the layman. The latter must . . . take these judgments and measures on "authority." . . . The doctor–patient relationship has to be one involving an element of authority—we often speak of "doctor's orders."[20]

Physicians' insistence on such authority over the needs and welfare of patients finds support in a related claim: that patients are incapable of understanding medicine's esoteric knowledge. As stated by Howard Becker:

> Professions . . . are occupations which possess a monopoly of some esoteric and difficult body of knowledge. . . This knowledge cannot be applied routinely but must be applied wisely and judiciously to each case.[21]

Or as recently argued by Thomas Duffy:

> The [patient] autonomy model fails to recognize the complex realities of medicine, the fashion in which diagnoses are made and the attractiveness of being able to trust another human being when one is ill. . . . Illness robs patients of their autonomy. . . . Paternalism exists in medicine, not as some evil perpetrated by the profession upon the patient but rather to fulfill a need created by illness. . . . The cry to install autonomy in its place appears to ignore the reality and sadness of illness.[22]

I have expressed my reservations about these all too sweeping contentions in my book *The Silent World of Doctor and Patient*, as well as in subsequent publications.[23] For now, I merely note that the idea of physicians making decisions *for*, rather than *with*, patients is still deeply embedded in the ideology of medical professionalism.

Similarly, the legal doctrine of informed consent has not significantly moderated the authority that physicians have traditionally exercised over medical decision-making. When it was first promulgated in 1957,[24] the medical profession seemingly embraced the doctrine because physicians found it difficult to reject judges' contention that patients had a right to know something about the risks and benefits inherent in diagnostic tests and therapeutic interventions. At the same time, physicians grumbled about judges' lack of appreciation of the complexities inherent in medical practice. Ultimately, informed consent became a siren call that made physicians and patients believe that they were communicating with each other when in fact they were not.

From the doctrine's beginnings, it has been insufficiently recognized that the newly created legal obligation to converse with patients about medical matters in therapeutic encounters is limited in scope. The legal precedents and objectives that shaped its promulgation make this inevitable. It is a tort doctrine that seeks to delimit physicians' *legal* liability, and how to escape it, whenever patients allege that *material* nondisclosures have vitiated their consent.[25] The doctrine was formulated subsequent to two lawsuits in which judges expressed concern that the employment of new, powerful medical technologies had exposed patients to significant risks of which they had not been apprised.[26] In their opinions, the judges primarily imposed a new duty on physicians to be more forthcoming about disclosing the material risks that their treatment recommendations might entail. While they also mentioned other disclosure obligations, *disclosure of risks* was the doctrine's central message that physicians took away and began to practice.

The doctrine did not explicitly address its underlying *idea*, which I believe is its central message: that from now on, patients and doctors must make decisions jointly. As I wrote elsewhere:

> [While] judges intended, in promulgating the doctrine of informed consent, to give patients a greater voice in decision-making, [they] largely undercut this intention with profound reservations that revealed their distrust of patients' capacities to make their own decisions. Thus the doctrine of informed consent allowed physicians to retain considerable "discretion" to make choices for patients. The doctrine has suffered from judges' convictions that doctors know better than patients what is good for patients. The promise to endow patients with the right to "thorough-going self-determination," which was to be the basis of the informed consent doctrine, remains largely unfulfilled. To distinguish between what judges have done and what they have aspired to, one must draw sharp distinctions between the legal doctrine, as promulgated by judges, and the idea of informed consent, based on a commitment to individual self-determination.[27]

Shared decision-making has not, and cannot, become a reality until doctors as well as judges accept this idea, which challenges medicine's ancient authoritarian ideology. Only then can physicians begin to address the difficult task of integrating disclosure and consent with the complex caretaking and being-taken-care-of transactions that take place between physicians and patients.

While it is true that patients now receive more information than before about the risks and benefits of *recommended* interventions, this change can obscure how little has fundamentally changed. Disclosure notwithstanding, the doctrine of informed consent has not substantially improved decision-making between physicians and patients in therapeutic settings. Thus, in the current climate of doctor–patient decision-making, the doctrine offers little support to those who claim that it can safeguard patients' choices when financial conflicts of interest are at stake.

Informed Consent and Medical Uncertainty

There are other problems with medical entrepreneurialism that a reliance on informed consent to safeguard patients from unnecessary tests and procedures leaves unconsidered. Earlier, I mentioned that the legal doctrine of informed consent was promulgated in the late 1950s as a direct consequence of the spectacular advances in medical technology spawned by the age of medical science. The proliferation of powerful diagnostic tests and therapeutic procedures promised patients relief from suffering that until then was beyond the reach of medicine. At the same time, these technologies could inflict considerable harm, and judges believed that patients ought to be given the opportunity to decide which interventions to accept and reject.

The possibility for patients to do so was aided by the radical transformation of medical practice during the twentieth century. Prior to the age of medical science, physicians did not have the capacity to discriminate satisfactorily between knowledge, ignorance, and conjecture inherent in their diagnostic and treatment recommendations. The introduction of scientific reasoning, aided by more precise scientific observations and experimentation, allowed physicians to get a better sense of what worked and what did not, and, in turn, to sort out with their patients the preferred options in light of known and unknown risks, benefits, and consequences to the patient's quality of life.

All these advances confronted physicians in new ways with an old problem: medical uncertainty.[28] Indeed, paradoxical as it may seem, the advances in medical science not only improved medical care (unheard of during the millennia of medical history); they also made physicians more aware of the extent of their ignorance.[29] What is new, as I have already suggested, is that physicians for the first time could discriminate better between knowledge and ignorance.

Physicians, however, have shown little inclination to learn how disclosures of medical uncertainty should be incorporated into their recommendations for diagnostic and therapeutic interventions that, in the prescientific past, they had expected patients to submit to on the basis of clinical judgment. Physicians, by and large, do not present all relevant options to their patients, even though medical uncertainty as to which treatment is best suggests that this be done in order to arrive at a mutually agreed-on decision. Physicians continue to be guided in their disclosures more by a conviction of certainty, in light of clinical experience, and less by uncertainty, in light of scientific evidence. Thus, it is not surprising that physicians have not learned how to communicate medical uncertainty to their patients and instead persist in choosing the appropriate treatment option first and then discuss its risks and benefits with their patients.

Physicians advance many reasons for not apprising patients of the ubiquitous uncertainties that stalk medical diagnosis and treatment, the most frequently invoked one being that patients cannot understand its complexity. This claim masks other issues: Physicians do not trust their patients to respond well to disclosures that reduce the omniscience that physicians have been accustomed to project; or they are concerned that patients will despair about their chances of cure, lose hope, and turn to quacks who promise so much more. As a consequence, the unwillingness to acknowledge medical uncertainty makes its own contribution to physicians' authoritarianism. Resort to "clinical judgment," apodictically asserted as in yesteryear, continues to substitute for a careful explanation of options.

Implications for Economic Conflicts of Interest

In highlighting medical uncertainty, I wanted to draw attention to two problems: First, until disclosure of medical uncertainty becomes an essential requirement of informed consent, information on risks, benefits, and alternatives remains largely meaningless in allowing patients to make well-considered choices. Thus, it is unwarranted to view informed consent as a safeguard for protecting patients from unnecessary tests. Dan Brock recognized this when he wrote that "[t]here is little reason to believe that disclosure [of financial interest] would have a significant effect on the ordering of excessive procedures . . . since the disclosure would give the patient no basis for questioning the physician's medical judgment that the procedure is necessary."[30] Second, the ubiquity of medical uncertainty gives physicians considerable discretion to order diagnostic tests and therapeutic procedures under the elastic standard of "due care."

Even before the age of medical entrepreneurialism, physicians were accused of performing too many unnecessary surgeries and being altogether too interventionistic.[31] They often felt unjustly accused, pointing to examples when delay caused harm and thus insisting that clinical judgment, not self-interest, motivated such conduct. To be sure, they said, an x-ray or a hysterectomy may have been unnecessary, but what if it had been otherwise?

Self-interest is inevitable in the practice of medicine. As the bioethicist Albert Jonsen has put it: "A profound moral paradox pervades medicine. That paradox arises from the incessant conflict of two most basic principles of morality: self-interest and altruism. Many of the social and economic features of medical care are, in some way, outgrowths of this paradox."[32]

I once wrote that too much may have been made of economic self-interest as an explanation for physicians' resort to unnecessary and more expensive procedures. Instead, I argued that "doctors' unwillingness to come to terms with their uncertainties about what properly falls within the domain of scientific medicine—whether to base their evaluation of a patient's condition on scientific or intuitive grounds, whether to delay or to intervene, and whether or not to share with patients their bafflement and even ignorance—influences their propensity to err on the side of intervention as much as do economic considerations."[33] I went on to say that "in not facing up to these issues, doctors and patients have become victims of too many unnecessary interventions. That there is money to be made out of all this is true, but it is not the whole story."[34] I was chided for having been too dismissive of economic considerations. My critics were probably correct that I had paid too little attention to the unholy alliance between medical uncertainty and economic gain. In today's world, however, with the technological innovations of endoscopy, mammography, magnetic resonance imaging, and other laboratory procedures, with facilities and equipment owned by physicians and from which they derive considerable financial benefits, medicine has moved closer to the world of commercialism than was true in the past.

There may never have been a time, as Talcott Parsons so confidently stated, when the practice of medicine was "[drastically different] from the usual pricing mechanisms of the business world . . . which for the most part cut off the physician from many immediate opportunities for financial gain which are treated as legitimately open to the business man."[35] Marc Rodwin recently gave an account of the history of financial conflicts of interest in American medicine from 1890 to 1992 and concluded that such conflicts "arising from fee splitting, self-referral, entrepreneurship, and other commercial practices are not new."[36] The AMA struggled with these problems early in this century, when it promulgated "a strict official position against fee splitting and various commercial practices [but] was unable to hold physicians accountable."[37] What is different in today's world, in contrast to the past, are three developments: (1) commercial practices have become much more widespread and legitimated by the medical profession; (2) thanks to the technological advances in medicine, much more money can be made from such entrepreneurial activities, contributing to the alarming rise in the percentage of the gross national product spent on medical care; and (3) the federal government has increasingly become involved in regulating the economic dimension of medical practice.

Medicine's historical claim, as Paul Starr put it, "to be above the market and pure commercializing" is increasingly being questioned as it had never been before, and so is physicians' claim that "public trust [can be justified since] professionals have set higher standards for themselves than the minimal rules governing the marketplace [and that therefore] they can be judged under those standards by each other, not by laymen."[38] I agree with Arnold Relman that "physicians serve their patients' interests best when they divorce themselves from financial interests in the medical marketplace."[39] Therefore, it may be the greater part of wisdom if the profession were to take the unprecedented step of prohibiting—to the extent allowed by federal and state statutes, regulations, and common law—all commercial practices beyond fee-for-service except under the rarest and most carefully defined circumstances. (It is beyond the scope of this chapter to specify, for example, the routine tests that physicians should be permitted to conduct as an integral part of their diagnostic work. Such tests are inexpensive and, more often than not, need not be billed separately.) As long as this policy recommendation cannot be implemented, other means must be found to curtail the exploitation both of patients through unnecessary procedures and of the state, as well as third-party payers, through unnecessary costs.

Informed consent, however, is not a suitable mechanism of control. Instead, it is a political ploy to stave off federal regulations and maintain physician autonomy. As I have already suggested, under the loose professional standard of due care, aided and abetted by medical uncertainty and the fear of malpractice suits, medical judgment can always justify the ordering of many diagnostic tests. And ownership of diagnostic laboratories, for example, makes it humanly impossible not only for physicians to trust themselves, but also for the public to trust physicians to keep economic interests from influencing, however unconsciously, their clinical judgments.

A few commentators have correctly pointed out that before disclosure and consent can ever become a meaningful barrier to abuse, a searching inquiry must be conducted into "what must be disclosed and to whom, the manner of presentation,"[40] and the quality of consent that must be obtained. If that were to happen, it would become apparent that the search for disclosure and consent standards to obviate the problems created by physicians' entrepreneurial activities is at present a largely futile quest.

Two Scenarios

Let me present two not so hypothetical scenarios in support of this assertion. In one, after the physician has examined the patient and formed a tentative impression of what ails her, he informs her that a series of laboratory tests are necessary to either confirm or rule out his preliminary diagnosis. He then tells her that he could refer her to a laboratory in which he has a financial interest or to another one. The choice is hers to make. After hearing this, the patient may silently ask herself: "Why is he telling me this? Is there something I should be concerned about? What should I be concerned about? Could he ever think of sending me to a second-rate facility?" She may not know how to respond but may feel forced to ask pro forma, and probably with some hesitation lest she offend her physician, whether his laboratory is a good one. He answers that "his laboratory is, of course, well known to him, and he can vouch for the competence with which the tests will be performed." To drive the point home, he may add, "It is as good as I am." The patient not only likes her physician but is also at a loss about what to ask him because his invitation to decide what laboratory to go to was not preceded by an explanation of which tests are essential and which are not, or by an invitation to decide together which procedures to perform and which to postpone. If a referral to his laboratory creates no undue hardships for her, she is likely to submit and to "consent" to an invitation that has all the earmarks of a command performance.

The physician did not tell her that studies have shown that when patients are sent to physician-owned laboratories, more tests as well as more expensive ones will be ordered than if they are referred to a facility in which physicians have no financial interest.[41] She was not told that, consciously and/or unconsciously, financial gain may influence his decision to order more tests. And she was not told that his doing so is not necessarily testimony to his lack of integrity but a consequence of the confluence of medical uncertainty and economic gain on the decision of how many tests to order. Had he disclosed these facts and concerns to his patient, she would most likely have been at a loss about how to respond. Perhaps after an awkward silence, she may have blurted out, "If all that is true, why do you complicate matters by owning a diagnostic facility?" She probably would have immediately apologized for being so rude. The doctor might now begin to worry about having a litigious person on his hands, and to consider either a recommendation that she see another physician or a referral to a laboratory in which he has no financial interests. From then on, however, both will be unsure as to whether their future relationship has been harmed.

In the second scenario, the physician is aware that financial gain may affect the extent of diagnostic testing and that by the time he discloses his financial interest—that is, after he has decided which tests to order—it is too late to reconsider should his patient decide to go elsewhere for the tests. Therefore, he posts a notice in his waiting room that informs patients of his financial interest in a laboratory. Beneath it, he includes a warning that his interest may unconsciously influence the tests ordered, followed by a reassuring comment that, since he is aware of this problem, he will exercise his best professional judgment to compensate for it. Finally, he invites his patients to decide before seeing him whether or not they want to be referred to his laboratory.

In presenting these scenarios, I ask the reader to pause and reflect on the disconcerting and disorienting aspects of such (or any) disclosures if they require a response from the patient. In customary medical practice, patients find it difficult to question physicians' professional recommendations. And this will remain a reality until physicians embrace shared decision-making as an alternative to beneficent authoritarianism. At least in these customary settings, patients can have some trust in their physicians' having their medical interests uppermost in mind. Though consent remains a formality, physicians and patients have become accustomed to such ceremonial practices. If consent, in situations when economic gain is an issue, is guided by the same ritual, it will be difficult for patients to do anything but consent out of fear that otherwise they would impugn the ethical integrity of their physicians. Thus, disclosure of conflicts of interest that require more than a perfunctory consent creates burdens for the physician and the patient that neither can assume.

Conclusion

Throughout this chapter, I have noted that proponents for disclosure of financial conflicts of interest generally say nothing about the quality of consent that patients must give to a referral to physician-owned facilities. This omission suggests some awareness, however dimly perceived, that in the present climate of physician–patient decision-making, obtaining informed consent is a charade. If the time ever comes when physicians are more willing to share the burdens of medical decisions with patients—being less reluctant for reasons of beneficence to discuss uncertainties, risks, benefits and alternatives—then informed consent may perhaps play a meaningful role in referrals to physician-owned facilities.

In all that I have said, I have talked about "informed consent," not "disclosure." And I do not wish to suggest that economic conflicts of interest should not be disclosed to patients *as long as patients' consent is viewed as mere acquiescence and not as an assumption of responsibility if patients agree to such a referral.* Calling such an agreement informed consent could readily be viewed as absolving physicians of responsibility for such practices under the guise of patients having made an autonomous choice. Thus, even with disclosure, physicians must be charged with the *sole* responsibility for resolving conflicts of self-interest and interest to patients, and for doing so as best they can. The doctrine of informed consent should not give physicians license to shift the responsibility for decision from themselves to their patients and, in turn, make both of them party to an unseemly charade. Faced with these responsibilities, physicians should, however, be mindful of Hippocrates' warning: "Life is short, the Art long, Opportunity fleeting, Experiment treacherous, Judgment difficult."[42] And I would add to his wise words: "Entrepreneurialism hazardous."

Notes

1. E. Haavi Morreim, Chapter 11 in this volume.
2. *See* text at notes 26–27 *infra.*
3. Arnold Relman, The New Medical–Industrial Complex, 303 *N. Engl. J. Med.* 963–970 (1980).
4. *Id.* at 963–964.
5. *Id.* at 967.
6. Arnold Relman, Dealing with Conflicts of Interest, 313 *N. Engl. J. Med.* 749, 751 (1985).
7. Note 3 *supra,* at 967.
8. *Id.* at 969.
9. *Id.* at 969–970.
10. Institute of Medicine, *For-Profit Enterprise in Health Care* (Bradford Gray, ed., 1986).
11. *Id.* at 163.
12. *Id.* at 164.
13. American Medical Association, Judicial Council Report: *Conflict of Interest—Guidelines* (adopted by the AMA House of Delegates, December 1984).
14. AMA Votes to Ease New Curbs on Physician "Self-Referral," *The Washington Post* A2 (June 24, 1992).
15. *See, e.g.*, AMA Rules Against Self-Referrals, *Chicago Tribune* N20 (December 9, 1992).
16. E. Haavi Morreim, Economic Disclosure and Economic Advocacy, 12 *J. Legal Med.* 275, 290 (1991).
17. *Id.* at 290, quoting Miller v. Kennedy, 522 P.2d 852, 860 (1974).
18. *Id.* 328.
19. *Id.* 318–320.
20. Talcott Parsons, *The Social System* 464–465 (1954).
21. Howard Becker, The Nature of a Profession, in *The Sixty-First Yearbook of the National Society for the Study of Education* (1962).
22. Thomas Duffy, Agamemnon's Fate and the Medical Profession, 9 *West. N. Engl. L. Rev.* 21, 27–28 (1987).
23. Jay Katz, *The Silent World of Doctor and Patient* (1984); Jay Katz, Physician Patient Encounters "On a Darkling Plain," 9 *West. N. Engl. L. Rev.* 207–226 (1987); Jay Katz, Duty and Caring in the Age of Informed Consent and Medical Science: Unlocking Peabody's Secret, 8 *Humane Med.* 187–197 (1992).
24. Salgo v. Leland Stanford Jr. University Board of Trustees, 317 P.2d 170 (Cal. Dist. Ct. App. 1957).
25. Note 23, *supra,* Duty and Caring, at 188.
26. Note 23 *supra* and Natanson v. Kline 350 P.2d 1093 (Kan. 1960).
27. Jay Katz, Preface to paperback edition of *The Silent World of Doctor and Patient* (1986).
28. Note 23 *supra, The Silent World* at 165–206.
29. Louis Thomas, *The Medusa and the Snail: More Notes of a Biology Watcher* 73–74 (1979).
30. Dan Brock, Medicine and Business: An Unhealthy Mix, 9 *Bus. Prof. Ethics J.* 20, 34 (1990).
31. Note 23 *supra, The Silent World* at 195–197.

32. Albert Jonsen, Watching the Doctor, 308 *N. Engl. J. Med.* 1531, 1532 (1983).
33. Note 23 *supra,* at 201.
34. *Id.*
35. Note 20 *supra,* at 464.
36. Marc A. Rodwin, The Organized American Medical Profession's Response to Financial Conflicts of Interest: 1890–1992, 70 *Milbank Q.* 703, 733 (1992).
37. *Id.*
38. Paul Starr, *The Social Transformation of American Medicine* 23 (1982).
39. Note 6 *supra,* at 751.
40. Marc Rodwin, Physicians' Conflicts of Interest, 321 *N. Engl. J. Med.* 1405 (1989).
41. Bruce Hillman et al., Frequency and Costs of Diagnostic Imaging in Office Practice—A Comparison of Self-Referring and Radiologist-Referring Physicians, 323 *N. Engl. J. Med.* 1604–1608 (1990); Jean Mitchell and Elton Scott, New Evidence of the Prevalence and Scope of Physician Joint Venture, 268 *JAMA* 80 (1992).
42. Hippocrates, *Aphorisms* 99 (Trans. W. Jones, 1967).

13

Physician Joint Ventures and Self-Referral: An Empirical Perspective

Jean M. Mitchell

Physician ownership of health care facilities and businesses to which they refer patients, but at which they do not practice or directly provide services, has become common in recent years.[1] Physicians have established such financial arrangements, known as "joint ventures," in a wide range of outpatient services such as diagnostic labs, radiological imaging centers, ambulatory surgical facilities, home health agencies, physical therapy clinics, medical equipment businesses, dialysis units, substance abuse treatment centers, and radiation therapy facilities. Although under existing federal law it is illegal for physicians to receive kickbacks for patient referrals, physician ownership of health care facilities is not per se illegal so long as any ownership compensation paid to each physician investor is not directly tied to the number of referrals made to the facility.

These ownership arrangements are controversial because they create a conflict of interest for referring physician investors.[2] Physician investors have a financial incentive to refer patients for treatment to facilities they own, even though such treatment may not be either medically necessary or cost-effective. Many critics have argued that these ownership arrangements are lucrative investments through which referring physician investors are able to earn legalized kickbacks for patient referrals. According to critics, the conflict of interest inherent in physician self-referral arrangements results in overutilization of services and increased costs to consumers. Critics also maintain that joint ventures limit access because they "cream skim", that is, treat patients only with good insurance. Uninsured and underinsured patients are generally not served by joint venture facilities because such individuals have only limited ability to pay. Moreover, critics note that these arrangements are anticompetitive because they create a captive referral system whereby physician investors send nearly all their patients to the facilities in which they have an ownership interest. Such "tying arrangements" insulate incumbent joint venture firms from new competition, make it difficult for existing non–joint venture providers to compete, and thus may subsequently lead to diminished quality and higher charges. In light of these considerations, these ownership arrangements have been the subject of extensive debate in the media, within the medical profession, in the medical literature, and by federal and state policy makers.[3]

Proponents have countered these criticisms with claims that physician self-referral arrangements are simply necessary adjustments to major changes that have occurred in the health care sector during the last decade. Perhaps the most noteworthy developments were the enactment of Medicare's prospective reimbursement system for inpatient services, managed care and preferred provider arrangements, a growing elderly population, and the development of new technologies that can be delivered in nonhospital settings. Proponents have noted that joint ventures have many benefits, including sources of venture capital, diversification of investment risks, economies of scale and scope,[4] and improved access to new technological procedures and services to persons residing in medically underserved or rural areas. It has also been argued that such self-referral arrangements give physicians more control over the quality of care provided to their patients.

Until recently, empirical evidence on the consequences of physician self-referral was limited because information on physician ownership of health care facilities, referrals of patients to such facilities, and financial and utilization data on these facilities were not reported to federal/state regulatory authorities, third-party insurers, or patients. Further, third-party insurers' claims data are generally not available to academic researchers or consultants. Instead, most of the literature on physician self-referral arrangements consists of commentaries and discussions of the pros and cons of joint ventures involving referring physicians. Examples include articles by Relman[5] and Todd and Horan.[6] Other studies have documented physicians' responses to other financial incentives, including fee-for-service, salaries, HMOs, and bonus payments. Recent studies that have surmounted the data limitations and evaluated the consequences of physician self-referral arrangements can be classified into two categories: self-referral within a physician's office and self-referral to free-standing, physician-owned facilities.

This chapter examines the empirical studies documenting the consequences of financial incentives, particularly physician self-referral arrangements. Following review of the empirical evidence, the strengths and weaknesses of legislative remedies, some already enacted and others being considered, are evaluated.

Evidence on Physicians' Responses to Other Financial Incentives

A number of studies have examined physicians' responses to financial incentives. The consensus of these studies is that physicians who stand to gain financially by ordering tests and procedures order more studies than physicians without this incentive.

Epstein, Begg, and McNeil[7] examined the influence of payment method on the use of ambulatory testing by internists by comparing the number of tests performed on patients with uncomplicated hypertension by ten physicians in large fee-for-service groups and seventeen physicians in large prepaid groups. After controlling for patient characteristics, the results indicate that physicians in fee-for-service practices ordered 50 percent more electrocardiograms and 40 percent more chest radiographs than doctors in prepaid groups. Both tests were associated with high profits and high patient charges. These findings suggest that physicians' ordering of diagnostic tests is influenced by the method in which they are compensated.

Hillman[8] points out the potential conflict of interest for physicians inherent in financial arrangements with HMO's, including capitation-based payments, fee-for-service contracts wherein the HMO withholds a percentage of payments, and salary-based payments. His analysis of approximately 300 HMOs implies that certain financial arrangements result in conflicts of interest that influence physician behavior and may adversely affect quality of care. Specifically, this situation is likely to arise when the HMO has established mechanisms to share profits with participating physicians.

More recently, Hillman, Pauly, and Kerstein[9] examined whether financial incentives affect physicians' clinical decisions and the operating performance of HMOs; the incentives under HMO arrangements are just the opposite of fee-for-service incentives. Their findings suggest that compensating physicians by either capitation payments or salaries was associated with lower hospitalization rates than compensating physicians on a discounted fee-for-service basis. Moreover, it appears that imposing penalties on physicians for any deficits in the HMOs' hospital funds results in fewer inpatient visits. The authors conclude that HMO type and certain financial incentives influence physician behavior.

Hemenway et al.[10] compared the practice patterns of physicians at a chain of ambulatory walk-in clinics over a one-year period. In the middle of the year, the clinics instituted a new compensation plan whereby physicians could earn bonuses tied to the gross revenues each physician generated. Prior to this change, physicians were paid a flat hourly wage. Under the new payment mechanism, physicians increased the number of laboratory tests performed per visit by 23 percent and the number of x-rays per visit by 16 percent. The total charges per month, adjusted for inflation, grew by 20 percent, primarily because of the significant increase in patient visits. Moreover, the wages of those physicians who regularly earned the bonus rose 19 percent. The authors conclude that significant monetary incentives may induce physicians to change their practices to increase office visits and utilization of diagnostic procedures.

Consequences of Within-Office Physician Self-Referral

Within-office self-referral occurs when a physician orders a test or diagnostic procedure for a patient that is performed in the physician's office. Examples of within-office self-referral include an orthopedic surgeon who orders a series of x-rays for a patient that are performed using equipment situated in his office; a neurologist who recommends a computed tomography (CT) scan for a patient, and the scanner is located in her office; a gynecologist who recommends a mammogram for a woman and the machine is located in his office. The alternative, which is not self-referral, occurs when a treating physician refers a patient to a hospital outpatient department or a radiology practice for diagnostic procedures. Three articles have documented the effects of within-office physician self-referral arrangements.

Childs and Hunter[11] analyzed claims data for an elderly population residing in California over a six-month period to examine the patterns of use of diagnostic x-rays among physicians. Nonradiologists providing direct x-ray services to their patients in their own offices performed x-rays almost twice as frequently as did physicians who referred their patients to radiologists. This finding suggests that nonradiologists who have a financial interest in radiological equipment perform more diagnostic x-rays than other physicians, although their choices of examination method suggest that they have limited knowledge of radiology in comparison to radiologists.

Hillman and colleagues[12] compared the frequency and costs of imaging examinations performed by physicians who conducted these diagnostic tests using equipment in their own offices (self-referring) with those ordered by physicians who referred their patients to radiologists (radiologist-referring). Their analysis is based on claims data for over 65,000 imaging procedures ordered by more than 6400 physicians for acute upper respiratory symptoms, pregnancy, low back pain, or difficulty in urinating (for men). The imaging procedures examined for each of the respective conditions were chest radiography, obstetrical ultrasound, radiography of the lumbar spine, and excretory x-rays or ultrasonography. The study found that, on average, doctors who owned the machines ordered 4.0 to 4.5 times more imaging tests than those who referred their patients to radiologists. Further, for chest radiography, obstetrical ultrasonography, and lumbar spine radiography, the self-referring physicians charged significantly more than the radiologists for imaging procedures of similar complexity. The combined effects of more frequent imaging and higher charges per procedure resulted in average charges per episode of care that were 4.5 to 7.5 times higher for the self-referring physicians. The authors concluded that the extreme differences in the charges between the two groups call into question the assumption that the financial interests of physicians do not influence medical decisions. The researchers question whether 4.0 times the utilization compounded by 4.0 times to 7.5 times the cost provide commensurate incremental benefits in health to these patients.

Hillman and colleagues[13] further analyzed the consequences of within-office self-referral arrangements in a more recent study. Here again, the researchers assessed differences in physicians' utilization of and charges for diagnostic imaging depending on whether the physicians performed imaging exams in their offices (self-referral) or referred their patients to radiologists (radiologist-referral). Using an established methodology, they generated episodes of medical care from an insurance claims database for an elderly population and within each episode determined whether diagnostic imaging had been performed. If so, they proceeded to classify each episode as either self-referring or radiologist-referring. The ten clinical presentations examined were (1) acute upper respiratory tract infections (plain films, fluoroscopy); (2) difficulty in urinating in men (excretory urography, cystourethrography, sonography); (3) low back pain (plain films, myelography, discography, CT scans, magnetic resonance imaging (MRI); (4) headache (CT, MRI); 5) transient cerebral ischemia (CT, MRI, sonography, angiography); (6) upper gastrointestinal bleeding (plain films, barium studies); (7) knee pain (plain films, arthrography, CT, MRI); (8) urinary tract infection (plain films, excretory urography, cystourethrography, sonography, CT, MRI); (9) chest pains (plain films, barium studies, radionuclide studies);and (10) congestive heart failure (plain films, echocardiography, real-time and Doppler sonography, angiography, radionuclide studies). For each of the ten clinical presentations, they compared mean imaging frequency, mean imaging charges per episode of care, and mean imaging charges per procedure, depending on whether the episode was self-referring or radiologist-referring.

Although the magnitude of the results differed for each clinical presentation examined, their analyses indicated that self-referring physicians employed diagnostic imaging 1.7 to 7.7 times more frequently than physicians who referred their patients to radiologists. Moreover, even after controlling for physician specialty, the ratio of frequency of imaging (self-referring to radiologist-referring) ranged from 1.5:1 to 4.8:1 for all the clinical presentations examined. Mean imaging charges per episode of care were 1.6 to 6.2 times higher for self-referring physicians compared to radiologist-referring physicians. Mean imaging charges per procedure were significantly greater for radiologists relative to self-referring physicians if the procedures were performed in a hospital outpatient department; this is attributable to the high technical charges of hospital outpatient departments. On the other hand, for imaging performed in radiologists' offices, mean imaging charges per procedure were significantly less than those of self-referring physicians. The authors conclude that nonradiologist physicians who operate diagnostic imaging equipment in their offices perform imaging exams more frequently than physicians who refer their patients to radiologists for these services. The greater frequency of imaging results in significantly higher imaging charges per episode of medical care. Although it was impossible for the researchers to determine whether any of the increased utilization associated with self-referral was inappropriate, there is no evidence to demonstrate that greater use of in-office ancillary procedures yields a commensurate benefit in improving patients' health. The researchers also discussed various policy options that insurers might adopt to mitigate the increased utilization accompanying the financial incentives linked to within-office self-referral. These include the denial of payment for self-referred imaging, reimbursing self-referred imaging at a lower rate than radiologist-referred imaging, and incorporating the payment for imaging in the reimbursement for an office visit.

Consequences of Physician Joint Ventures and Self-Referral

Before the Medicare prospective payment system started in 1983, physician joint ventures were essentially nonexistent. The only empirical evidence on the effects of such ownership arrangements in the pre-prospective payment period is from a demonstration project funded by the Robert Wood Johnson Foundation in which fifty-four hospitals sponsored joint ventures with physicians in primary care group practice. Shortell, Wickizer, and Wheeler[14] evaluated what happened when acute care hospitals oriented to providing high-technology services attempted to diversify into providing primary care, low-technology services. Importantly, the types of hospital-physician joint ventures established under this demonstration project differed substantially from the types of physician joint ventures that have been established in the past ten years. For this reason, the results of this demonstration project have only limited implications for physician self-referral arrangements established in the late 1980s and early 1990s.

Despite these limitations, the results of this pre-prospective payment demonstration project suggest that joint ventures can have substantial financial impacts for hospitals. The joint ventures accounted for an average of 9 percent of hospital admissions; participating hospitals increased their market shares by approximately 4 percent. Inflation-adjusted revenues from hospital laboratory charges increased by 15 percent; revenues generated from hospital radiology services rose by 14 percent. Many of the joint-venture group practices attracted high percentages of self-pay and privately insured patients. As to the impact on physician charges to patients, costs per visit were lower for both emergency room visits and outpatient department visits, while costs per visit were slightly higher than for private-practice fee-for-service physicians.

Governmental Studies

Two studies have been conducted by the federal government to document the consequences of physician joint ventures in the post-diagnosis related group (DRG) period. The first was conducted by the Office of the Inspector General (OIG) and was cited by Rep. Pete Stark during congressional hearings in May 1989 in his efforts to win support in Congress for new legislation restricting the practice of physician self-referral. The other study, conducted by the General Accounting Office (GAO), was never completed; therefore, only preliminary findings from the GAO report will be reviewed.

The OIG Report. The OIG conducted two surveys of health care providers in eight states—Arkansas, California, Connecticut, Florida, Michigan, New York, West Virginia, and Kansas City, Missouri—to determine the prevalence, nature, and impact of physician ownership of medical businesses to which they make referrals, but at which they do not practice or directly provide services.[15] One survey involved approximately 4000 physicians; the other focused on ownership and/or compensation arrangements between physicians and three types of health care businesses: free-standing clinical labs, durable medical equipment suppliers, and free-standing physiological labs. Physiological or imaging facilities perform noninvasive diagnostic testing such as MRI scans, CT scans, and ultrasound exams.

Estimates derived from the data reported by the 2690 physicians who responded to the survey imply that, nationwide, 12 percent of the physicians who bill Medicare have ownership interests in facilities to which they make referrals, and that about 8 percent of the physicians who bill Medicare have some type of compensation arrangement with one or more health care facilities to which they make referrals. National estimates calculated from the surveys of health care entities imply that at least 25 percent of free-standing clinical labs, 8 percent of durable medical equipment suppliers, and 27 percent of free-standing physiological labs or imaging centers are owned, either partially or wholly, by physicians.

The findings indicate that Medicare patients of referring physicians who have a financial interest in a clinical lab received 45 percent more clinical lab services than all Medicare beneficiaries, irrespective of place of service. The results further show that Medicare patients of referring physicians who have investment interests in free-standing clinical labs received 34 percent more tests directly from these labs than the general population of Medicare patients. The latter group is comprised of patients treated by both physician owners and physicians who have no investment interests in health care facilities. Medicare patients of physicians who reported investment interests in diagnostic centers received about 13 percent more tests than all Medicare beneficiaries in general. Although the results indicated no overall significant differences between the Medicare patients of physician owners and all Medicare beneficiaries with respect to the utilization of durable medical equipment items, significant variation was found on a state-by-state basis. The OIG report estimated that the costs of the additional clinical lab testing amounted to $28 million in 1987. It is important to recognize that the actual effects of referring physician ownership are even greater because the control group (all patients) includes the comparison group (patients treated by physician owners).

The GAO Study. Michael Zimmerman, director of Medicare and Medicaid issues for the GAO, presented preliminary results from a study focusing on physician referrals to clinical laboratories and diagnostic imaging centers in Maryland and Pennsylvania.[16] Eighty-seven percent of the facilities in each state had responded to the questionnaire. Preliminary estimates suggest that about 18 percent of the free-standing clinical labs and imaging centers in Maryland are owned by one or more physicians in a specialty unrelated to the services rendered at either of these health care entities. In Pennsylvania, about 29 percent of the free-standing labs and imaging facilities are owned, in part or entirely, by referring physicians.

With respect to overall utilization of laboratory services, physician owners in Maryland ordered more tests, and more costly tests, than physicians with no investment interests. A breakdown by specialty indicates that cardiologists who owned labs ordered fewer tests than nonowners specializing in cardiovascular disease. In contrast, both family practice and internal medicine physicians with investment interests in clinical labs ordered significantly more tests per visit than nonowners. The data for diagnostic imaging procedures show that physician owners ordered fewer, but more expensive, tests than physicians without ownership interests. Analysis of the data on utilization patterns of physician-owned labs and imaging centers in Pennsylvania is still incomplete.

The AMA Survey

A 1990 survey by the AMA suggests that about 8 percent of the 4000 physicians surveyed had an ownership interest in a private, free-standing health care facility to which they referred patients for services.[17] The AMA survey also reveals that physician owners were more likely to be surgical specialists and to have incomes in excess of $150,000. Other findings indicate that physicians residing in the South, as well as those practicing in states with either regulation or legislation affecting ownership, were more likely to have investment interests in health care facilities to which they referred patients. Physicians were most likely to have an investment interest in MRI, radiology or clinical laboratory services.

The Florida Study

Under a mandate by the 1989 Florida legislature, my colleague Elton Scott and I conducted a comprehensive study to document the effects of physician joint ventures on access, costs, charges, and utilization of health care services in Florida for the Florida Health Care Cost Containment Board.[18,19] "Joint venture" was defined as any ownership or investment interest between referring physicians (or any health care professional who makes referrals) and a business providing health care goods or services. Surveys to obtain ownership, financial, and utilization data from Florida health care providers regarding the 1989 fiscal year were mailed to over 3500 free-standing health care facilities: ambulatory surgical facilities, clinical laboratories, diagnostic imaging centers, durable medical equipment suppliers, home health agencies, hospitals, mental health treatment centers, nursing homes, physical therapy and rehabilitation centers, and radiation therapy centers. Physicians' practices were not surveyed. Telephone follow-up was conducted to obtain missing data and to correct inconsistent information reported on the facility questionnaires. The final overall response rate was 82.4 percent; 2200 of the 2669 eligible facilities submitted a survey with usable and consistent information to classify each facility as joint venture or nonjoint venture. Nearly all facility types had individual response rates exceeding 80 percent. Durable medical equipment suppliers had the lowest response rate—just under 70 percent. The majority of the nonrespondents were concentrated in the Southeast peninsula region. The telephone follow-up of nonresponding facilities indicated that they were more likely to be involved in joint ventures.

Ownership by referring physicians of health care businesses providing diagnostic testing or other ancillary services is pervasive in Florida. For example, over three-fourths of the ambulatory surgical facilities and more than 90 percent of the diagnostic imaging centers are owned by referring physicians. In contrast, physician ownership of hospitals and nursing homes is less common. Only 5 percent of the acute care hospitals and 12 percent of the nursing homes have physician owners. Our findings indicate that at least 10,000 owners of the health care facility types surveyed are health care professionals or health care entities; more than 80 percent of these owners are physicians. Of approximately 8100 physician owners, more than 20 percent were identified as indirect investors through parent corporations and holding companies. About 91 percent of the physician owners are specialists who are likely to refer patients to their own facility for surgery, diagnostic testing, and other ancillary services or equipment. We estimate conservatively that at least 40 percent of the physicians involved in direct patient care in Florida are owners of joint venture health care facilities to which they refer their patients for services but at which they do not practice.

Proponents contend that joint ventures increase geographic access to services and new technological procedures to persons residing in rural, medically underserved areas. This is not the case in Florida, however, as none of the joint venture facilities is located in a rural area. Furthermore, with the exception of some hospitals and nursing homes, few of the joint venture businesses are located in less densely populated regions. The concentration of all types of health care facilities in urbanized areas is not surprising, however, because it is unlikely that less urbanized areas could generate the volume of patients necessary to achieve a break-even point for the business.

Our analysis evaluated the effects of physician joint ventures on access, costs, charges, and utilization. We tested the null hypothesis that there are no differences (or that differences are beneficial to consumers) in average values for joint venture and non-joint venture facilities. The alternative hypothesis assumed that differences in averages are detrimental to Florida consumers. In these comparisons, we controlled for obvious systematic influences such as the type of service provided and geographic factors.

The comparisons of joint venture and non-joint venture facilities enabled us to classify each facility group into one of three categories. We found that joint venture ownership arrangements had no apparently negative effects on access, costs, charges, or utilization of health care services for acute care hospitals and nursing homes. For ambulatory surgical centers, durable medical equipment suppliers, and home health agencies some problems were found, but the data did not allow us to draw definitive conclusions. Joint venture ownership had significant negative effects on access, costs, charges, and utilization of health care services for clinical laboratories, diagnostic imaging, and physical therapy-rehabilitation facilities. For these three types of health care facilities, we found that joint venture facilities cream-skim patients with good insurance and treat relatively few patients with limited ability to pay. Also, for the three problematic facility types, both utilization rates and charges per patient were significantly higher at joint venture facilities in comparison to their otherwise similar non-joint venture counterparts.

We also explored the complex ownership structures of physician joint ventures.[20] This analysis shows that, compared with other health care business arrangements, physician-owned joint ventures are significantly more likely to choose complex ownership structures. Multiple levels of incorporation or partnership can make it difficult to identify the individual owners of the parent organization. Failure to obtain information on the owners of the parent organizations means that both the prevalence and scope of physician joint ventures will be understated.

These results have important implications for policymakers who must design regulations to address the problems associated with physician self-referral. If the objective of the regulation is to prohibit self-referral to free-standing health care facilities, then the legislation must clearly define investment interests, ownership structures, and compensation relationships to include both direct and indirect ownership arrangements. Failure to acknowledge indirect ownership and compensation arrangements will limit the impact of any regulation that attempts to prohibit physician self-referral.

In another article, Scott and I[21] evaluated the effects of physician ownership of free-standing physical therapy and rehabilitation facilities on utilization, charges, profits, and three measures of service characteristics for physical therapy treatments. Statistical comparisons of each of these indicators between joint venture and non-joint venture facilities were performed using data from 118 outpatient physical therapy clinics and 63 comprehensive rehabilitation facilities providing services in Florida during 1989. Visits per patient were 39 to 45 percent higher in joint venture facilities. Both gross and net revenue per patient were 30 to 40 percent higher in facilities owned by referring physicians. Percent operating income and percent markup were significantly higher in joint venture physical therapy and rehabilitation facilities. Licensed physical therapists and licensed therapist assistants employed in non-joint venture firms spend about 60 percent more time per visit treating patients than their counterparts working in joint venture facilities. Joint venture facilities generate more of their revenues from patients with well-paying insurance, and the increased utilization and charges that characterize joint venture facilities cannot be attributed to the economic and health characteristics of the Florida population. Finally, the authors present data documenting physician-owned physical therapy services nationally. In many states, the proportion of therapists working in physician-owned clinics is comparable to that in Florida. This suggests that the Florida findings can be generalized and that physician self-referral for physical therapy services is a national concern.

Sunshine and I[22] examined physician joint ventures in radiation therapy, evaluating the effects of such arrangements on access, use of services, costs, and quality. Specifically, we compared Medicare data for Florida with similar data for the remainder of the United States because, in 1989, 44 percent of the free-standing radiation therapy facilities were joint ventures compared with 7 percent elsewhere. We also compared joint venture and non-joint venture radiation therapy facilities in Florida.

No joint venture facilities providing radiation therapy were located in inner-city neighborhoods or rural areas. In contrast, 11 percent of non-joint venture free-standing facilities and hospital-based facilities were located in such areas. Among the free-standing facilities, joint ventures generated 39 percent of their revenues from well-insured patients compared with 31 percent for facilities that were not joint ventures. The frequency and cost of radiation therapy treatments performed in free-standing centers were 40 to 60 percent higher in Florida relative to the rest of the United States, which cannot be attributed to underutilization of radiation therapy at hospitals or differences in cancer incidence. Radiation physicists employed at joint venture facilities spent 18 percent less time per patient than their counterparts in non-joint venture facilities. Finally, since mortality among patients with cancer in Florida was not lower than the U.S. average despite the high percentage of joint ventures in Florida, any improvement in quality is subtle, at best. The authors conclude that joint ventures in radiation therapy have adverse effects on access, utilization, costs, and quality, and recommend legislation to ban such self-referral arrangements.

Other Studies

Dyckman[23] analyzed private health insurance claims data, as well as Medicare Part B data, to evaluate whether the conclusions of the Florida Joint Venture Study by Mitchell and Scott,[24] as related to diagnostic imagining services, were consistent with other data. Mitchell and Scott found that nearly all free-standing diagnostic imaging facilities in Florida were physician joint ventures, and that utilization of imaging services was significantly higher than elsewhere due to such financial incentives. Analyzing data from twelve Blue Cross-Blue Shield plans, Dyckman found that both charge levels and utilization rates were higher in Florida relative to other states. His analyses of Medicare Part B data corroborate the findings using the private insurance data. Regardless of the place of service, Florida ranked fourth among the forty-eight states for which data were available in terms of the number of MRI tests per 1000 Medicare beneficiaries; the difference between Florida (27.4) and the United States as a whole (18.8) was 45 percent. Nearly all of this difference can be attributed to the volume and total charges for MRI scans performed in free-standing imaging centers, virtually all of which are joint ventures. The average charge per MRI scan performed in Florida's free-standing centers was 14 percent higher than the national average ($812 versus $711). The number of MRI scans per 1000 Medicare enrollees performed in Florida's free-standing centers was 92 percent above the national average (17.1 for Florida compared to 8.9 for the United States as a whole). Total charges per 1000 Medicare beneficiaries (including price and volume effects) were $13,856 in Florida free-standing centers compared to $6,354 for the United States. Thus, total charges for MRI scans performed in nonhospital imaging centers in Florida exceed the national average by 118 percent. In contrast, Florida charge and utilization experience for MRI scans performed in hospitals were similar to the national experience. Moreover, Dyckman found no evidence that the substantially higher utilization and total charges for MRI scans in Florida compared to the national average was due to the substitution of MRI tests for CT scans, since the volume and total charges for CT scans in Florida were also higher than the averages for the United States as a whole.

In another unpublished study, Dyckman[25] analyzed the effects of physician joint venture activity on the costs of diagnostic imaging services in California. Using data from the 1989 Part B Medicare Annual Data (BMAD), Dyckman compared the Medicare utilization experience in California with the remainder of the United States. His analyses indicate that the number of MRI procedures per 1000 Medicare beneficiaries was 27 in California compared to 17.9 for the remainder of the country, a difference of 51 percent. California ranked sixth among the states for which data are available. One possible explanation for this utilization difference might be a possibly greater incidence of serious illnesses or conditions requiring MRI scans among California Medicare enrollees than among those residing elsewhere. This appears unlikely, as the number of Medicare hospital admissions per 1000 beneficiaries in California is 10 percent below the national admission rate, and the volume of outpatient services is 19 percent below the national average. Dyckman concludes that a likely cause of the higher MRI utilization rate among Medicare enrollees in California is the greater prevalence of joint ventures involving referring physicians. Evidence reported by Mitchell and Scott corroborates this. They found that of the 198 free-standing MRI centers in California, at least 85 percent were owned by referring physician investors. Employing a moderate estimation approach, Dyckman estimates that the cost of the excess MRI scans performed (56 percent) due to physician joint ventures in California is $215 million. Using an extremely conservative approach, Dyckman estimates a volume effect of 34 percent at a cost of $130 million.

Swedlow and colleagues[26] analyzed 6581 California workers' compensation cases to evaluate the effects of physician self-referral on three high-cost medical services: physical therapy, psychiatric evaluations, and MRI scans. They compared the costs per case for all three services, measured the frequency with which physical therapy was performed, and evaluated the medical appropriateness of MRI scans, depending on whether the case was self-referred or independently referred.

Physical therapy was prescribed 2.3 times more often by the physicians in the self-referral group (68 percent) relative to the physicians in the independent referral group (30 percent). The mean cost per case was significantly lower for the self-referral group: $404 for self-referral cases compared to $440 for independent referral cases. The mean cost for psychiatric evaluations was significantly higher for the self-referral group. For psychometric testing, the mean cost was $1165 for self-referral cases and $870 for independent referral cases. The average cost of psychiatric evaluation reports was $2056 for the self-referral group compared to $1680 for independent referrals. Thus, the total cost per case for psychiatric evaluation services was on average 26 percent higher for self-referral cases ($3222) relative to independent referral cases ($2550). The authors also found that 38 percent of the MRI scans ordered by self-referring physicians were deemed medically inappropriate compared to 28 percent of the MRI scans recommended by physicians without such financial interests. There was, however, no difference in the cost per case. The authors conclude that physician self-referral significantly increases the costs of medical care for workers' compensation cases.

Conclusions from Empirical Evidence on Physician Self-referral

This review of the empirical evidence on physician self-referral indicates that these ownership arrangements have negative effects on utilization, costs, access and quality. Specifically, the consensus of all the evidence is that the financial incentives in self-referral arrangements result in increased utilization of services and higher costs to patients. Moreover, physician joint venture facilities appear to target patients with good insurance and treat relatively few indigent and under-insured patients. Regarding geographic access, all physician joint ventures are located in metropolitan areas, and do not increase access to services and new technologies to persons residing in medically underserved or rural areas. Finally, there is limited evidence suggesting that joint ventures have adverse effects on quality. None of the studies has been able to evaluate whether the increased utilization that accompanies the practice of physician self-referral represents inappropriate or unwarranted services, but there is no evidence demonstrating that physician self-referral arrangements have any benefits for consumers.

Conclusions and Recommendations

Physician self-referral arrangements have proliferated during the last decade. Both within office-self-referral and physician joint ventures are controversial because these arrangements create a conflict of interest for the referring physician investors. This review of the empirical studies on physician self-referral indicates that the financial incentives inherent in such arrangements are associated with increased utilization of services and higher costs to consumers. Although none of these studies could determine whether any of the higher utilization associated with self-referral was inappropriate, there is no evidence indicating that this increased utilization resulted in commensurate improvements in patients' health. Furthermore, my research on Florida shows that physician joint ventures cream-skim patients with good insurance. In addition, joint ventures do not increase geographic access to persons in medically underserved and rural areas, as all joint ventures are located in metropolitan areas.

Despite the substantial empirical evidence on the negative consequences of physician self-referral, proponents of these arrangements have been very critical of these studies. For example, the Florida Medical Association commissioned Lewin-ICF, a consulting firm, (1) to evaluate the strengths and weaknesses of the Florida study and (2) to determine if the Florida study provides an adequate basis for imposing regulatory controls on physician joint ventures.[27] Not surprisingly, Lewin-ICF criticized and disagreed with the conclusions of the Florida study for three reasons. First, the economic theory of the potential effects of joint ventures is ambiguous. Second, key comparison variables used in the analysis are often misleading or incomplete. And third, the statistical analysis failed to discover any strong evidence that joint ventures are significantly different from non-joint ventures. The authors of the Florida study wrote a detailed response to the Lewin-ICF critique refuting each of the criticisms raised.[28]

It should also be noted that the validity of the Florida results was confirmed by testimony presented to Congress in April 1993 regarding the findings of a GAO follow-up of the original Florida physician joint venture study.[29] The GAO analyzed 1.3 million claims for imaging service, representing over 55 percent of all Florida Medicare referrals for imaging in 1990, to determine if physician owners of imaging services refer more of their patients for imaging services than nonowners. The results indicate that physician owners had higher referral rates for all types of imaging services than nonowners. The differences in referral rates were greatest for costly, high-technology imaging services: Physician owners had 54 percent higher referral rates for MRI scans, 28 percent higher referral rates for CT scans, and 25 percent higher referral rates for ultrasound and echocardiography. These estimates are conservative because the control group of non-owners includes some owners not identified because the imaging center failed to comply with the mandated survey.

Although existing federal and states laws are likely to have some impact on this problem, these laws have some loopholes that may limit their effectiveness. For example, the current federal prohibition applies only to clinical laboratory services for Medicare patients. Moreover, it does not explicitly include all indirect ownership arrangements, and it exempts group practices. State self-referral prohibitions also have some potential weaknesses. First, some of the state laws contain "grandfather" clauses or extended divestiture periods during which existing self-referral arrangements are still legal. Second, some state laws apply only to specific designated health services. Thus, the potential for abuse still exists for other ancillary services not covered by the prohibition. Third, all of the existing state laws exempt physician group practices from the self-referral prohibition.

At its 1991 annual meeting in December, the AMA House of Delegates adopted new guidelines regarding the practice of physician self-referral: "In general, physicians should not refer patients to a health care facility outside their office practice at which they do not directly provide care or services when they have an investment interest in the facility" (Council on Ethical and Judicial Affairs, AMA, 1992). An exception was made for facilities established because there is a demonstrated need in the community and alternative financing is not available. In adopting this policy, the AMA emphasized that a physician's professional obligation is to the well-being of his patient and that the financial interest created by joint ventures results in at least the appearance of a conflict of interest.

But in June 1992, the House of Delegates reversed this action and voted to support self-referral if the patient is fully informed about both the physician's ownership interest in the facility to which he is referred and the existence of any alternative facilities. Despite the action of the House of Delegates, the Council on Ethical and Judicial Affairs refused to reverse its opinion that self-referral is unethical. As a result, the House of Delegates reconsidered the issue in December 1992 and voted to reaffirm the guidelines against self-referral.

Indeed, the substantial evidence on the negative consequences of physician self-referral, the conflict of interest inherent in it, and the considerable variation in state laws prohibiting it all point to the need for additional legislation. Various federal and state laws directly and indirectly regulate self-referral. These laws differ in many respects—for example, the types of services, practice arrangements, and time periods covered. Legislatures should enact laws that prohibit physicians from referring patients to health care facilities in which the physician (or an immediate family member) has either a direct or an indirect investment interest; this prohibition should apply to all types of health care facilities and to both public and privately insured patients. Prohibitions on payments for self-referrals should be included in such legislation. To ensure that this legislation is effective, the prohibitions on self-referrals, as well bans on third-party reimbursement for such referrals, must impose severe penalties for violations. If such prohibitions are to be effective, there must be a requirement for reasonably prompt divestiture or dissolution of existing joint ventures. For example, the federal law prohibiting referrals to clinical laboratories allowed a two-year period for divestiture or dissolution.[30] Any form of midrange or long-term grandfathering provisions for existing joint ventures only perpetuates their deleterious effects. Such laws must include provisions to preclude new abusive arrangements.

If joint ventures are clearly outlawed and actively prosecuted, one would expect to see attempts to achieve the same inappropriate financial gains through yet another organizational form. For some types of ancillary services, referring physicians could simply skirt a prohibition on self-referral to free-standing facilities in which they have invested by providing the service within their group practice. Thus, to preclude new abusive arrangements, the law must narrowly define group practices to recognize such potential loopholes. Finally, to monitor compliance with these prohibitions, all direct as well as indirect ownership arrangements should be disclosed to federal and state authorities, third-party insurers, and patients. Penalties imposed on facilities that fail to comply with such disclosure requirements should be severe enough to work.

Many critics of self-referral contend that the new prohibitions on self-referral to free-standing facilities should apply to within-office self-referral arrangements as well. But extending the self-referral prohibitions as such may not be desirable, especially if many within-office arrangements are established for patients convenience. Alternatively, other mechanisms are apt to be more effective in limiting the financial incentives to engage in within-office self-referral. Such policy options include the denial of payment for self-referred within-office service, reimbursement of self-referred imaging or physical therapy at a lower rate than that paid for referred diagnostic tests or physical therapy, or for bundling the payment for clinical lab tests, diagnostic imaging, or physical therapy as part of the reimbursement for an office visit.

Notes

1. Jean Mitchell and Elton Scott, New Evidence of the Prevalence and Scope of Physician Joint Ventures, 268 *JAMA*. 80, 84 (1992).
2. For more details on this debate, see John Iglehart, The Debate Over Physician Ownership of Health Care Facilities, 321 *N. Engl. J. Med.* 198, 204 (1989); Arnold Relman, Dealing with Conflicts of Interest, 313 *N. Engl. J. Med.* 749, 751 (1985); Arnold Relman, The Health Care Industry: Where Is It Taking Us? 325 *N. Engl. J. Med.* 854, 859 (1991).
3. Examples of articles in the media include Michael Waldholz and Walt Bogdanich, Doctor-Owned Labs Earn Lavish Profits in a Captive Market, *Wall Street Journal* A1 (March 1, 1989); Robert Pear and Erik Eckholm, When Healers Are Entrepreneurs: A Debate Over Costs and Ethics, *New York Times* A1, A16 (June 2, 1991). Examples of articles and commentaries in the medical literature include Relman, Dealing with Conflicts of Interest, *supra* note 2; E. Haavi Morreim, Conflicts of Interest: Profits and Problems in Physician Referrals, 262 *JAMA* 390, 394 (1989); Relman, The Health Care Industry, *supra* note 20. For a discussion of the debate among policymakers, see Iglehart, *supra* note 2.
4. A firm is said to have economies of scale if long-run average costs decline as output increases and diseconomies of scale if long-run average cost increase as output increases. Specialization and technological change factors enable producers to reduce long-run average costs by expanding the scale of operation. The concept of "economies of scope" is unique to multiple-output entities such as the hospital. This term refers to cost differences arising from joint production of outputs by the same firm rather than separate production specializing firms. Economies of scope are said to exist when the cost of joint production is less than the total costs of producing the same outputs separately.
5. Relman Dealing with Conflicts of Interest, *supra* note 2; Relman, The Health Care Industry, *supra* note 2.
6. James Todd and Janet Horan, Physician Referral—the AMA View, 262 *JAMA*. 395, 396 (1989).
7. Arnold Epstein, Colin Begg, and Barbara McNeil, The Use of Ambulatory Testing in Prepaid and Fee-for-Service Group Practices: Relation to Perceived Profitability, 314 *N. Engl. J. Med.* 1089, 1094 (1986).
8. Alan Hillman, Financial Incentives for Physicians in HMO's: Is There a Conflict of interest?, 322 *N. Engl. J. Med.* 1059, 1062 (1987).
9. Alan Hillman, Mark Pauly, and John Kerstein, How Do Financial Incentives Affect Physicians' Clinical Decisions and the Financial Performance of Health Maintenance Organizations?, 321 *N. Engl. J. Med.* 86, 92 (1989).
10. David Hemenway, Alice Killen, Suzanne Cashmen, Cindy Parks, and William Bicknell, Physician Responses to Financial Incentives: Evidence from a For-Profit Ambulatory Care Center, 322 *N. Engl. J. Med.* 1059, 1063 (1990).
11. Alfred Childs and E. Diane Hunter, Non-medical Factors Influencing Use of Diagnostic X-Ray by Physicians, 10(4) *Med. Care* 323, 335 (1972).

12. Bruce Hillman, *et. al.,* Frequency and Costs of Diagnostic Imaging in Office Practice: A Comparison of Self-Referring and Radiologist-Referring Physicians, 323 *N. Engl. J. Med.* 1604, 1608 (1990).

13. Bruce Hillman, *et. al.,* Physicians' Utilization and Charges for Outpatient Diagnostic Imaging in a Medicare Population, 268 *JAMA* 2050, 2054 (1992).

14. Stephen Shortell, Thomas Wickizer, and John Wheeler, *Hospital-Physician Joint Ventures* (1984).

15. U.S. Department of Health and Human Services, Office of the Inspector General, *Financial Arrangements Between Physicians and Health Care Businesses,* (May 1989).

16. Michael Zimmerman, *Referring Physicians' Ownership of Laboratories and Imaging Centers,* Testimony before the Health Subcommittee, Committee on Ways and Means, 101st Congress, 1st Session, May 1989.

17. American Medical Association. Physician Ownership of Health Care Facilities, in *Physician Marketplace Update* (1991).

18. Jean Mitchell and Elton Scott, *Joint ventures among health care providers in Florida: Volume II, Contract report for the Florida Health Care Cost Containment Board,* September 1991, State of Florida, Tallahassee, Florida.

19. For more details on the prevalence and scope of physician joint ventures see Jean Mitchell and Elton Scott, New Evidence of the Prevalence and Scope of Physician Joint Ventures, 268 *JAMA* 80, 84 (July 1992).

20. Jean Mitchell and Elton Scott, Evidence on Complex Structures of Physician Joint Ventures, 9 *Yale Journal of Regulation* 489, 520 (Summer 1992).

21. Jean Mitchell and Elton Scott, Physician Ownership of Physical Therapy Services: Effects on Charges, Utilization, Profits and Service Characteristics, 268 *JAMA* 2055, 2059 (1992).

22. Jean Mitchell and Jonathan Sunshine, Consequences of Physicians' Ownership of Health Care Facilities: Joint Ventures in Radiation Therapy, 327 *N. Engl. J. Med.* 1497, 1501 (1992).

23. Zachary Dyckman, *Joint Ventures Among Health Care Providers in Florida: Impact on MRI Services and Costs* (September 1991).

24. *See* note 18 *supra.*

25. Zachary Dyckman, *Impact of Physician Joint Venture Activity on Costs of Diagnostic Imaging Services in California* (February 1992).

26. Alex Swedlow et al., Increased Costs and Rates of Use in the California Workers' Compensation System as a Result of Self-Referral by Physicians, 327 *N. Engl. J. Med.* 1502, 1506 (1992).

27. Lewin-ICF, *Review of Joint Ventures Among Health Care Providers in Florida: Volume II,* (April 1992) (on file with author).

28. Jean Mitchell & Elton Scott, *Responses to Lewin-ICF Review of Joint Ventures Among Health Care Providers In Florida, Vol. II* (May 1992) (on file with author).

29. Janet Shikles, *Physicians Who Invest in Imaging Centers Refer More Patients for More Costly Services,* Testimony of the General Accounting Office before the Committee on Ways and Means, U.S. House of Representatives, April 1993.

30. John Iglehart, Congress Moves to Regulate Self-Referral and Physicians' Ownership of Clinical Laboratories, 322 *N. Engl. J. Med.* 1628, 1687 (1990).

Part III

THE PHARMACEUTICAL INDUSTRY'S INFLUENCE ON CLINCICAL PRACTICE AND RESEARCH

14

Conflicts of Interests in Relationships Between Physicians and the Pharmaceutical Industry

David S. Shimm, Roy G. Spece, Jr. and

Michelle Burpeau DiGregorio

Relations between physicians and pharmaceutical or medical device manufac-turers present many opportunities for conflicts of interest. Manufacturers employ physicians directly; they contract with physicians to perform the clinical testing required for drug or device approval by the Food and Drug Administration (FDA); they are regulated by bodies (like the FDA) directed in part by physi-cians; and they rely on practicing physicians to use or prescribe their products. Manufacturers can try to influence physicians by offering gifts, payment for con-sulting, honoraria for presentations, and subsidies or hospitality for physicians attending conferences; sponsoring continuing medical education; making direct payments to clinician–investigators for performing research; marketing products via advertisements and personal detailing; and lobbying regulators and legislators. They can also issue direct orders to their employed physicians. In this chapter, we will survey the major practices used by manufacturers to influence physician behavior and discuss how this introduces conflicts of interest into relationships among patients, physicians, the biomedical industry, and the public. We will use the manufacture of coagulation factor concentrates for hemophiliacs (espe-cially during the advent of the AIDS epidemic) as a case study that illustrates the pervasive influence of pharmaceutical companies. Finally, we will suggest reforms to be considered in response to these conflicts of interest.

The British Analogy

Dr. Joe Collier has strong views on pharmaceutical company influence on the British health care system:

> [I]n Britain the largesse of the pharmaceutical industry has resulted in a position where the information given by doctors about medicines is not necessarily reliable, not necessarily relevant, not necessarily clear and rarely complete, and where patients have their understanding artificially distorted by the intellectual atmosphere to which they are subjected.
>
> How has this come about? The position becomes clear when it is recognized that through its largesse the pharmaceutical industry determines the content and direction of the bulk of medical research and much postgraduate information and education, influences the publication and distribution of medical research data and attitudes of the opinion formers and undermines critics, curries favor with patients/public and finally has a special (favorable) relationship with government. This being so, the main requirements of informed consent, and so of patients rights, are undermined.[1]

Dr. Collier goes on to explain that the pharmaceutical industry (1) pays for 60 percent of Britain's medical research; (2) initiates most drug research; (3) determines the direction of much basic academic research and the terms of all early (and many late) clinical research protocols; (4) creates a climate in which it is difficult to undertake research that does not relate to or might even lessen the use of drugs; (5) spends a large part of its budget on producing papers, bulletins, books, slides, and videos to educate and promote its products to physicians; (6) funds physicians' attendance at symposia on industry products; (7) influences the content of so-called independent medical journals through its substantial outlays for advertising space; (8) "is selective about the data it chooses to make public, being secretive about selective aspects of its own research;" (9) forges links with prominent physicians who are "opinion formers," as well as members of medical advisory committees that counsel the government and concomitantly attempts to undermine the influence of potential critics; (10) provides the country with needed revenue from sales abroad; (11) promotes its role as a benefactor and works to ensure that doctors endorse its products by sponsoring charities, publishing leaflets and public health posters, facilitating campaigns, and advertising in national newspapers about its contributions to society; (12) constitutes the major funder of postgraduate medical education and funds a large majority of the prizes in medicine (particularly pharmacology and clinical pharmacology); and (13) advertises drugs, often in disregard of seldom enforced statutes that require ads to be clearly written, not misleading, and consistent with product licenses.[2]

We shall see that much of what Dr. Collier says about the pharmaceutical industry in Britain is applicable to the pharmaceutical industry in the United States.

Manufacturer Conduct and Sponsorship of Clinical Research

Collier notes that the British pharmaceutical industry pays for 60 percent of that country's medical research. In 1990, federal, state, and local governments and philanthropic organizations in the United States spent $12.4 billion on medical research.[3] The Pharmaceutical Manufacturer's Association reports that its members spent $6.4 billion on U.S.-based human drug research alone in the same period.[4] Although the U.S. pharmaceutical industry does not fund as large a proportion of our country's medical research, it is nevertheless a significant proportion that gives the industry corresponding power over the direction of research.

Although much of this budget is spent on the development of new drugs and devices that are synthesized and tested on animals in-house, a drug or device can be marketed in the United States only after undergoing extensive testing on humans. This requires large numbers of patients, and pharmaceutical manufacturers commonly contract with clinician-investigators in academic centers as well as in private practice to perform this testing. The precise percentage of the industry's total research budget devoted to "extramural" funding is not known. It has been reported, however, that "[i]ndustry support for biotechnology research, which perhaps is more likely than most research to be based in medical centers, is becoming quite substantial. For example, funds from industry account for 16% to 24% of all university-based research in biotechnology."[5] In any event, it is obvious that the pharmaceutical industry greatly influences the direction of research through the sheer magnitude of its expenditures, be they intra- or extramural.

To obtain a sufficient number of patient-subjects in an acceptable period of time, manufacturers offer clinician-investigators financial inducements to enter patients into studies, typically $2000 to $5000 per patient. By contrast, when a patient is entered into a National Institutes of Health–sponsored study, the clinician-investigator receives capitation of approximately $1000 per patient to cover the cost of the physician-investigator's time, the data manager's salary, and additional expenses (secretarial, photocopying, etc.) incurred in participating in the study.[6] These payments offer a mechanism to receive severalfold greater reimbursement for patient care than Medicare or third-party carriers will pay.

While institutional safeguards generally prevent the academic physician from personally appropriating the amount of capitation payment in excess of costs, these excess funds represent a source of money to pay for travel to meetings, books, computer equipment, or salaries for fellows. For academic investigators coping with a shrinking pool of peer-reviewed grant money to compete for, as well as an increasing number of competitors, these funds also offer a means to fund research that is unable to compete successfully for peer-reviewed grant funding.[7] There is always a conflict of interest between patient-subjects' interests and those of researchers, consisting of the researchers' desire to enroll a sufficient number of patients/subjects to meet the requirements of study protocols so that projects will be funded. Moreover, although NIH does not offer capitation payments as large as those supplied by pharmaceutical companies, its payment of substantial overhead expenses represents a benefit to the institution that will at least indirectly benefit the principal investigator. The larger capitation payments by pharmaceutical companies arguably make the financial conflict of interest greater. The availability of drug company funding, with its greater potential for excess payments, introduces another conflict of interest because it is an enticement for researchers to plan projects that are beneficial to pharmaceutical companies when alternative projects might be of more benefit to patients or society.[8]

The conflicts of interest presented by capitation payments share some qualities with those inherent in any fee-for-service situation but have some additional pernicious aspects. Where a purveyor of a service stands to receive more money for providing more services, there is an inherent conflict between the provider's interest in maximizing income and the client's interest in receiving no more services than are necessary. This is true whether the service is automobile repair or cardiovascular surgery. While provision of excess fee-for-service medical care is relevant to the debate on the cost of health care, the conflict of interest in this setting is one so familiar to patients that in many cases they would be on guard. (However, compare Hall's discussion of the dangers of unnecessary care in Chapter 10.) On the other hand, with the unique incentives of capitation payments to researchers (especially the large payments by drug companies), there is greater likelihood that patient/subjects may be taken advantage of.

With fee-for-service medicine, the patient is aware that his physician is being paid only by him and by his third-party carrier. This is important because the patient can be sure that his own motivations and those of the third party are similar; both are interested in the patient's receiving the most appropriate medical care at the lowest cost (although the relative importance of these two factors may be different for the patient and his insurance company). On the other hand, when the clinician-investigator is receiving capitation payments from a pharmaceutical manufacturer, there is a financial interest acting on the patient-subject's physician, and the patient-subject is ignorant of this interest. Moreover, this interest deviates from the primary concerns of the patient and his third-party payer.

The industry-funded research setting is also different from the fee-for-service situation in the sheer magnitude of the payments. While patients may not know exactly how much an office visit or a coronary artery bypass procedure costs, they do understand that the surgery is far more expensive than the office visit. What they do not understand, unless they are explicitly told, is that the capitation payment for entering a patient into a clinical study rivals the professional fee for a major surgical procedure.

Here the situation is one of hard conflict of interest, where the clinician-investigator's self-interest conflicts with that of the patient-subject. The clinician might enroll a patient into a study when no treatment or an alternative would be in the patient's best interest. Some commentators believe that the clinician-investigator's professionalism will prevent abuse of this situation. They also believe that patient-subjects are not really interested in knowing the funding details of a clinical study.[9] We find it more reasonable to handle this situation with two approaches.[10] First, the patient should be informed fully of the source, amount, and mechanism of the clinician-investigator's funding and of whether the clinician-investigator is a major stockholder, a corporate officer, or a paid consultant for the sponsoring corporation. The physician should also inform the patient that some reasonable persons believe that these arrangements might induce a physician to enroll a patient in a study. Second, to minimize investigator self-interest, capitation funds should not be administered by the investigator but rather by the institution. The institution would pay the direct and indirect costs of study participation (the data manager's salary, photocopying and telecommunication, costs, secretarial services, investigator's time—if unsalaried—etc.), and the excess would be placed in a pool for all members of the institution to compete for, instead of allowing the investigator or his department to reap the excess personally. (Brody argues in Chapter 18 that all excess payments should simply be eliminated.)

Manufacturer Sponsorship of Continuing Medical Education

Continuing medical education (CME) courses represent an important means for physicians to continue learning after completing their formal training, and often represent a requirement to retain hospital privileges and medical licensure. CME can be done on the cheap locally, with intramural speakers. However, the expenses and honoraria required for national or international authorities to participate can make CME a costly endeavor. Furthermore, with the participation of recognized authorities, CME activities can draw audiences nationally or even internationally, with correspondingly high travel, lodging, meal, and registration expenses for attendees. While CME has the laudable goal of educating physicians after they have completed training and are in the business of caring for patients, its expenses, and the need for funds to defray them, provide an opportunity for pharmaceutical manufacturers to influence prescribing behavior. Further, unlike gift giving or advertising, CME usually takes place under the aegis of a legitimate and supposedly neutral academic or professional institution or organization, so that physicians listening to presentations are much less likely to suspect bias in the information. CME programs also offer the pharmaceutical companies opportunities to forge ties with prominent physicians or opinion formers. (Recall Dr.

Collier's point about the British pharmaceutical industry's courting of "opinion formers.") They can hire these physicians to present programs, often at prime resorts, for substantial fees.

Evidence suggests that pharmaceutical manufacturer sponsorship does affect the content of CME. One study examined the content of two courses describing the use of calcium channel blocking agents, each sponsored by the manufacturer of a different agent.[11] Verbatim transcripts were reviewed to identify the number of times each of three calcium channel blockers (one made by the sponsor of one course, one made by the sponsor of the other course, and a third made by yet another manufacturer) was mentioned. In addition, the clinical effects (beneficial or adverse) attributed to each drug, and comparative or evaluative comments, were recorded. In one course, the drug made by the course sponsor was more likely to be mentioned (60 percent of total drug mentions, compared with 12 percent and 28 percent for the other two calcium channel blockers), while in the other course, drug mentions were fairly evenly distributed among the three calcium channel blockers. However, in both courses, the sponsor's drugs were more likely to be mentioned in connection with positive clinical effects, and less likely to be mentioned in connection with adverse clinical effects than the other two drugs. Since the two courses were judged by the author to cover the same topic and very similar drugs, she judged the differences in assessment of the three drugs to be biased as a result of the funding of the two courses.

Although this study suggests that the funding source biases CME, it did not examine whether this bias was reflected in attendees' prescribing patterns. This question was addressed in another study of three CME courses, chosen so that a single sponsor supported each course and so that the topic of the course was related to a single set of closely related drugs, with similar activities, toxicities, and costs.[12] Two of the courses concerned calcium channel blockers, and the third covered beta blockers. Attendees were surveyed before and six months after each course to determine their prescribing habits for the drugs discussed in each course. Although physicians increased their prescriptions of beta blockers and calcium channel blockers, respectively, after attending the courses, the greatest increases were seen in the two calcium channel blockers and the beta-blocker made by the course sponsors. These self-reported data indicate that a bias in content in favor of the sponsor's product might well be reflected in changes in physician prescribing practices.

Because of concerns reflected by these data, several organizations have formulated guidelines regulating CME.[13] The FDA issued a draft of its own guidelines, discussed at the Second Conference on Industry–CME Provider Collaboration in CME.[14] Although similar to the guidelines issued by the AMA and the Accreditation Council on CME, they reflected the FDA's concern about the intrusion of marketing into CME. The FDA was concerned that corporate sponsors covertly exerted nearly total control over CME course content. The draft guidelines required that the drug company have no overt or covert control over the scientific content of the program or the selection of the presenters. They required that the financial relationships between presenters and companies be disclosed. They specified that any data regarding drugs made by the sponsor, and those made by other manufacturers, be selected and presented objectively to reflect the entire body of valid evidence, including favorable and unfavorable information, as well as alternate therapies. Discussion of unapproved uses of drugs would be permitted, with appropriate scientific rigor.

Manufacturers' hostility to these mild guidelines seems to indicate that they do in fact regard the sponsorship of CME programs to be largely promotional rather than educational.[15] While there is nothing inherently evil in promoting one's product, to do so under the guise of an unbiased educational program raises questions of conflict of interest with regard to the manufacturers as well as the physicians who shill for them. The FDA's proposed guidelines represent a good approach to promoting scientific objectivity in industry-sponsored CME, and to making the line between informing and promoting more distinct.

Gifts to Physicians from Pharmaceutical Manufacturers

It is common for pharmaceutical and medical device manufacturers to give gifts to physicians, with an estimated value of approximately $165 million annually.[16] These can be of minor value, like pens or pads embossed with the name of a product, or they can be more substantial, although related to patient care, like textbooks or stethoscopes. Gifts can also include hospitality and other subsidies, ranging from sandwiches and pizza at grand rounds and other hospital conferences to lavish meals at professional conferences and air fare, room, and board to attend conferences located at resorts.[17]

Gift giving has some arguably defensible aspects: (1) it provides a means for pharmaceutical manufacturers to promote new products, and thereby to recoup research and development costs; (2) it helps new manufacturers enter the market (an important goal in trying to maintain competition and reduce prices); (3) certain gifts provide physicians with information on new products and technologies;[18] and (4) gifts that are related to patient care—but not necessarily to a specific product, like equipment or textbooks—may improve the recipient physician's practice of medicine. However, gift giving raises ethical issues.[19] First, gifts, hospitality, and subsidies can be costly and therefore can indirectly increase the cost of pharmaceuticals.[20] Second, gifts, especially if expensive, may be perceived as underhanded, essentially bribes to use the givers' products. This may undermine patients' faith in their physicians' integrity and may degrade the medical profession in the eyes of physicians themselves. Finally, although personal and marketplace interactions are not identical, giving and accepting gifts establishes a certain relationship with specific obligations in our culture. These last two issues raise questions of conflict of interest.

In our culture, as well as many others, offering a gift represents the offer of friendship, and rejecting a gift often implies rejection of that relationship. Conversely, accepting a gift carries tacit obligations, including gratitude and reciprocation.[21] For example, the physician may reciprocate by devoting more time to the representative's sales presentation than he would otherwise, or he might unconsciously (or even consciously) favor the use of that company's products. This contrasts with the physician's ethical responsibility to study each potentially useful drug, device, or treatment to the extent necessary to articulate intelligent choices based on the patient's best interests.

There is circumstantial evidence that industry gift giving may affect physicians' judgment. Internal medicine faculty and residents were surveyed at several hospitals in Wisconsin and Minnesota.[22] Seventy-seven percent of faculty and 85 percent of residents believed that receiving a gift would compromise a physician's judgment, and 24 percent of faculty and 15 percent of residents believed that judgment could be compromised by a gift as small as $5. This study only examined whether physicians thought that gift giving would influence their judgment rather than whether it really did affect their judgment. Since in this study physicians, rather than third parties, were opining about physicians' practice patterns, the conclusions are quite suggestive.

In another study, the opinions of the directors of all approved internal medicine residency training programs in the United States were surveyed regarding pharmaceutical company interaction with their house staff; 45 percent were "moderately concerned" or "very concerned" with the effect of pharmaceutical manufacturer representatives on residents' prescribing behavior.[23] These studies indicate that, at least in some academic centers, physicians have concern, though unproven, that pharmaceutical company gift giving may affect a physician's judgment. This concern is based on two potential consequences. The first is that if the public becomes aware of these gifts and perceives them as a problem, this could further erode public trust in the medical profession. A second apparent consequence appears to be physicians' self-concept, and the consequences this would have on physician morale and the self-policing practices of the profession.

Because of these issues, several organizations have formulated codes regulating the acceptance of gifts from manufacturers by physicians, and the Pharmaceutical Manufacturer's Association has adopted a Code of Pharmaceutical Marketing Practices.[24] These guidelines lack precision; a physician who wanted to behave ethically could have difficulty in determining what behavior was permissible, and a physician who wanted to behave unethically would have little difficulty in squaring practically any activity with these guidelines. Furthermore, all of these guidelines lack teeth. The guidelines issued by

the American College of Physicians and the AMA have no force other than persuasion. Nevertheless, the AMA guidelines have generated heated debate,[25]
many physicians indicating that they see no reason why they should not benefit
from drug company largesse.

The data compiled by the studies mentioned above and the resistance to the
AMA guidelines indicate that gifts to physicians from pharmaceutical manufacturers are a problem with potentially important effects on the practice of
medicine. It is helpful to analyze gift giving under the agency cost theory perspective described by Hall in Chapter 10. The patient is the principal, and the
physician is his agent. (Any third-party payer can also be conceived of as a
coprincipal and/or a coagent). The job of the agent is to purchase medical
devices and drugs that are effective and efficient. When physicians accept gifts,
they are essentially accepting bribes meant to influence them as agents to favor
the sellers' products over alternative products. There is generally no benefit in
this for the principal. Indeed, this is why most manufacturing businesses prohibit
their purchasing agents or employees from accepting "gifts."[26]

The agency cost theory perspective leads to the question: Should a practice
routinely condemned in the manufacturing sector be accepted in the medical
field? For example, should purchasing agents for hospital consortiums accept
gifts from sellers of products such as hospital beds? The answer is obviously
"no." Even more so, physicians should not accept gifts (except perhaps small
items such as book marks and cheap pens) from sellers of drugs and devices. The
sacrifice of such largesse is a small price for a profession to pay for self-respect
and public trust.

Advertisement and Promotion of Pharmaceutical Products

Like any other business, the pharmaceutical industry must sell its product to
make a profit, and it uses advertisement and other forms of promotion in order
to increase sales. Manufacturers are increasingly advertising directly to patients
in popular magazines such as *Newsweek*, and they have found that this has led
patients to often request (or at least inquire about) specific drugs from their
physicians.[27] Here, however, we will focus on advertising directed to physicians. If drug companies can influence or mislead physicians, it is obvious that
consumers are much easier targets.

Where advertisements seek to persuade physicians to use one manufacturer's
product instead of another manufacturer's comparable product, does this raise no
greater ethical issue than that created by General Motors trying to convince consumers to buy Chevrolets instead of Fords? When the information transmitted to
physicians via advertisement and other promotional activity is factually accurate
and helpful to physicians in their medical practices, advertisement and promotion

serve valuable functions. On the other hand, while pharmaceutical advertisements have not yet reached the level of beer advertisements featuring the "Swedish bikini team," some studies have indicated that the information featured in some advertisements stretches the facts and that, moreover, physicians sometimes rely on information in advertisements that is flatly contradicted by the scientific medical literature.

One study used expert reviewers to evaluate pharmaceutical advertisements in nine leading specialty journals and one leading general medical journal.[28] A total of 109 advertisements were reviewed by 113 physician reviewers and 54 clinical pharmacist reviewers; all but one advertisement was reviewed by 2 or, in a few cases, more reviewers. The featured products related to a wide variety of medical specialties, with the majority pertaining to infectious disease, cardiology, psychiatry, gastroenterology, and neurology. In 30 percent of the advertisements where a drug was claimed to be the "drug of choice" for a particular condition, at least two of the reviewers disagreed. In 40 percent of advertisements, at least two reviewers did not feel that there was a fair balance in the advertisements between efficacy, on the one hand, and side effects and contraindications, on the other. Two or more reviewers felt that 57 percent of the advertisements had little or no educational value; in fact, in 44 percent of the advertisements, two or more reviewers felt that the information could lead to improper prescribing.

Although this study indicates that pharmaceutical advertisements often play fast and loose with the data, it does not address the question of whether physicians rely more heavily on data from advertisements or from the scientific medical literature. One study that addressed this issue, albeit indirectly, involved a survey of twenty-nine primary care physicians at an HMO.[29] When asked to list the most frequently used general sources of information about drugs, twenty-four mentioned various scholarly sources and none mentioned drug industry–based sources. However, when these physicians were queried about their earliest sources of information about two specific drugs, at least half mentioned drug industry–based sources like advertisements or pharmaceutical service representatives. Although first-source information is not necessarily relied on, the study nevertheless suggests a problem.

Another study has addressed this issue more directly.[30] These investigators chose two types of drugs where advertising claims differed greatly from published data on efficacy. The ads were for peripheral and cerebral vasodilators, which were promoted for use in peripheral vascular insufficiency and senile dementia, respectively, despite evidence in the scientific medical literature that they were not useful for these conditions; and propoxyphene, which was promoted for use in moderately severe pain, despite evidence that it had no more analgesic efficacy than aspirin. The authors surveyed eighty-five randomly chosen physicians practicing in Boston for their attitudes regarding these two drugs.

Although 68 percent of the physicians stated that drug advertisements had a minimal effect on their prescribing patterns, and although an equivalently high proportion stated that they formed their opinions based on articles in medical journals, nearly one-third of the sample believed cerebral vasodilators useful in managing confused elderly patients, and nearly one-half believed propoxyphene to be more potent than aspirin. That such a high proportion of physicians' prescribing practices are congruent with advertisements, rather than with the scientific medical literature, indicates that physicians may not be doing a good job of sorting out fact from advertising claims.

Considering again the agency cost theory perspective, another way in which pharmaceutical advertisements differ from beer advertisements is that they are not aimed at the product's consumer but rather at the consumer's agent. In the case of an advertisement directed at the product's consumer, the consumer decides whether the benefits promised by the advertisement are congruent with his own interests; the beer drinker can decide for himself whether the participation of the Swedish bikini team in an advertisement renders a particular brand of beer more appealing. On the other hand, when the promotion is directed at the consumer's agent, conflict between the consumer's and the agent's interests can arise. For example, physicians who falsely pride themselves on being current with the most recent developments in drug therapy but in fact rely on advertisements could be manipulated into using a newer, and possibly more expensive and more toxic drug, even where the literature shows a more established medication to be less expensive, safer, and just as effective. This could occur if the advertisement stressed that its featured drug was the newest, most current treatment for the condition in question.

Although we have focused on published advertisements, we must say a few words about detailing. This is a complex and much studied area.[31] Detailing could provide a legitimate educational function, and it could provide a means for new companies and products to enter the market and foster competition. Given the above data concerning published advertisements, however, we are skeptical. We agree with one commentator who has advocated that Congress pass enabling legislation explicitly allowing the FDA to regulate detailing, and that the FDA adopt regulations, including a requirement that detailers provide a fair balance of information about products.[32] This commentator conveys the typical salesmanship tenor of detailing practices by quoting Merck's instructions to its detailers during its Indocin campaign: "Tell'em [doctors] again, and again, and again. Tell'em until they are sold and stay sold. . . . Take off the kid gloves. . . . Now every extra bottle of 100 Indocin you sell is worth an extra $2.80 in incentive payments. Go get it. Pile it in!!!"[33]

Although the evidence indicates that pharmaceutical advertisements often contain inaccurate information, and that this information influences physician behavior, does this represent any conflict of interest? We believe so. First, physicians deviate from their expected roles as trusted agents by unreasonably favoring their own time and convenience. They read ads or listen to detail representatives rather than study journals. Additional conflicts of interest lie with the pharmaceutical manufacturers who commission the advertisements, the prominent physicians who allow their names to be associated with the products, and the medical journals that publish the advertisements—a conflict between their corporate or personal interests, on the one hand, and the interests of health care consumers and the medical profession, on the other.

This assumes, of course, that pharmaceutical manufacturers and the journals that sell advertising space have higher obligations over and above their commercial relationships. Some would undoubtedly argue that it would be counterproductive to treat pharmaceutical companies differently from other businesses. These persons would argue that the duty of these companies is to their shareholders, and that the rigors of the marketplace will sufficiently protect consumers. Undue regulation will simply inflate the costs of drugs and devices and further exacerbate our health care crisis.

On the other hand, lobbyists for pharmaceutical companies are quick to argue for unique treatment of their industry when this means *exclusion* from rules that govern other enterprises. For example, pharmaceutical companies invariably contend that they should be exempt from products liability rules that govern other manufacturers. Although products liability law is extremely complex, it essentially allows consumers to collect damages caused by a product whenever there is a defect in the product, its design, or information provided to the consumer. Providers of services, on the other hand, can be held liable only if they were negligent, a concept explained in Chapter 3. Pharmaceutical manufacturers contend that they should only be subject to negligence rather than product liability rules because of the unique importance of their products.

We agree that their products are uniquely important, but we draw radically different conclusions from this observation. Pharmaceutical products and devices are so essential to consumers, consumers so rely on these products, and consumers are so uninformed about the utility and risks of these products that pharmaceutical companies should be subject to products liability rules. Moreover, we advocate that courts impose on them a fiduciary duty to consumers (which we explain below in the coagulation factor concentrates case study). Fiduciary duty is discussed, insofar as it applies to individual physicians, by Morreim in Chapter 11.

It can be argued that such a fiduciary duty would be unfair to investors in pharmaceutical companies and that it is unnecessary because, as already admitted, physicians are agents of patients. Physicians, not patients, purchase these products. And physicians, as "learned intermediaries," are knowledgeable and are independent of pharmaceutical companies. Our discussion here illustrates, however, that pharmaceutical companies have a pervasive influence on physicians, many of whom rely on ads and detail representatives for their prescribing information. Many HMOs and hospitals have found this influence so potent that they have implemented "counterdetailing" by their own representatives.[34] As to investors, they *choose* to invest in health care, and, in so doing, they assume obligations to consumers. Moreover, most pharmaceutical products depend for their development largely on the publicly or governmentally funded research and education complex. Having benefitted from these public resources, they must provide the quid pro quo of public responsibility. We wish to make explicit that our position is informed by the assumption that basic health care is *not* just another commodity. Rather, it is a necessity or "social good."

Rather than offering the quid pro quo of public responsibility, pharmaceutical companies have been criticized for exploiting the public by charging excessive prices. Some legislators have argued that price controls might be a remedy.[35] Although we will not explore that issue here, it is obvious that, if applied, product liability and fiduciary duty principles would encourage pharmaceutical companies to devote larger parts of their budgets to research to improve the safety of their products. This might leave less money available for promotional activities that create false demand with slanted claims and thus drive up costs.

Turning to the obligations of journals, while journal editors feel an obligation to ensure the veracity of the articles featured in their publications, their sense of obligation does not appear to extend to the advertisements that support them. They contend that they do not have the resources to review advertisements, that to do so would place journals in the position of appearing to endorse (or not) specific pharmaceuticals, and that the FDA already has statutory authority to regulate pharmaceutical advertising.[36] They also point out the importance of advertisements in holding down the price of journal subscriptions.[37] While these are legitimate sentiments, it troubles us that medical journals, with their strict peer review procedures for manuscripts that are widely held to ensure bias-free publication, are so deeply in the thrall of pharmaceutical manufacturers' support, and that their editors are so confident that he who pays the piper does *not* call the tune. As the editors state, it would be difficult for their journals to stay solvent without advertiser support. With this sort of leverage, it is difficult to imagine an editor standing up to an advertiser regarding the factual accuracy of an advertisement; one can even imagine subtle pressure being placed on an editor either to print data favorable to an advertiser's product or to suppress unfavorable data.

A number of solutions can be proposed, none ideal. It is easier to propose better or more accessible CME courses and journal articles or informative "drug fairs" than it is to carry these to fruition. One appealing, though costly, solution that should be explored is for the FDA (either on its own or through organized medicine) to institute a system of "pharmaceutical agents" similar to agricultural agents. These individuals would be available to physicians for consultation regarding the proper indications for drugs and devices, just as the county agricultural agent provides consultation to the farmer whose crops are infested by nematodes. Another solution is for journal editors to subject advertisements to the same rigorous peer review process applied to articles. This process is already in place with respect to articles, and it is feasible and advisable to extend it to ads.

Employing and Lobbying Physicians: Blood Products and Infectious Diseases as a Case Study

The Blood Products Industry: For- and Not-For- Profit Sectors

Conflicts of interest also ensnare physicians who regulate pharmaceutical companies or who are directly employed by companies. Consider the manufacture of coagulation factor concentrates. The blood industry is broken into two major sectors under our "National Blood Policy": the nonprofit or voluntary blood sector and the for-profit plasma sector.[38] The nonprofit sector obtains fresh blood from nonpaid donors and then distributes it in the form of red blood cells, platelets, fresh frozen plasma, and cryoprecipitate, with gross revenues exceeding $1 billion a year.[39] The for-profit sector collects plasma from fresh blood of paid donors, and it manufacturers and distributes products such as albumin, gamma globulin, and coagulation factor concentrates, with gross revenues exceeding those of the voluntary sector.

Treatments for Hemophiliacs Before the Advent of AIDS

This section focuses on the manufacture of coagulation factor concentrates used by hemophiliacs. A major event for hemophilia A patients was the development of factor VIII–rich cryoprecipitate in 1964, followed by fairly widespread production and use shortly thereafter.[40] Each dose of cryoprecipitate is prepared from fresh (frozen) plasma of one donor, and it was and is a product of the voluntary sector.[41] At about the same time, new methods of producing coagulation factor concentrates were being discovered and later developed.[42] Significantly, the process used to make factor concentrate in the United States involves pooling the clotting factors of thousands (2000 to 20,000 or more) of sellers of blood in large pools or "lots."[43] Therefore, each injection of a factor concentrate exposes a hemophiliac to thousands of sellers, ironically called "donors." The coagulation products manufactured by the commercial sector are reduced to powdered form. They can be stored at room temperature and prepared at home by mixing with water when needed for injection. While cryoprecipitate can be stored at home, this is less convenient because of its limited shelf life and the need for large refrigerator storage space.[44]

That these products posed the threat of transmission of various infectious diseases was known very early in their use. Indeed, the manufacturers distributed a warning—albeit insufficient—about the hepatitis risk.[45] It was also known many years before 1980 (and the recognition of AIDS) that the risk of transmitting hepatitis via coagulation factor concentrates could be reduced by (1) exclusion of male bi- and homosexuals and prisoners as donors because they had a high incidence of hepatitis B; (2) use of the hepatitis B core antibody test *as well as* the hepatitis surface antigen test;[46] (3) use of smaller pools or lots of donors, so that one infected person would taint a smaller quantity of product; and (4) use of a heat treatment process to reduce infectivity by destroying hepatitis viruses (or use of other viral inactivation methods).[47]

Why were these safety measures not employed? First, the production of the major factor concentrate—factor VIII—was controlled by four major pharmaceutical companies.[48] They were regulated by a division within the FDA, but they in fact exercised tremendous influence over the regulators. This group was, then, a cartel of quasi-competitors not too anxious to force each other to adopt costly safety measures but very anxious to present a united front to government regulators. Moreover, these manufacturers had been successful in convincing legislatures and courts to exempt them from products liability rules even when those rules would be applied in some respective jurisdictions to drugs and devices.[49] As pointed out earlier in this chapter, products liability rules generally allow consumers injured by products to recover damages if there are defects in the products, their design, or information provided to consumers. For example, failure to use the hepatitis B core antibody test and failure to adapt known heat treatment processes to the U.S. manufacturers' processes would have been considered defects. In the absence of exposure to products liability rules, however, the industry was singularly successful in defending against claims of negligence because it controlled the actual practices that courts usually relied on when determining the expected standard of care.[50]

The failure to exclude male bi- and homosexual and prisoner blood donors can also be attributed to politics and convenience. Their plasma was needed for production of hepatitis immune globulin, and excluding homosexuals from donating blood for factor products, but not for immune globulin, was judged too expensive and would have risked offending them. Similarly, prisoners were a stable, available, willing, and convenient source of supply that the manufacturers were loath to relinquish. (Interestingly, donors were excluded if determined to be IV drug abusers because of the high incidence of hepatitis B in that group.)[51]

To summarize, then, many years before the beginning of the AIDS epidemic in the early 1980s, hepatitis already posed a substantial safety threat to the users of coagulation factor concentrates. At least four methods of reducing this risk—

heating factor products, using smaller donor pools, excluding all groups of high-risk donors, and implementing the hepatitis B core antibody test—were not vigorously pursued because of financial and political considerations.

The Advent of AIDS and the Safety of Blood Products

The Connection Between AIDS and Blood Products, and Safety Measures to Reduce the Risks. AIDS blood-borne transmission was readily apparent by mid-1982. AIDS was first identified in 1981, predominantly among male bi- and homosexuals. Its incubation period and pattern of spread resembled those of hepatitis B, and it had been known since 1975 that male bi- and homosexuals (and prisoners) had a high incidence of hepatitis because of anal intercourse and the resulting exchange of blood and bodily fluids.[52] Another early identified high-risk group was IV drug abusers. Here too the passage of blood, this time through shared needles, was the source of infection.[53] Additional evidence was supplied when hemophiliacs (users of coagulation factor products) and recipients of whole blood transfusions began to develop AIDS. The epidemiological pattern among transfused patients—as among male bi- and homosexuals—resembled that of hepatitis B transmission. By January 1983 there were almost 1000 persons with AIDS in the United States, 75 percent of whom were male bi- or homosexuals and 40 percent of whom had already died.[54]

Initially, manufacturers claimed to be uncertain that AIDS was a blood-borne disease.[55] However, in August 1982 the FDA requested that the manufacturers not use plasma collected at centers with a high male homosexual donor base to make coagulation factor products.[56] At the end of 1982 and the beginning of 1983, the four major manufacturers met and agreed among themselves to form a consensus strategy concerning whether, when, and how to screen donors in high-risk groups, issue warnings to physicians and patients, and use surrogate tests such as the hepatitis B core antibody test.[57]

A crucial meeting was held on January 4, 1983, in Atlanta, Georgia, the headquarters of the Centers for Disease Control (CDC), including thirty to forty representatives from the for-profit and nonprofit sectors (including each of the four manufacturers of coagulation factor products), the National Gay Task Force, and other groups.[58] The CDC is the government agency primarily responsible for dealing with epidemics. Its infectious disease experts, particularly Dr. Don Francis, were the most knowledgeable persons concerning the appropriate response to AIDS.[59] However, they had to "sell" their position to physicians—primarily hematologists—who treated hemophiliacs, as well as to gay activists, politicians, and entrepreneurs in the for-profit and non-profit sectors.[60]

Tracing donors of the eight hemophiliacs and five blood transfusion recipients who were known to have contracted AIDS, in each case CDC investigators found a male bi- or homosexual donor. CDC scientists studied thousands of blood samples from homosexuals who had AIDS, who had swollen lymph glands, and who had not exhibited any symptoms of AIDS whatsoever.[61] Almost 90 percent of the first two groups had the hepatitis B core antibody and 80 percent of the latter group had the antibody, while only 5 percent of the general population had it. They concluded that approximately 90 percent of the carriers of AIDS could be excluded from blood donations by using the hepatitis B core antibody test, which they were convinced could be immediately implemented using the same equipment, processes, and facilities already in use with the hepatitis surface antigen test.[62]

Dr. Francis was adamant about the need to exclude homosexuals from the donor pool and to implement the hepatitis B core antibody test (or a similar "surrogate test"). He indicated to the assembled group at the January 4, 1983, meeting that they would be guilty of negligent homicide if they did not take immediate precautions.[63]

In a January 6, 1983 memorandum to Dr. Jeff Koplan of the Public Health Service, who had chaired the January 4 meeting, Francis urged that the CDC promulgate the following recommendations, with or without the FDA's concurrence: (1) use cryoprecipitate or coagulation factor concentrates made with small pools of donors, at least until the other measures were implemented; (2) implement the hepatitis B core antibody test; (3) exclude active homosexuals and other high-risk donors (and those who had had sex with any of the same); and (4) spend an additional $10 million on epidemiological, etiological and clinical studies of AIDS.[64] Dr. Francis concluded his memorandum: "I understand that these recommendations will be controversial and that there will be objections by industry and blood bankers. I think we should get comments from these groups and should keep them informed of our to-be-published recommendations. However, to wait for their approval of our recommendations will only endanger the public's health."[65]

Hemophilia specialist Dr. Oscar Ratnoff announced at the January 4, 1983, meeting that he had already recommended that his patients use cryoprecipitate instead of coagulation factor concentrates because of the risk of AIDS.[66] At the same meeting, representatives of Alpha Therapeutics Corporation, one of the four major manufacturers of coagulation factor concentrates, reported that they had just begun a program to identify and screen male homosexual donors through verbal and written questioning.[67] The other manufacturers implemented various verbal and written screening programs within months, but many experts considered them amateurish and ineffective. For example, answers to sensitive questions about AIDS symptoms and sexual behavior were asked or collected in much less than private settings, often by clerical personnel.[68]

The manufacturers initially did not implement the hepatitis B core test, move to small pool production, or warn physicians and patients about the AIDS risk to physicians and patients, arguing that the government never required small pool production, a warning, or use of a surrogate test.[69] However, the government response was mediated in part by the manufacturers. For example, according to an internal memorandum of the largest manufacturer (the Cutter Biological Division of Miles, Inc.), Dennis Donohue, the head of the FDA division primarily responsible for regulation of coagulation factor products, "requested that we send him some official notification of our plans so that he could use this as ammunition that voluntary efforts of the industry precluded the need for any further regulation or activities in the FDA compliance area" (December 1982).[70] Another of Cutter's memos states: "A series of meetings will be held in Europe to review the screening process in the U.S., and Donahue [sic] stated that his mission was to defend our current procedures. He asked assistance from the manufacturers to convince those overseas that we are doing an acceptable job of screening out any AIDS donors" (June 1983).[71] Also in early 1983, an internal Cutter memo stated that the manufacturers had agreed to deflect issues from the CDC (Dr. Francis' organization) to the FDA (Dr. Donohue's organization).[72]

The Failure to Warn Physicians and Patients About the Danger and Efforts to Trivialize the Danger. The manufacturers avoided a warning about the dangers of AIDS until December 1983.[73] Yet, in December 1982, one of Cutter's in-house counsel, Mr. Ed Cutter, wrote: "It is advisable for us to send a warning to both physicians and to patients."[74] A December 1982 draft *Morbidity and Mortality Weekly Report*, published by the CDC, contained such a warning to physicians, but it was deleted.[75]

In March 1983, Dr. Bruce Evatt of the CDC made a presentation to a meeting attended by representatives of the manufacturers. He stated that according to the latest epidemiological data, approximately half of the nation's hemophiliacs would develop AIDS because of their use of coagulation factor concentrates, no matter what was done at this point.[76] Nevertheless, the manufacturers still did not issue a warning, use a small lot process, or implement the hepatitis B core antibody test. In fact, they took steps to convince physicians, patients, and the public that, if there was a risk, it was exceedingly small. At least one employee of Cutter cited a figure of 1 in a million risk from a single-unit blood transfusion, a figure he attributed to a prominent hemophilia specialist and member of the board of the National Hemophilia Foundation (NHF), speaking at the National Hemophilia Meeting in Memphis, Tennessee, in October 1983. He claimed she "indicated that the potential for harm faced by an individual engaged in bike riding was one in fifty, while the potential risk the individual faced of contracting AIDS from a blood transfusion was one in a million."[77] Indeed, in a November 1983 press release issued by Cutter when it recalled lots of factor products known to contain plasma from a suspected AIDS victim, the company stated that any risk was "exceedingly remote."[78] By early 1983, Cutter had hired a prominent public relations firm (Hill and Knowlton) to advise it on how to communicate with donors and the public.[79] Cutter's in-house staff did market surveys and teleconferences with physicians and patients to discover why many of them were using less factor concentrate or switching to cryoprecipitate.[80] This was a prelude to a campaign to encourage continued use of the products.

In addition, Cutter sponsored a seminar in Stockholm, Sweden, on the safety of coagulation factor concentrates from June 27 to July 1, 1983. It arranged presentations by prominent hemophilia specialists, including the medical director and another official of the NHF.[81] This seminar resulted in a publication—the *Cutter Forum*—distributed to hemophilia specialists throughout the United States. Selected quotes give the flavor of the publication's message:

> Frightened by the heavy media coverage of AIDS, many hemophilic patients are apparently cutting down on their treatments—sometimes with serious results. . . . Another MD added, "With the anxiety our fellow physicians are causing patients, we're going to see more fear of AIDS than actual cases of AIDS." . . .
>
> A physician who has dealt with AIDS directly also doubted the validity of T-cell tests. . . . I think, too, if one looks at people who have common colds, he will see a lot of reversal in the T-4 and T-8.[82]

The message of the *Cutter Forum* seemed to be: The media has created false fear about AIDS; there is no reason to use inconvenient and sometimes hard to obtain cryoprecipitate; the benefits of factor concentrates vastly outweigh their risks; altered T-cell counts do not really indicate an AIDS problem; and patients should be reassured rather than warned.

The Conspiracy to Delay the Hepatitis B Core Antibody Test. Perhaps the most cynical of the missteps taken by the manufacturers concerned the hepatitis B core antibody test. Just before a meeting with FDA officials in late 1983, the manufacturers got together and forged a consensus strategy—essentially the same strategy they had agreed on a year earlier. In the words of an internal Cutter memorandum:

> Donohue recommended that Anti-core Hepatitis B testing be incorporated for routine plasma screening (in addition to current requirements) since it would identify 90 percent of all potentially infectious (or high risk) donors. The Anti-core testing would add a further measure of confidence in product safety at a relatively low cost for the products involved. . . . Mike Rodell of Armour [one of the four large manufacturers] proposed a Task Force to deliberate the details of the recommendation and provide further information in 3 months. This proposal was one that had been agreed upon by all the fractionators the previous evening. The general thrust of the task force is to provide a

delaying tactic for the implementation of further testing. It was generally agreed that core testing would eventually become a requirement . . . . The fractionators met with Donohue following the meeting and, although Donohue was not completely satisfied with the task force approach, he agreed to it. Rodell was named chairman of the Task Force and a meeting will be scheduled in January. John Hink, in a prescient move, has already begun core testing at Cutter centers. We recommend that the implementation of core testing be accelerated to the maximum degree possible to obtain a competitive advantage in the market place. The approval of our heat-treat submission, in conjunction with core-screened plasma, could present us with a potent marketing advantage. We made no mention of our plans to others.[83]

Summary. To summarize, the manufacturers were conspiring to further delay the hepatitis B core antibody testing, which could have been implemented to reduce the risk of hepatitis years before the advent of AIDS. Cutter, however, stabbed its coconspirators in the back by not telling them that it had already begun core testing and would accelerate it. The company was, in effect, encouraging its competitors to continue marketing an unsafe product so that it could gain a market advantage. The outcome of the task force was equally astounding. About a year later, the task force recommended that hepatitis B core testing not be implemented, for one, because "The incidence of AIDS has declined markedly in the last 6 months. This appears to herald a containment of the AIDS epidemic."[84] During this time, a Cutter in-house doctor's standard response to concerned physicians, patients, and family members who communicated with the company was: The risks are not known, but *everything possible* has been and will be done in cooperation with others to deal with this crisis.[85] Dr. Thomas Drees, chief executive officer of Alpha Therapeutics (one of the four manufacturers of coagulation factor products) from 1978 to November 1983, had direct access to the thinking of the manufacturers. He states in a December 15, 1988, affidavit submitted in the case of *Doe v. Cutter Biological:*

> To a very large degree, the safety standards in the fractionator industry are influenced by the ABRA [American Blood Resources Association] of which all fractionators were members from 1980 to 1985. . . .
>
> I was severely criticized by my competitors for taking the immediate actions that I did [in December 1982] regarding screening for high risk donors. Further, my superiors at Alpha were highly critical of my actions. It is my firm belief that the actions I took in late 1982 in good conscience to protect the public from the AIDS virus were in large part the reason for my being terminated from Alpha as its CEO in November 1983.
>
> Although I was not aware of the goings on at various meetings that were attended by my subordinates of the BPAC [Blood Products Advisory Committee], NIH, CDC, ABRA, NHF and AABB [American Association of

Blood Banks], specifically Penny Carr, our regulatory representative, it is now apparent to me after reviewing the documents in this case that there was a "conspiracy" at work among the various fractionators to avoid using the surrogate test known as the HB Core Antibody Test. . . .

Had I been properly advised by my medical advisors at Alpha regarding the correlations between HB [hepatitis B] and Non A Non B [hepatitis], I would have implemented the HB Core Antibody Test at the same time I began using the screening for high risk groups at our donor centers (December 26, 1982). . . .

It is now clear to me that the HB Core Test should have been used from the time it became available through Abbott Laboratories in 1975. If it had been used from 1975, countless deaths from HB and Non A, Non B, would have been avoided. Further, . . . thousands of . . . hemophiliacs would not have AIDS today, as this disease would have never been allowed into the blood supply in any great degree.

The fact that there was such resistance to the use of the HB Anti Core Test by the blood industry, and the blood industries [sic] resistance to take the most obvious and needed precautions to the AIDS epidemic convinces me that there was a concerted effort by the influential leaders of the blood industry to save dollars at the expense of lives, even when it was clear beyond any doubt that there was widespread contamination of the blood supply in November, 1982.[86]

Focusing on Conflicts of Interest in the AIDS Crisis. Here let us examine the conflicts of interest in our case study. Focusing first on the pharmaceutical manufacturers, they have conflicting duties to their shareholders and customers (i.e., physicians and patients). Physicians who work for manufacturers or bodies that regulate them become entwined in these conflicts. Ideally, manufacturers serve the financial interests of shareholders by producing and distributing the best products and information, while regulators simply fine-tune the process in the public interest.

The real falls short of the ideal in several ways. Patients are generally uninformed about pharmaceutical products, so their choices do not necessarily direct manufacturers to favor the best mixture of safety, effectiveness, and cost. Although physicians should inform patients about the safety, effectiveness, and costs of alternative therapies, they rely strongly on the information supplied by the pharmaceutical companies. The companies have superior information, especially about risks, from their ongoing research and collection of data regarding the national and international use of their products.[87] They are not anxious to share information because it might be proprietary or might discourage the use of their products. Moreover, physicians do not necessarily pass relevant information on to patients. They often fail to take the time necessary to attempt a reasonable exchange of information.[88]

This "market failure," in which consumers and often their physicians do not have sufficient information to make intelligent choices, is manifest in our case study. The manufacturers were privy to unpublished data provided by the CDC in early January 1983. The biggest manufacturer was urged by one of its own counsel to provide a warning even before if obtained formal access to these data. Yet a warning was not given until December 1983. At the same time, physicians were being advised to downplay any risk.[89]

That patients are not necessarily protected by reliance on their physicians is also shown by our case study. The coagulation factor concentrate manufacturers exercised influence over prominent hemophilia specialists, including members of the leadership of the NHF.[90] Approximately 80 percent of all severe hemophiliacs alive in the early 1980s contracted the AIDS virus from coagulation factor concentrates.[91] When patients or their survivors began to sue because of the tainted products, specialists associated with the NHF testified for the defendant manufacturers.[92] This was a conflict of interest and was inappropriate for several reasons. First, the purpose of the NHF is to advance the interests of hemophiliacs. When hemophiliacs went to court to press alleged grievances, the NHF should have at least remained neutral. Instead, some of its leaders testified for the defendants, whose attorneys were able to argue: "Our experts are affiliated with the NHF, the body responsible for defending hemophiliacs."[93] This scandal went on for years, until in December 1992 the NHF belatedly prohibited NHF-affiliated physicians from testifying against hemophiliacs in a manner that would imply NHF endorsement.[94]

Testifying against the group of patients one is responsible for treating was inappropriate, moreover, because prominent hemophilia specialists at certain major medical centers had a vested interest in minimizing any alleged negligence, since they were involved in prescribing coagulation factor concentrates for their patients. They themselves therefore faced possible liability. Even more apparent, these few prominent physicians had a psychological investment in denying that they failed to heed warnings given by epidemiological experts like Dr. Francis.

Having focused on the conflicts of interest of the coagulation factor concentrate manufacturers and hemophilia specialists, let us examine the physicians responsible for regulating the manufacturers and those who worked for them. The Division of Blood and Blood Products within the Bureau for Biologics of the FDA—directed by Dr. Dennis Donohue—was most directly involved in regulating the coagulation factor concentrate manufacturers. Its job is to ensure that products are safe and effective, and to encourage dissemination of accurate information to physicians and consumers.[95] FDA personnel, however, are often subject to conflicting interests. The highest officials are political appointees and must support administration policies or face removal. Politicians with the power of removal are often subject to the lobbying efforts of the manufacturers. The political philosophy implicitly embraced by most citizens is one that requires politicians to act in the public interest.[96] Given the pluralistic interest group philosophy that actually reigns, however, politicians often attempt to influence regulatory officials within the FDA and elsewhere to "go light" on their constituents (i.e., campaign contributors).[97]

In addition, some fear that 1992 federal user-fee legislation will further entangle the FDA in conflicts of interest.[98] This legislation provides for implementation of a program that will be phased in over five years. The FDA will charge $60,000 annually ($138,000 in the fifth year) to each facility that manufactures prescription drugs, as well as $6000 annually ($14,000 in the fifth year) for each of its prescription products. In addition, one-time fees for new drug applications that include human clinical data will start at $100,000 and rise to $233,000 by the fifth year. The program is expected to raise $300 million over five years, which will be used to increase staff and speed up decisions on new drug applications.[99] Supporters tout the program as a way to get better products to consumers more quickly, with little cost to taxpayers.[100] However, others fear that the program will, at least subtly, influence FDA personnel to be more solicitous of drug company interests. The argument is that persons are naturally disinclined to bite the hand that feeds them, and that industry will be perceived as the FDA's benefactor, to be treated with kindness and concern rather than firmness and skepticism.[101]

In addition, FDA personnel are subject to less tangible influences. The tendency of regulatory bodies to become captured by their regulatees is recognized by most scholars.[102] One of the principal means by which this takes place is regulators' contemplation of lucrative or secure employment with regulatees. Professional reputation is, moreover, forged in the field where one does one's daily business. If one is a regulator, one's primary field of interaction is among regulatees. One can earn a good reputation by being thought of favorably by regulatees. Thus, there are strong financial and emotional interests that potentially conflict with the regulator's responsibilities. These influences might help explain the conduct attributed to Dr. Donohue by the internal Cutter memos.

Physicians who work in the pharmaceutical industry are subject to even greater conflicts than physicians working in regulatory bodies. They have obligations to shareholders, the public, and their employers. If they feel that an action is detrimental to shareholders or the public, they are not necessarily able to convey this to anyone other than their employers. To do otherwise might compromise proprietary information and make them personally liable to their companies. At the very least, it might lead to unpopularity, reprimand, or dismissal.

On the other hand, at a certain point—as noted in Chapter 3—physicians' duties to the public outweigh duties to specific third parties or even patients. At the very least, for example, no physician should have ensured inquirers that Cutter was doing and would do everything possible to cooperate with others to minimize the risk of its product if he had any clue about what was actually happening. Moreover, all physicians should demand to know what is actually happening if they are assigned the task of communicating with third parties or the public on the subject of product safety and efficacy.

Remedies. What might be done to ameliorate the conflicts of interest described above? We propose the following reforms. First, the AMA should form committees (with representatives from industry and consumer groups) to promulgate codes of ethics for physicians who work for, consult or testify for, and regulate pharmaceutical, blood product (or other biologicals), and medical device manufacturers (a primary element of which must be a paramount concern for consumer safety and well being). Second, for-profit and nonprofit drug, biological, and device manufacturers should be subject to products liability rules that require them to adopt, and inform the public about, all feasible safety measures. Third, antitrust laws should be developed to make clear that the answer is unequivocally "yes" to a question whose answer is now probably "yes": Is it a violation of the antitrust laws to impede competition in regard to efficacy and safety as well as to the price of products?[103] Such a change would make the above-described agreement among the coagulation factor concentrate manufacturers concerning delay of the hepatitis B core antibody test a clear violation of the antitrust laws. As the law now stands, it was certainly immoral and tortious but only probably a violation of the antitrust laws. Fourth, for-profit and nonprofit drug, biological, and device manufacturers should be held to owe a duty of utmost good faith and concern ("fiduciary duty") for consumers' safety and well-being. Fifth, additional laws should be passed that encourage whistle blowing and protect whistle blowers. We will add a few words about proposals four and five. First, as to fiduciary duty, Morreim briefly discusses the concept in Chapter 11, and Rodwin argues in Chapter 9 that "conflict of interest," as a legal term, requires the existence of a fiduciary duty. We also offered a general definition of fiduciary duty in Chapter 1 and explained in Chapter 3 that the California Supreme Court reasoned that the physician in the *Moore* case had breached a fiduciary duty by failing to inform his patient that he had a conflict of interest consisting of an intent to use the patient's tissue to develop a commercial product. But what is a fiduciary duty? From the moral perspective, most authorities characterize the physician–patient relationship as a fiduciary one. This is because physicians (1) have special knowledge (2) that is relatively inaccessible to patients (3) who are usually in desperate need of help and (4) therefore have little choice but to rely on their physicians.[104]

From the legal perspective, there is a split of authority concerning whether the physician–patient relationship is a fiduciary one.[105] In the eyes of the law, the paradigm of a fiduciary relationship is that between a guardian and an incompetent ward. Here there is abject dependency by the incompetent, and the very purpose of the guardian is to act in utmost good faith, eschewing self-interest and acting for the exclusive benefit of the ward.[106] The authorities that refuse to characterize the physician–patient relationship as a fiduciary one argue that patients are not the equivalent of incompetent wards.[107] Some argue that the relationship is a quasi-fiduciary one because of the incomplete analogy between wards and patients.[108] Our position is that the analogy is close enough to combine with obligations rightfully placed on physicians because of their special benefits and status provided by society to justify requiring them to act in utmost good faith, eschewing undue self-interest and presumably acting for the exclusive benefit of their patients (the presumption being overridden when, as described in Chapter 3, invocation of the good citizen model allows or requires physician action to protect third persons or society).

We do not propose that physicians in pharmaceutical companies have fiduciary duties to patient-consumers. They may not have sufficient opportunity or power to direct company policy. We propose, however, that the *companies* be deemed to have a fiduciary duty to patients-consumers.

It will undoubtedly be argued that no such duty is appropriate because physicians, as "learned intermediaries,"[109] protect patients from the companies; the incentives of the market and negligence law are adequate to encourage product efficiency, responsible cost, and safety; and it is nonsensical to speak of corporate entities having fiduciary duties. We have already explained, however, that pharmaceutical companies have more knowledge about their products than physicians do; that the companies influence physicians through multiple methods; that physicians often do not adequately share the information they possess; and that government regulation is not adequate. Moreover, the corporate structure is amenable to imposition of moral and legal duties and, indeed, can be adequately bridled only by imposition of such duties. Corporations have complex decision-making structures, so a harmful decision can emerge because of the structure itself. It might be virtually impossible to identify the person(s) responsible for a decision. In this sense, the corporation has a mind of its own. It is sensible to recognize this capacity and bridle it with moral recognition and control.[110]

Negligence law requires plaintiffs to demonstrate, by a preponderance of evidence, that unreasonable decisions were taken and that these decisions caused their harm. In theory, a plaintiff could show that a corporation was negligent in developing its decision-making processes. This is, however, a massive undertaking and is not within the capacity or resources of the vast majority of plaintiffs. What is needed, therefore, are mechanisms to encourage corporations to be self-conscious about and to police their decision structures. The imposition of a fiduciary duty to consumer-patients is precisely such an incentive. Much work remains to be done to fill out this and similar concepts. The new federal criminal sentencing guidelines, for example, allow sanctions to be applied to corporations

when they fail to carry out quality assurance or moral audits of their decision-making processes.[111] Others have called for members of the public to sit
on boards of directors and moral audits by external bodies.[112] These and other
mechanisms must be studied and perfected so that we can prevent mass
tragedies such as the hemophiliac/AIDS crisis.

Although direct imposition of fiduciary duties on company physicians is not
appropriate, we do propose greater incentives to encourage whistle blowing by
these physicians, including stronger protections for them when they do so.
Consider what would have been the rights and obligations of a physician
employee of the coagulation factor concentrate manufacturers, who, in January
1983, totally agreed with Dr. Don Francis and other CDC epidemiologists about
the danger of AIDS in blood products. We have noted that Cutter in-house attorney Ed Cutter advocated warning physicians and patients in December 1982.
The American Bar Association's Model Rules of Professional Conduct bind
lawyers (when acting as lawyers) to keep confidential any internal information
about risks and responses thereto, with the following exception: "A lawyer may
reveal such information to the extent the lawyer believes necessary . . . to prevent the client from committing a criminal act that the lawyer believes is likely
to result in death or bodily harm."[113]

There is an apparent consensus that this *permissive* policy of disclosure
becomes obligatory when "it appears beyond a reasonable doubt that the client
has formed a firm intention to inflict serious personal injuries on an unknowing
third person."[114] It is probable that attorney Cutter could have gone public, without risk of liability or discipline, in reliance on the position advanced by the CDC
epidemiologists such as Dr. Francis that thousands would die if their warnings
were not heeded. He reasonably *might* have concluded that there was knowing,
and thus criminal, endangerment of hemophiliacs.

On the other hand, he could probably have defended himself successfully
against the charge that he had an affirmative obligation to blow the whistle. He
could have argued that it was not evident *beyond a reasonable doubt* that his
client, Cutter, or one of the other manufacturers (1) was about to commit a criminal act and (2) this would inflict serious bodily harm. After all, months after
attorney Cutter's advice regarding issuing a warning, a prominent hemophilia
specialist allegedly stated that the risk of developing AIDs from a single-unit
blood transfusion was 1 in a million—hardly beyond a reasonable doubt (even
though use of coagulation factor products—especially heavy use—posed greater
risks than individual transfusions because of the large pool manufacturing process). In any event, even Dr. Francis had characterized the risk from blood and
blood products as a "reasonable medical certainty" rather than beyond a reasonable doubt.[115] Generally, an attorney cannot be expected to resolve such apparent disputes between experts.

But what about company physicians, if any, who had all the information available to attorney Cutter, as well as that presented by the CDC at the January 4, 1983, meeting? Confidentiality and the duty to warn intended victims were discussed in Chapter 3. There, however, the duty of confidentiality was discussed in the context of the physician–patient privilege. The justification there is that confidentiality encourages full disclosure by patients and resulting optimum care by physicians. Similar reasoning grounds the attorney–client privilege applicable to in-house counsel. However, the only source of a duty of confidentiality by in-house physicians who worked for coagulation factor concentrate manufacturers is that arising from the principal–agent or employer–employee relationship. That duty has never been considered as weighty as duties arising from professional–patient or professional–client relationships. The courts have not been uniform in ruling when a mere agent must or can blow the whistle. Suffice it to say that employees can be personally liable for certain misrepresentations (even nondisclosures) made on behalf of their employers,[116] and that some authorities have protected from retaliation employees who have blown the whistle on unethical, albeit not illegal, conduct.[117]

We suggest the following reforms in this area: (1) the legal profession should reexamine its position with respect to permissive and obligatory disclosures, with the intent to give more weight to the interests of large groups—such as hemophiliacs—who might be placed at substantial physical risk; (2) the medical profession and our civil liability system must *require* physicians to go public whenever there is a clinically significant risk of serious bodily injury to one or more persons; and (3) the medical profession and our civil liability system must protect from discipline, liability, or retaliation physicians who go public because of a significant risk of bodily injury to one or more patients/consumers. Consistent with our position in Chapter 3, the risk at issue need not be imminent if its magnitude and probability are sufficiently severe to reasonably require or allow a response. Particular attention should be paid to the risks of infectious diseases because they exhibit a "multiplier effect" whereby each new victim can generate several others.

None of the above remedies will be effective without sufficient education of physicians regarding their rights and duties in this complex field. Here is an area where physicians can profitably borrow from lawyers. Law schools and bar associations now require courses and examinations on professional responsibilities and ethics in which students and lawyers tackle problems similar to those discussed in the last several pages. Medical schools and boards of medical examiners should do the same.

Moving back to a broader perspective on the entire blood industry, as pointed out above, the United States is one of the few developed countries that allow the sale of blood.[118] The World Health Organization has adopted the goal of eradicating the sale of blood and its components throughout the world. The reasoning against the sale of blood is that it leads to poor, desperate, and probably less healthy and more infectious donors.[119] The contention is that there is an inherent industry conflict of interest between the goal of profit, on the one hand, and maximum safety of patients, on the other hand.

As also pointed out above, the United States has reached a compromise position that divides the blood industry into for-profit and nonprofit sectors. It is interesting to mention in passing, therefore, that the nonprofit sector was, in some respects, more culpable than the for-profit sector during the early days of the AIDS epidemic. The criticism of the for-profit sector may disguise very similar conflicts of interest in the nonprofit sector. This error has been well documented in comparisons between for-profit and nonprofit hospitals.[120] The authorities have demonstrated that nonprofit entities behave much the same way as for-profit entities in the cutthroat competition of the marketplace.[121]

The largest organization in the nonprofit sector is the Red Cross.[122] It is tax exempt, presumably because it offers society the quid pro quo of special attention to public safety and welfare. The Red Cross and other entities in the nonprofit sector refused to implement questioning and mandatory exclusion of homosexual donors early in 1983, when the coagulation factor concentrate manufacturers did so because the entire blood industry was warned that male homosexuals were a high-risk group for carrying AIDS.[123] The Red Cross issued joint statements with the American Association of Blood Banks and the Council of Community Blood Centers suggesting that the risk of transmission of AIDS through blood transfusion was minuscule—on the order of 1 in 1 million.[124] It repeated this statement in 1984, even after it became privy to the results of preliminary tests of donors for antibodies to the AIDS virus. This testing was done with kits for testing AIDS antibodies obtained before such kits were licensed for universal use, and it demonstrated that the 1 in 1 million risk figure was grossly understated.[125]

Moreover, although the Red Cross minimized the risk of AIDS transmission in blood, it urged its affiliates throughout the country to prepare to produce large quantities of cryoprecipitate in case physicians and patients switched from coagulation factors products because of the AIDS risk.[126] It did not minimize the risk of AIDS when it spoke of marketing cryoprecipitate. Instead, it reasoned that cryoprecipitate would be safer, since it was prepared from the blood of only one or a few donors. This obviously reduced the risk of being exposed to high-risk donors inherent in coagulation products manufactured using pools of blood from thousands of donors. Yet, while recognizing the greater risk inherent in coagulation factor concentrates, the Red Cross cooperated with the for-profit sector to prepare and sell those concentrates using plasma donated to the Red Cross. It shipped its plasma to the for-profit sector for production of factor VIII and then disseminated the product though its own distribution system. It also sold some of the plasma it collected to the commercial manufacturers so that they could use it to produce their own coagulation factor concentrates. In 1986, sales of plasma derivatives represented 15 percent of the Red Cross's gross revenues.[127] The Red Cross's position has always been that its coagulation factor concentrates are safer because they are made from the plasma of volunteer donors.[128] In reality, these donors were less well screened to exclude members of groups at higher risk of AIDS than paid donors.[129]

The culprits here are not just the large for-profit and nonprofit companies. Individual hospital blood banks and certain hospital-based physicians share the blame. The January 13, 1983, "Joint Statement on Acquired Immune Deficiency Syndrome (AIDS) Related to Transfusion" of the American Association of Blood Banks, American Red Cross, and Council of Community Blood Centers was inadequate because it did not (1) recommend screening out homosexuals and members of other high-risk groups through written and oral questioning, and it did not (2) call for implementation of surrogate testing. However, the Statement did observe: "Blood banks and transfusion services should further extend educational campaigns to physicians to balance the decision to use each blood component against the risks of transfusion, be they well-established (e.g., hepatitis, cytomegalovirus, malaria) or under investigation (e.g. AIDS)."

One can get some indication of how individual hospital blood banks and physician heads of hospital transfusion services responded to the call for education of physicians about the need for more judicious use of blood components by considering part of a speech given the following year by the president of Blood Systems, Inc., the second largest company in the nonprofit sector:

> We estimate that in 1983 some 2,150,000 units of FFP [fresh frozen plasma] were used for direct patient care. Experts have indicated that probably only 5% of that volume is truly medically indicated. I have mentioned the problem to a number of blood bankers and they are hesitant about educational programs to correct this problem—I quote one of them, a physician; "I need that revenue for my bottom line." [130]

We do not suggest that intentional misconduct explains all overuse of blood. Rather, an article published in 1990 in the *Journal of the American Medical Association* indicates *continued widespread physician ignorance* regarding both the risks of transfusions and guidelines designed to limit the inappropriate use of blood.[131]

The cynicism and ignorance displayed by the for-profit and nonprofit companies, individual hospital blood banks, and certain hospital-based physicians lead us to conclude that the nonprofit companies should be subject to the same restrictions we propose for the for-profit sector. It also strengthens our conviction that the entire health care sector must be much better educated and regulated to be sensitive to conflicts between personal or institutional concerns, on the one hand, and the safety and well-being of patients and the public, on the other hand.

Finally, it convinces us that neither the companies, nor individual blood banks, nor physicians should be protected by a deferential negligence standard under which jurors are instructed to give great weight to customary practice when determining the reasonableness of practices questioned by plaintiffs injured by blood components. (Consistent with the authors' positions regarding the standard of care for physicians staked out in Chapter 3, Shimm believes that physicians' practices should presumptively set the standards.) The companies and individual blood banks cannot even claim to possess the dedication to excellence and dominant commitment to serving others described by Buchanan in Chapter 5 as necessary to "professionalism" and the privilege of self-regulation that this label entails. Buchanan questions whether physicians themselves merit the label "professional," particularly because of their poor record of self-regulation. Deference to customary physician practices is a form of self-regulation. One need not go as far as Buchanan, however, to advocate nonuse of a professional standard of care concerning use of blood components. Rather, it has been demonstrated that, in this specific area, physicians rely substantially on the suppliers of blood components for information concerning efficacy and safety. This reliance and ignorance about the need for cautious use of blood cited above in the *Journal of the American Medical Association* undercut any justification for deference to the customs of physicians in this area.[132]

Conclusion

We began this chapter by summarizing the thesis of Dr. Joe Collier that the British pharmaceutical industry has "distorted the intellectual atmosphere" of British medicine and thus "undermined" the rights of patients by, among other behavior, paying for a large portion of the country's research, spending a large amount of money on promoting its products, funding physician attendance at symposia concerning its products (essentially gift giving), influencing medical journals with large outlays for advertising, forging links with opinion formers among the physician community, and advertising in misleading ways. We have demonstrated that the pharmaceutical industry in the United States has engaged in the same behavior, and we have studied this behavior in some detail, using the production of coagulation factor concentrates as a case study. We have described various attempts to deal with the conflicts of interest presented by the pharmaceutical industry's relationship with physicians, and we have suggested several reforms to further blunt the deleterious effects of the pharmaceutical industry's pervasive influence: prohibit direct capitation payments to academic researchers;

prohibit gifts to physicians beyond those of trivial value; explicitly empower the FDA to regulate detailing and to specify that detailers must supply balanced information; subject journal ads to scholarly review; apply products liability rules to pharmaceutical companies; impose a fiduciary duty to consumers on pharmaceutical companies, as well as on for-profit and nonprofit blood banks and companies; develop antitrust laws to make absolutely clear that concert of action to impede competition in regard to efficacy and safety, as well as price, is illegal; explore the feasibility of a system of pharmaceutical agents analogous to the present system of agricultural agents; create stronger protections for whistle blowers; reexamine the legal profession's position with respect to permissive and obligatory disclosures, with the intent to give more weight to the interests of large groups—such as hemophiliacs—who might be placed at substantial physical risk; have the medical profession and our civil liability system *require* physicians to go public whenever there is a clinically significant risk of serious bodily injury to one or more persons; have the medical profession and our civil liability system *protect* from discipline, liability, or retaliation physicians who go public because of a significant risk of bodily injury to one or more patient–consumers (the risk at issue need not be imminent if its magnitude and probability are great enough to reasonably require or allow a response); and not insulate blood component companies, individual blood banks, or (according to author Spece) physicians from liability by inappropriately applying a professional standard of care in lawsuits brought by persons who have been injured by blood components.

Notes

1. Joe Collier, Conflicts Between Pharmaceutical Company Largesse and Patients' Rights, 60 *Medico-Legal J.* 243, 244 (1992).
2. *Id.* at 244–246.
3. U.S. Department of Commerce, *Statistical Abstract of the United States* 98 (1990) ($11.537 billion government; $827,000,000 private).
4. *The Pharmaceutical Manufacturers Association Fact Book* 2 (1991).
5. American Medical Association Council on Scientific Affairs and Council on Judicial and Ethical Affairs, Conflict of Interest in Medical Center/Industry Research Relationships, 263 *JAMA* 2790 (1990), citing D. Blumenthal, University Industrial Research Relationships in Biotechnology: Implications for the University, 232 *Science* 1361 (1985).
6. David Shimm and Roy Spece, Industry Reimbursement for Entering Patients into Clinical Trials: Legal and Ethical Issues, 115 *Ann. Intern. Med.* 148 (1991).
7. D. R. Hathaway, Revitalizing The Federal Commitment in Support of Biomedical Research, 36 *Clin. Res.* 475 (1988); Wittenberg, NCI Budget Tapped for AIDS Care, 80 *J. Natl. Cancer Inst.* 1523 (1988); and American Federation for Clinical Research, Conflicts of Interest and Biomedical Research, 38 *Clin. Res.* 239 (1990).

8. This conflict of interest is arguably exacerbated by the pharmaceutical companies' practice of not paying the large overhead expenses covered by NIH grants. A researcher might prefer the direct subsidy to his lab through capitation payments over the indirect benefit from payment of large indirect costs. This could skew his choice of projects from that expected given his role as a searcher for and professor of the truth.

9. Robert Levine, Response to IRB's and Pharmaceutical Company Funding of Research, 4 *IRB* 9 (October 1982).

10. David Shimm and Roy Spece, Conflicts of Interest and Informed Consent in Industry-Sponsored Clinical Trials, 12 *J. Legal Med.* 477 (1992).

11. Laura Bowman, The Impact of Drug Company Funding on the Content of Continuing Medical Education, 6 *Mobius* 66 (1986).

12. Laura Bowman, Changes in Drug Prescribing Patterns Related to Commercial Company Funding of Continuing Medical Education, 8 *J. Cont. Ed. Health Prof.* 13 (1988).

13. American College of Physicians, Physicians and the Pharmaceutical Industry, 112 *Ann. Intern. Med.* 624 (1990); ACCME, *Guidelines for Commercial Support of Continuing Medical Education*, approved March 16, 1991; and AMA Council on Ethical and Judicial Affairs, Gifts to Physicians from Industry, 265 *JAMA* 501 (1991).

14. A. Skolnick, FDA Issues Draft "Concept Paper" on Drug Company Funding of CME, 266 *JAMA* 2947 (1991).

15. Leigh Page, Drug Makers Hit FDA Proposal on CME Restrictions, *American Medical News* 5 (December 2, 1991).

16. D.R. Waud, Pharmaceutical Promotions— A Free Lunch, 327 *New Engl. J. Med.* 351 (1992).

17. *Id.*

18. Susan Heilbronner Fisher, The Economic Wisdom of Regulating Pharmaceutical "Freebies," 1991 *Duke Law J.* 206, 238.

19. Chren, Doctors, Drug Companies, and Gifts, 262 *JAMA* 3448 (1989).

20. *Id.*

21. Paul Camenisch, Gift and Gratitude in Ethics, 9 *J. Relig. Ethics* 1 (1981).

22. W. Paul McKinney, Attitudes of Internal Medicine Faculty and Residents Toward Professional Interaction With Pharmaceutical Sales Representatives, 264 *JAMA* 1693 (1990).

23. Lichstein, Impact of Pharmaceutical Company Representatives on Internal Medicine Residency Programs —A Survey of Residency Program Directors, 152 *Arch. Intern. Med.* 109 (1992).

24. GMC's Doctor-Industry Code, *Scrip* No. 802 at 8 (1983); Royal College of Physicians, The Relationship Between Physicians and the Pharmaceutical Industry, 20 *J. R. Coll. Phys. Lond.* 235 (1986); American College of Physicians, Physicians and the Pharmaceutical Industry, 112 *Ann. Intern. Med.* 624 (1990); AMA Council on Ethical and Judicial Affairs, Gifts to Physicians from Industry, 265 *JAMA* 501 (1991); and D. S. Greenberg, Washington Perspective—All Expenses Paid, Doctor, 336 *Lancet* 1568 (1990) (discussing the Code of Pharmaceutical Marketing Practices).

25. David Page, Reaction to AMA Gift Code Shows Rumblings in the Ranks, *American Medical News* 2 (March 16, 1992).

26. National Association of Purchasing Management, *Principles and Standards of Purchasing Practice*, Principle 4 (January 1992).

27. Business Briefs: Consumer Drug Ads Working, *American Medical News* 17 (March 1, 1993) (". . . 93 percent of physicians surveyed in 1992 said patients had raised the subject of drug alternatives, up from 53 percent in 1989. Almost half the 37,700 physicians surveyed in 1992 said patients started discussions by bring on [sic] direct-to-consumer ads").

28. W. S. Wilkes, Pharmaceutical Advertisements in Leading Medical Journals: Experts' Assessments, 116 *Ann. Intern. Med.* 912 (1992).

29. D. B. Christensen, Sources of Information and Influence on New Drug Prescribing Among Physicians in an HMO, 13A *Soc. Sci. Med.* 313 (1979).

30. James Avorn, Scientific versus Commercial Sources of Influence on the Prescribing Behavior of Physicians, 73 *Am. J. Med.* 4 (1982).

31. *See, e.g.*, Note, *supra* note 18.

32. *Id.* at 237.

33. *Id.* at 226.

34. Counter-Detailing: Not "Counter" Anymore, *American Medical News* 14 (May 17, 1993). *See also* Annica Burns, Reinventing the Detailer, *American Medical News* 15 (May 17, 1993) (drug reps being given more training so that they can become "consultants" who might be more trusted, especially in light of counter-detailing efforts).

35. Charles Culhane, GAO Study Confirms It: Drug Prices Higher in U.S., *American Medical News* 6 (March 8, 1979).

36. Arnold Relman, Who Reviews the Ads?, 301 *N. Engl. J. Med.* 999 (1979).

37. R. H. Moser, Advertising and Our Journal, 87 *Ann. Intern. Med.* 114 (1977).

38. Office of Technology Assessment, U.S. Congress, *Blood Policy and Technology* 3, 51, 63 (1985).

39. Andrea Rock, Inside the Billion-Dollar Blood Industry, *Money* 153 (March 1986).

40. David Aronson, The Development of the Technology and Capacity for the Treatment of Factor VIII for the Treatment of Hemophilia, 30 *Transfusion* 748, 749 (October 1990); Harold Roberts and Marsha Jones, Hemophilia and Related Conditions, in *Hematology* 1459, 1463 (William Jones et al., eds, 1988). While hemophilia A patients are deficient in factor VIII, hemophilia B patients are lacking in factor IX. Hemophilia A patients can be treated with either cryoprecipitate or factor VIII concentrate, and hemophilia B patients can be treated with either fresh frozen plasma (from one or a few donors) or factor IX concentrate (from thousands of donors).

41. *Id.* at 1459.

42. Aronson, *supra* note 40, at 749; Roberts and Jones, *supra* note 40.

43. Roberts and Jones, *supra* note 40, at 1459.

44. *Id.*

45. Aronson, *supra* note 40, at 751–752. The hepatitis B core antibody test was widely implemented as a surrogate test starting in 1986. Ross Eckert, The AIDS Blood-Transfusion Cases: A Legal and Economic Analysis of Liability, 29 *San Diego L. R.* 203, 281 and 282 ns. 311 and 312 (1993). The hepatitis warning was insufficient because it did not make clear that virtually all users of factor VIII and factor IX would be exposed to blood borne hepatitis, and that there is a significant morbidity and mortality with both hepatitis B and what was then known as non-A, non-B hepatitis. The latter was known to exist even though the virus that caused it had not yet been identified. It is now known that non-A, non-B hepatitis is caused by a group of viruses, the primary one being hepatitis C. Hepatitis C has been identified, and hepatitis C is now known to be the primary hepatitis risk associated with use of blood and blood products.

46. Interview with Dr. Donald P. Francis, San Francisco, California, January 8, 1993 (hereafter "Francis interview").

47. *See, e.g.*, internal memorandum of Cutter Division of Miles, Inc., October 27, 1983, from Pete DeHart to Willi Ewald, in regard to the "National Hemophilia Foundation Meeting, Memphis, Tennessee 20–22 October 1983" (Behring [Germany] representative states that "large scale production using large pools of human plasma is unsafe," and that his company has marketed

a heat-treated product since 1978); and December 15, 1988, Affidavit of Dr. Thomas Drees, former CEO of Alpha Therapeutics, submitted in Doe v. Cutter Biological, U.S. District Court, District of Hawaii, Civ. No. 87-8232.

48. *Id.*

49. Doug Irish, Transfusion Liability, in *Blood Bank Risk Management* (M. Clark-Gilbert, ed., 1988), 107, 110–112 (1988); and Eckert, *supra* note 45 (describing parallel success of the voluntary sector and advocating products liability for that sector).

50. *Id.* all citations in *supra* notes 48 and 49. *See also* United Blood Services v. Quintana, 827 P.2d 509, 521–524 (Colo. 1992).

51. Video Deposition of Dr. Donald P. Francis, in Quintana v. United Blood Services, District Court, Denver County Colorado, Case. No. 86-CV-11750, July 3, 1992, at 68 (hereafter "Francis deposition").

52. Francis interview; Francis deposition at 62, 78, 83-84, 107, 109.

53. Francis interview; Francis deposition at 79.

54. Francis deposition, at 29, 41.

55. *See generally* Lorraine Day, *AIDS: What the Government Isn't Telling You* (1991); and Randy Shilts, *And the Band Played On* (1987).

56. Charles Perrow and Mauro Guillen, *The AIDS Disaster* 40 (Table 2-1) (1990).

57. January 17, 1983, Inter-Company Memorandum authored by S. J. Ojala, Cutter Biological Division of Miles, Inc., to "Those Listed" *re* "National Hemophilia Foundation/Industry Strategy Meeting on AIDS," January 14, 1983 New York City."

58. Francis Deposition at 37–38.

59. Shilts, *supra* note 55, 93–97, 118–119, and 220–224.

60. Francis interview.

61. Francis deposition, at 37, 55–58.

62. *Id.* at 56–66.

63. Shilts, *supra* note 55, 220–224; Francis interview; Francis deposition, at 44–45.

64. Francis deposition, at 67–73.

65. *Id.* at 2.

66. Inter-Office Memorandum of January 6, 1983, from John Hink, Cutter Biological Division of Miles, Inc., to Dr. K. Fischer et al. re "AIDS meeting of January 4th at CDC Atlanta."

67. Francis Deposition, at 112.

68. *Id.* at 145–146.

69. Author Spece was assistant counsel in an AIDS case tried against Miles, Inc., in April and May 1991 —Doe v. Miles Inc., et al., Pima County (Arizona) Superior Court, No. 264072. He has also been a member of the AIDS Litigation Group of the American Trial Lawyers Association and a consultant and assistant counsel to plaintiffs' attorneys in blood cases. As such, he has firsthand knowledge of the manufacturers' defenses. Ross Eckert has scrupulously detailed the parallel excesses of the voluntary sector; *see supra* note 45. The manufacturers did belatedly increase their efforts to develop heat-treated factor products, but they suggested that this was done in response to hepatitis, not AIDS. The "less than aggressive" approach toward blood safety, pre- and post- AIDS, by both the voluntary and for-profit sectors is well-documented in, Institute of Medicine, *HIV and the Blood Supply: An Analysis of Decisionmaking* (1995).

70. December 21, 1982, from S. J. Ojala to "Those Listed" re "More AIDS and FDA."

71. Inter-Office Memorandum of June 13, 1983, from S. J. Ojala, Cutter Biological Division of Miles, Inc., to "Those Listed" re "FDA Recall Recommendation Meeting, June 9, 1983."

72. Inter-Office Memorandum of January 17, 1983, from S. J. Ojala to "Those Listed" re "National Hemophilia Foundation/Industry Strategy Meeting on AIDS, Jan. 14, 1983, New York City."

73. *See, e.g.,* Cutter package insert for "Antihemophilic Factor (Human) Koate," revised December 1983.

74. Inter-Office Memorandum from Ed Cutter, December 29, 1982, to Jack Ryan et al. re "AIDS."

75. Draft 4 (December 3, 1982) ("In addition the number of cases [of AIDS] continues to increase and the illness may pose a significant risk for patients with hemophilia. Patients receiving therapy should be advised of that possible risk" (bracketed text added).

76. Inter-Office Memorandum, March 14, 1983, from John Hink, Cutter Biological Division of Miles, Inc., to S. J. Ojala [*et al.*] re "American Blood Resources Assn. Meeting—Las Vegas, 3/10-3/11—A Summary of the More Significant Information Discussed" (bracketed text added).

77. Inter-Office Memorandum, October 29, 1983, from Pete DeHart to Willi Ewald re "National Hemophilia Foundation Meeting—Memphis Tennessee 20-22 October 1983."

78. Press Release on Hill and Knowlton, Inc., Stationery, "For: Cutter Laboratories Contact: . . . *FOR IMMEDIATE RELEASE* . . . EMERYVILLE, CA, November 1, 1983."

79. *See, e.g.,* February 10, 1983, Memorandum on Hill and Knowlton stationery from Hill and Knowlton's Jim Musslewhite to Cutter's Bud Modersbach re "Packets for Managers of Cutter Affiliated Centers."

80. *See* Inter-Office Memorandum, August 24, 1983, from Kathy Larkin, Marketing Research, Cutter Biological Division of Miles, Inc., to Jan Peterson re "AIDS Physicians Teleconferences."

81. Cutter Forum: AIDS and Hemophilia Treatment, July 1, 1983, at 2.

82. *Id.* at 3–6. We sought permission to quote more extensively from the Forum, but Miles Inc. (of which Cutter was a division) said "no."

83. Inter-Office Memorandum, December 19, 1983, from S. J. Ojala, Cutter Biological Division of Miles, Inc., to W. F. Schaeffler [President] [et al.] re "Trip Report, FDA/NIH Non-Specific Testing Meeting December 15–16, 1983" (bracketed text added).

84. Majority Position Paper Opposing the Implementation of Anti-Core Testing for Source and Recovered Plasma, forwarded from Dr. Michael Rodell of the Revlon Health Care Group to Dr. John C. Petricciani, Director of the Division of Blood and Blood Products, Center for Biologics, FDA, July 16, 1984, at 1.

85. *See, e.g.,* March 8, 1983, and January 7, 1983, letters of Cutter's Director of Medical Services, G. M. Akin, M.D., to the parent of a hemophiliac and to Joel Spalter, M.D.

86. U.S. District Court, District of Hawaii, Civil No. 87-8232. For additional analysis of the AIDS/blood product crisis, see, e.g., Perrow and Guillen, *supra* note 56, at 38–44, 148–151; Shilts, *supra* note 56; Day, *supra* note 55; Rock, *supra* note 39; Report of the Presidential Commission on the Human Immunodeficiency Virus Epidemic, submitted to the President of the United States, June 24, 1988; and Eckert, *supra* note 45.

87. *Id.* at 283–288 (regarding the similar superior knowledge of blood banks); M. S. Madden, 2 Products Liability § 23.11, at 366 (2d ed., 1988) and R. E. Cartwright and J. J. Phillips, 3 Product Liability § 6.22, at 715 (1986).

88. *See, e.g.,* Jay Katz, *The Silent World of Doctor and Patient* (1986).

89. *See* notes 80–84 and text thereat.

90. *See* notes 77–81 and text thereat.

91. Telephone interview with Anne M. King, Public Relations Office, National Hemophilia Foundation (NHF), June 11, 1993; *see also* NHF Hemophilia Information Exchange, *Med. Bull.* No. 137, July 1, 1991 (statistics on all hemophiliacs).

92. Spece was assistant counsel in one of those cases: Doe v. Miles Inc. *et al.*, Pima County Superior Court, No. 264072. *See also* note 78.

93. *Id.*

94. National Hemophilia Foundation, Chapter Advisory No. 169, Medical Bulletin No. 167, December 3, 1992: MASAC Statement on Testimony Provided By Physicians and/or Other Associated with the National Hemophilia Foundation. Subsequently the NHF was named as a defendant along with the manufacturers in a national class action on behalf of hemophiliacs. Conflict of interest and breach of fiduciary duty were the central claims against the NHF. The gist of the claims was that the NHF purported to give objective advice concerning coagulation factor concentrates when in fact it was influenced by a Medical Advisory Committee composed of physicians who did research or related work for the manufacturers. Wadleigh vs. Rhone-Poulenc, Rorer, Inc., U.S. District Court for the Northern District of Illinois, No. 93C 5969, filed September 30, 1993.

95. James T. O'Reilly, *Food and Drug Administration*, Chapter 15 (1992).

96. Scott Bice, Rationality Analysis In Constitutional Law, 65 *Minn. L. Rev.* 1, 17–21 (1980).

97. *Id.*

98. Susan Dickinson, FDA User Fees to Speed Drug Review, *The Scientist* 3 (December 7, 1992).

99. Charles Culhane, FDA, Drug Makers Enter Era of Good Feelings Over User Fees, *American Medical News* 5 (March 1, 1993).

100. *Id.*

101. *Id.*

102. Bernard Schwartz, *Administrative Law* § 1.14 at 24 (3d ed., 1991).

103. Regarding the antitrust laws and "nonprice" competition, see, e.g., Thomas Sullivan, On Non-Price Competition: An Economic and Marketing Analysis, 45 *U. Pitt. L. R.* 771 (1984).

104. *See, e.g.*, Tom Beauchamp and James Childress, *Principles of Biomedical Ethics* 73 (3d ed., 1989).

105. E. Haavi Morreim, Economic Disclosure and Economic Advocacy, 12 *J. Legal Med.* 275, 296–301 (1991).

106. *Id.* at 296–297. Note the overlap between the criteria defining "professions" discussed by Buchanan in Chapter 5 of this volume and the criteria listed in the text as defining "fiduciary relationship." However, although there is sufficient justification to apply a fiduciary duty to pharmaceutical companies, they are not close enough to professionals to justify application of the "professional" standard of care. *See* text between notes 131 and 132.

107. *See, e.g.*, Stephen Feldman and James Ward, Psychotherapeutic Injury: Reshaping the Implied Contract or an Alternative to Malpractice, 58 *N.C. L. Rev.* 54, 79 (1979).

108. *See, e.g.*, Deborah DeMott, Beyond Metaphor: An Analysis of Fiduciary Obligation, 1988 *Duke L.J.* 879, 900.

109. S. M. Speiser *et al.*, 5 *The American Law of Torts*, § 18.100 at 997 (1988).

110. Peter French *et al.*, *Corporations in the Moral Community* 44–46 (1992).

111. United States Sentencing Guidelines Manual (28 U.S.C. §§ 991-98), Section 8 (2.5 CF) (November 1992) (compliance program requisite for mitigation credit).

112. *See, e.g.*, Peter French *et al.*, *Corporations in the Moral Community* 100–106 (1992); and Christopher Stone, *Where the Law Ends: The Social Control of Corporate Behavior* 152–183 (1975).

113. Rule 1.6 (b)(2) (1983).

114. *Problems, Cases and Materials in Professional Responsibility* 282 (Robert H. Aronson *et al.*, eds., 1985).

115. Francis deposition at 123.

116. Stuart M. Speiser, *et al.*, *The American Law of Torts* § 32:90 (1992).

117. Wagenseller v. Scottsdale Memorial Hospital, 710 P.2d 1025 (Ariz. 1985) (allegation that nurse was fired for refusing to "moon" enough to state public policy–wrongful dismissal

claim regardless whether mooning constitutes technical violation of statute). *But see* Campbell v. Eli Lilly & Co., 413 N.E.2d 1054 (Ind. App. 1980) (employee of drug company could not defend himself against dismissal because he had neither a statutory right nor a duty to report the erroneous nature of safety and efficacy data regarding drugs manufactured by the company); Buethe v. Britt Airlines Ind., 787 F.2d 1194 (7th Cir. 1986) (a copilot could not refuse to fly a plane simply because it was not "airworthy" within the meaning of state statutes); and Balla v. Gambro, Inc., 584 N.E.2d 104 (Ill. 1991) (an attorney could not defend himself against discharge resulting from telling his employer that he would do all in his power to prevent the sale of a defective kidney dialysis machine because public policy of protection of patients was adequately protected by an ethical rule requiring attorneys to reveal information necessary to prevent clients from committing acts that would result in serious bodily injury or death).

118. Sanford Kurtz, The Blood Collection System, in *Transfusion Medicine* 1, 5–6 (W. Halowell Churchill and Sanford Kurtz, eds., 1985).

119. Resolution WHA 28.72 of the Twenty-Eighth World Health Assembly, 29 May 1975, reprinted in W. N. Gibbs and A. F. H. Britton, *Guidelines for the Organization of a Blood Transfusion Service* ix (1992).

120. *See, e.g.*, National Academy of Sciences, *For Profit Enterprise in Health Care* (1986).

121. Dan Brock and Allen Buchanan, Ethical Issues in For Profit Health Care, in *For-Profit Enterprise in Health Care* 224, 247, 248 (1986).

122. Rock, *supra* note 39, at 153, 154.

123. *Id.* at 162.

124. Eckert, *supra* note 45, at 225–231.

125. *See, e.g.*, June 4, 1984, internal American Red Cross memorandum from Dr. Dodd to Dr. Katz and Dr. Sandler re "San Jose: MAC."

126. American Red Cross, BSL No. 83-12, Attachment III (cryoprecipitated AHF and AHF concentrates), disseminated to Executive Heads, Directors, and Medical/Scientific Directors from Dr. Katz, January 26, 1983.

127. Rock, *supra* note 39, 137n.

128. Affidavit of S. Gerald Sandler, M.D., Chief Medical Officer, Blood Services, American National Red Cross, submitted April, 1991, in Doe v. Miles, Inc., *et al.*, Pima County (Arizona) Superior Court, No. 264072.

129. Deposition of Dr. Tom Asher of HemaCare Corporation, April 23, 1990, in Doe v. South Florida Blood Service, Inc., Circuit Court of the 11th Judicial District, County of Dade, Florida, No. 8917674, pp. 4–40.

130. Speech submitted as attachment 6 to materials submitted by the Phoenix law firm, Meyer, Hendricks, Victor, Osborn and Maledon, to Senator Cindy L. Resnick of the Arizona Legislature on March 27, 1991, in connection with hearings on Arizona legislation designed to characterize litigation against licensed blood banks as medical malpractice actions.

131. Susanne Salem-Schatz et al., Influence of Clinical Knowledge, Organizational Context, and Practice Style on Transfusion Decision Making, 264 *JAMA* 476 (1990).

132. *See* our positions regarding the appropriate *general* standard of care for physicians in Chapter 3 of this volume.

Part IV

CLINICAL RESEARCH

15

An Introduction to Conflicts of Interest in Clinical Research

David S. Shimm and Roy G. Spece, Jr.

Part IV of this book focuses on clinical research,[1] which presents some particularly troublesome conflicts of interest. The major ones result from the magnitude of the financial and other rewards that ride on the results of the research and from the explicit diversion of the clinical researcher's loyalty from the interests of the patient to the requirements of the scientific study.

Comparing Conflicts and Interests in the Practice and Research Settings

General Comparison

In fee-for-service medical practice, conflict can arise between the physician's interest in maximizing income by performing additional procedures and the patient's interest in avoiding unnecessary procedures. Although the information asymmetry between physician and patient can permit the physician to talk the patient into tests and procedures, in principle this resembles an everyday situation like negotiating with automobile dealers. Managed care is a more opaque situation, since the patient may not recognize that the gatekeeper physician can increase income by withholding medical care, but the conflict is essentially the same as in the fee-for-service setting—physician's financial interest versus duty to the patient.

361

With clinical research, in addition to the conflict between the clinical investigator's fiduciary duty as a physician and his financial interest, the clinical investigator is also a scientist, which adds other conflicting obligations—to science, society, the sponsor, and the host institution. Contrast Dr. Anthony Fauci's (director of the National Institute of Allergy and Infectious Diseases) description of the goals of the Phase III randomized clinical trial—"It's not to deliver therapy. It's to answer a scientific question"[2]—with the findings of a study indicating that even after supposed informed consent, half of the adult subjects receiving placebo in a nonblind, nonrandomized placebo trial still believed that they were definitely receiving active medication.[3] Clinical trial subjects' inclination to believe that clinical investigators are treating them in accordance with Marquis's "therapeutic obligation"[4] in the setting of a clinical trial designed "not to deliver therapy, [but rather] to answer a scientific question" creates a situation not only characterized by numerous conflicts of interest but one in which clinical trial subjects, by virtue of their vulnerability, their ignorance of the nature of a clinical trial, and the diverse influences acting on the investigator, are ill-equipped to defend their own interests.

We realize that varied conflicts of interest arising from obligations to multiple parties are not unique to clinical research. For example, a managed-care gatekeeper physician in the practice setting might unduly limit care to an individual patient to benefit society, as he sees it, rather than because of his own pecuniary or emotional interests. The research setting is unique, however, in several respects. First, the conflict between the patient's best interests and the interests of science is virtually always present. Second, the research setting adds institutional and individual interests, in the form of pride, grand accomplishment, and fame, that are usually not present in clinical practice. Third, the degree of conflict between the interests of patients and other interests is stark in clinical research. This extreme conflict is exemplified, once again, by Fauci's description of clinical research in comparison to Marquis's concept of the therapeutic obligation.

This conflict is highest in randomized clinical trials (RCTs), the gold standard for clinical research. Indeed, some commentators have argued that RCTs are flatly inconsistent with the physician-patient relationship.[5] Samuel and Deborah Hellman have argued that RCTs and their casting of the doctor in the role of "physician-scientist" "do serious damage to the concept of physician as a practicing empathetic professional who is primarily concerned with each patient as an individual."[6] RCTs, they argue, require the physician to withhold information (suspicions, hunches, and beliefs about which therapeutic alternative is best) in the interest of science that they have an obligation to share with their patients. Moreover, once again in the interest of science, RCTs bar physicians from preliminary data about the efficacy of treatments that they should share with patients. The counterargument is essentially that RCTs are done only when there is "clinical equipoise," that is, when no treatment has been shown to be preferable. Therefore, no useful information is being withheld from patients, who, in any event, give consent monitored by the Institutional Review Board (IRB) process and substantive regulations.[7] We will not resolve this dispute here, but it certainly shows the stark conflicting interests in clinical research. We observe that significant amounts of clinical research are solely to the benefit of science, scientists, society, institutions, and industry and at the expense of subjects who do not realize that their chances of personally benefitting from the research are *extremely* remote.

A fourth difference between the practice and research settings is that since research is disproportionately (and appropriately) directed to serious medical problems, clinical research subjects are typically sicker and more desperate than patients seen in routine medical practice.

Fifth, and related to but broader than the second difference mentioned above, the practice and research settings are characterized by similar but distinct involvements of parties and interests external to the physician-patient relationship. This last point of difference demands explanation. In Chapter 2, Erde created taxonomies of conflicts and of interests at a very general level. It is instructive, however, to explore and compare in more detail the types of conflicts and interests that arise in the practice and research settings.

Some Specific Comparisons Between Practice and Research Settings

More specific comparison of the practice and research settings can be done, in part, by identifying the various parties, conflicts, and interests involved in industry-sponsored clinical research and then comparing them to the parties, conflicts, and interests implicated in clinical practice.

The former task is performed in Chapter 17 by Edward Huth. He lists the parties most directly interested in the outcome of industry-sponsored clinical research—the clinical investigator, the sponsor, the host institution, the scientific community, the public, and the clinical trial subjects—as well as their interests. He also describes a rough, ordered array of interests that must be respected: (1) research leading to safe, effective, and inexpensive diagnostic methods and treatments; (2) information available to enable all parties to judge how effectively their interests are being protected; (3) low risk/benefit ratio for patients or other research subjects; (4) adequate information for decisions by the sponsor regarding further development or marketing; (5) fair compensation for the investigator and the host institution for their participation; (6) minimal cost to the sponsor; (7) time-efficient conduct of research; (8) protection of the scientific community's need for esteem by the public and government; and (9) rapid dissemination of new information derived from the research.

Huth formulates metaprinciples to judge research guidelines and to help reconcile the various parties' competing interests in the research setting. He then describes a number of institutional research guidelines and judges these according to his metaprinciples. Finally, he proposes an ideal set of guidelines that incorporate the strengths of the Canadian National Council's guidelines while ensuring that responsibility for contractual arrangements is spread satisfactorily.

The parties interested in a practice situation can be just as varied as in the clinical research setting described by Huth: the patient; the physician; family members and close friends; the provider group of which the physician is a member; the insurer, HMO, or government entity, which reimburses or hires the physician group; the hospital where the physician provides care to the patient; and individuals or groups who are responsible for or hired to do quality assurance or utilization review concerning the situation. The major interests of these parties are their own health, privacy, autonomy, and financial well-being as well as the quality, cost, accessibility, and equitable distribution of health care.

Although many of the same parties and interests interact and clash in the practice and research settings, it is instructive to compare and contrast these intersections. The major conflicts of interest in clinical research—identified above as patient-subjects' interests versus companies' desire to develop treatments and investigators' desire to advance knowledge and their own prestige—lead to the possibility that patients might be subjected to unnecessary procedures. Here the several parties with direct or indirect financial interests—the investigators, the sponsor, the host institution—all stand to gain by a patient's participation. To prevent such abuse, research must be prescreened by IRBS. There is usually no equivalent prior review in the practice setting. On the other hand, in the practice setting there is possible subsequent review: for example, review of medical necessity for reimbursement purposes, institutional quality assurance and utilization review, and possible license or medical malpractice liability proceedings (such proceedings are extremely rare in the research context). Moreover, these and other incentives can either encourage or discourage additional diagnosis or treatment.

The most direct problem in clinical research thus seems to be the improper enlistment of subjects, and the primary protective mechanism is *prior* committee review. In clinical practice, problems of both over- and underutilization are present, sometimes simultaneously, and they are primarily bridled by post hoc mechanisms. It is interesting to note that there has been a renewed call for increased *ongoing* review of clinical research by IRBs or a similar institution,[8] and that *prior* reviews and control of clinical practice through protocols, second opinions, and preadmission screening are being used more frequently.[9] This perhaps reflects a practical judgment that prior review and post hoc review are necessary and useful to confine conflicts of interest in both practice and research settings. Here scholars should systematically study the lessons (1) prior review of research might teach in the practice setting and (2) post hoc review of practice might teach in the research setting. For example, if prior review of experimental protocols often uncovers poor communication with experimental subjects, this might indicate the need for prior intervention into the informed consent process in the practice setting. If post hoc review in the practice setting indicates frequent failure to follow protocols, this might signal the need for ongoing monitoring of compliance with research protocols.

Moving to long-term problems presented in the practice and research settings, the greatest long-term problems presented by specific research studies are erroneous findings leading to foregoing beneficial care or to unnecessary, costly, and even harmful treatment in future patients. In the practice setting, the major long-term problem from physician–patient interactions is the "bloating" of practice standards, driving up the cost of health care and preventing access and equity for those who cannot afford to purchase adequate care. (We recognize the dangers of underutilization discussed by Rodwin in Chapter 9, but they do not seem to threaten a *general* attenuation of practice standards.)

It is also helpful to recognize that values usually thought essential in either the practice or research setting might be important in both settings. For example, the values of access and equity often stressed in the practice setting apply to research as well. Indeed, several commentators have decried as unfair denying certain groups participation in clinical studies.[10] Similarly, Buchanan argued in Chapter 5 that although physicians decry it, loss of status trust in physicians is not bad in the practice setting. Huth thinks that one of the important values in the research context is "protection of the scientific community's need for esteem by the public and government." Extending Buchanan's reasoning in the practice setting, however, one could conclude that it might be good for patient–subjects and government to be skeptical about *researchers'* proposed actions.

Conflicts of Interest Common to Industry, Academic, and Government Research

Industry and Government–Funded Research

In Chapter 18 Baruch Brody addresses both industry-funded and government-financed research, advocating close attention to conflicts of interest in both settings. It is his view that the appropriate attention directed to industry–academic ties, and particularly to equity interests of academic investigators in companies whose products they are investigating, has diverted attention from the conflicts of interest created by *grants* from both industry *and* the government. Brody distinguishes between conflict of interest and scientific fraud. He believes that while clinical trials are designed to minimize the risk of fraud, there are still opportunities for investigators' conflicts of interest to affect the design, conduct, and analysis of trials. He identifies eight types of decisions in which conflicts of interest can affect clinical research and illustrates them through application to clinical trials of thrombolytic agents.

Although Brody gives a brief recent history of the development of thrombolytic therapy and demonstrates how controversy arose in the trials of thrombolytic agents, he does not identify any specific flawed decisions. One commentator raises possibilities that illustrate the conflicts of interest in these thrombolytic trials: (1) Some critics argued that the first published findings comparing t-PA and streptokinase (SK) failed to report results unfavorable to t-PA because five of the investigators owned stock in the company (Genentech) that manufactured t-PA; (2) Scientists with stock in Genentech participated in decisions to increase significantly the dosages and consequent risks of t-PA given to patients participating in the study, and these decisions may have been influenced by the stock ownership. ("At one facility, the dosage increases caused severe intracranial bleeding in 5 of 311 patients. As a result, three patents died and 41 suffered extra-cranial bleeding"); and (3) Others have alleged that physician-researchers involved in the trials may have violated patients' rights to informed consent (e.g., the consent form failed to mention that t-PA was an experimental treatment not yet approved by the FDA).[11]

Brody describes two approaches to conflicts of interest of the type presented by the t-PA trials: (1) disclose the equity holdings and financial relationships between researchers and the companies whose products are being evaluated, and (2) prohibit certain holdings and relationships. Although Brody endorses some mixture of these approaches, he argues that they are both incomplete. He states that conflicts of interest arise whenever (1) discretionary decisions are to be made, and (2) these decisions might be biased by researchers' financial interests. Brody's argument is that situation (2) can be created even when researchers have no equity holdings in, or consulting or other financial relationships with, commercial entities. It can be created simply by grants from industry *or* government. Brody therefore agrees with the British Royal College of Physicians, which has indicated that per capita payments to clinical investigators should not exceed the true direct and indirect costs of a study and should not include any profit to the investigator, the investigator's academic department, or the investigator's institution. Here he goes beyond our writing, which has suggested that captation payments in excess of true direct plus indirect costs are acceptable, provided that they do not flow to the clinical investigator.[12] Whether all capitation payments in excess of true direct and indirect costs should be banned, as advocated by Brody and the Royal College, or whether the excess should just be taken out of the control of the clinical investigator, is an important question that cannot be resolved here but that deserves further study.

Brody advocates prohibition of excess payments to ameliorate the risk that the financial conflict of interest they represent might skew any one of the eight types of questions he identifies as inevitably arising in the design and conduct of clinical trials. Moreover, he points out that many of these eight types of questions are amenable to independent policy formulation. Room for discretion and operation of conflicts of interest can be restricted through explicit policies on these questions.

Research By Government Scientists

Brody goes beyond the problems created by industry-sponsored academic research to discuss government-sponsored extramural research as well. In Chapter 16, Thomas Kurt compares the situations of scientists working in corporate, academic, and government settings. His analysis includes government scientists in regulatory as well as research roles. He concludes that government scientists have traditionally been less subject to conflicts of interest than academic or corporate scientists, since, until recently, they were unable to participate in any financial developments from their work. He notes that government scientists are, paradoxically, more highly regulated than academic or corporate scientists, and he asks whether this degree of regulation should be extended to nongovernmental scientists as well. He briefly summarizes the major provisions of 1995 Public Health Service regulations that bring private but government-funded scientists under closer scrutiny, yet still leave the greatest responsibility for regulating conflicts of interest with investigators' institutions.

Kurt points out that the traditional perception of government scientists as independent searchers for truth for the public good has been called into question by Congress's authorization and encouragement of Cooperative Research and Development Agreements (CRADAs), a mechanism by which private institutions—academic as well as commercial—may enter into joint ventures with federal government laboratories. Kurt summarizes the arguments for and against CRADAs. He notes that objections to CRADAs are similar to fears expressed when industry–academic research relationships were first being formed. Kurt argues that, on the whole, industry–academic relationships have been beneficial for society. Properly regulated, they should be encouraged. He suggests that the same is true of CRADAs. One additional danger not inherent in the industry–academic setting, however, is presented by CRADAs: They can compromise government agencies' regulatory missions. For example, if a Food and Drug Administration (FDA) or National Institute of Health (NIH) scientist enters into a CRADA regarding a product that must be approved by the FDA, the FDA will be called on to approve or disapprove studies submitted by one of its own or by a sister agency. This presents opportunities for personal and institutional relationships and loyalties to influence decisions and for skepticism by the public.

Just such a situation is presented by the taxol CRADA between the National Cancer Institute and Bristol Myers, where the manufacturer provides Pacific yew bark, seeks alternative renewable sources for taxol, and pursues a New Drug Application (NDA) with the FDA; and the NCI provides exclusive access to pre-clinical and clinical data.[13] Here a conflict of interest can arise when the FDA, a branch of the Department of Health and Human Services (DHSS), is required to evaluate the NDA. Should there be questions about the data supporting the NDA, one branch of DHHS could find itself actively questioning the scientific validity of data derived by another branch of DHHS in an issue with serious financial consequences for DHHS.

Nevertheless, Kurt concludes that, to date, CRADAs represent an ethically acceptable means for retaining talented scientists at government laboratories and for encouraging scientific and economic advancement. They should be carefully monitored and regulated, but they should not be eliminated.

Conflicts of Interest in IRBs

Leslie Francis outlines the history, structure, membership, and functions of the Institutional Review Board (IRB, or Human Subjects Committee) in Chapter 19. She describes a number of conflicts of interest that can involve an IRB member. She also draws attention to the conflicts of interest peculiar to free-standing IRBs, whose continued existence might depend on pleasing their clients by giving favorable reviews.

Francis notes that there exist little comprehensive data concerning IRB membership (other than domination by physicians), affiliation (e.g., university hospital versus nonprofit hospital versus for-profit hospital versus free-standing) or deliberative process. By analogy to empirical data on hospital ethics committees and scientific fraud investigations, she suggests that conflicts of interest may affect IRB decisions more frequently than we would like to believe. Francis concludes by arguing that IRB members with interests that might affect their evaluation of a particular study should disqualify themselves from evaluating that study, and she calls for more research on conflicts of interest involving IRBs.

Common Themes

Although the authors in this part address different topics from different perspectives, common themes run throughout the chapters. Brody, Huth, and Kurt believe that the overall purpose of research—development of safe, effective, and inexpensive methods of diagnosing and treating medical conditions—should not be overlooked in the effort to minimize the effects of conflicts of interest. Brody, Huth, and Francis also indicate the importance of non–financial conflicts of interest. They point out that investigators can be influenced by their own, or their allies', desire for renown, professional advancement, and power, rather than by financial considerations alone, and that attempts to manage conflicts of interest will fail unless these nonfinancial conflicts are addressed as well. Finally, all four authors stress the need for further empirical study to adduce the factual data necessary for sound policy choices about conflicts of interest presented in clinical research.

Although these chapters shed considerable light on a murky area, they raise questions as well. In general, although they identify problems accurately, solutions prove more elusive. Compared with nonfinancial conflicts of interest, financial conflicts are, in principle, easier to identify, and formal guidelines and regulations can address these problems or, at least, eliminate ignorance as a defense. For example, if certain types of equity holdings are judged to represent unacceptable conflicts of interest, statutes or regulations can be devised that describe the forbidden financial activity, prescribe an acceptable means of and timetable for divestiture, and provide specific penalties for noncompliance. Nonfinancial conflicts are more pervasive and subtly nuanced, and therefore represent a more difficult issue to address. While guidelines and regulations can catalog prohibited financial relationships, it is difficult to imagine a similar catalog of interpersonal relationships, classifying some as representing an impermissible conflict of interest, except perhaps at the margin (e.g., current spouses, ex-spouses). To that extent, minimizing the effects of these nonfinancial conflicts of interest depends more strongly on the willingness of individual clinical investigators to recognize them, declare them, and disqualify themselves from situations where these could prove troublesome. Unfortunately, it is not clear how frequently clinical investigators recognize conflicts of interest and how frequently they would behave responsibly in the presence of a conflict of interest. This is another area for empirical study. Moreover, education is clearly a key issue. Investigators must develop expertise in recognizing conflicts of interest, and must cultivate the fortitude to disclose such conflicts and disqualify themselves when appropriate.

The Cumulative Impact of Conflicts of Interest in the Research Setting

The individual chapters cannot portray the cumulative impact of the distinct conflicts of interest that they discuss. We fear that the many conflicts discussed in this part represent a privatization and instrumentalization of science that threatens to debase our scientific culture, skew our national research priorities, and further expose patient–subjects to exploitation.

As Huth points out in Chapter 17, clinical research as we know it today emerged in the aftermath of World War II. Initially, government was virtually the only source of clinical research funding at universities and colleges. Academic research institutions and researchers viewed themselves as public servants, and were largely unconcerned with industry goals and financially disinterested in their own findings. They freely shared information to enable others to replicate research findings and thereby facilitate the advance of science. The reward for discovery, and for prompt sharing and publication of findings, was recognition by colleagues and the public.

Now that private industry has become a significant source of research funding (e.g., $9.26 billion for all health research and development in 1989),[14] research institutions and researchers can gain either direct or indirect financial rewards, depending on the outcome of their research. There is greater interest in applied research than in basic research, and applied research is often tied to the agendas of private companies. Findings have become proprietary information to be protected rather than shared. Indeed, the conflicts of interest posed by interlacing relationships between academic scientists and private companies have sometimes resulted in actual fraud. It is therefore appropriate to mention the connection between conflicts of interest and concerns about scientific fraud and university–industry interactions. We believe society benefits from the existence of a tenured professoriate that searches for and professes the truth. Competition for money and prestige has become so fierce in the academy, however, that it has occasionally displaced the search for truth. Moreover, interlacing relationships between professors and private businesses have heightened the emphasis on financial productivity and, at the same time, have undercut the professoriate's claims for a secure niche in which academicians can independently and unselfishly search for the truth. For example, the very notion of academic freedom is confused and thereby threatened when it is invoked by professors to resist academic administrators' good-faith attempts to police professors' relationships with industry.[15]

Until recently, intramural government research and funding served as a counterpoint to the possible weakening of academic researchers' objectivity. Now, however, industry, academic, *and* government scientists are encouraged to enter into CRADAs and jointly undertake research studies. We fear that the various partnerships among professors, government scientists, and private industry are coalescing to privatize and particularize the search for truth. Perhaps no institution or group of individuals will remain dedicated solely to the search for truth independent of particular concerns of specific companies or industries. On the other hand, our fears might be born out of a naive nostalgia for a past that never was. An analysis similar to that presented by Buchanan in Chapter 5—suggesting that there is no medical profession because physicians have traditionally exhibited selfishness and that selfishness is anathema to a true profession—might be extended and lead to the conclusion that, similarly, government and university scientists have always been interested in prestige, power, and a quick buck.

Additional "Institutions" That Pose Potential Conflicts of Interest

CRADAs are not the only institutions that represent potential coalescence of power. Consider Contract Research Organizations (CROs)—private companies or academic consortia that provide a range of services for pharmaceutical companies that need to comply with FDA-required studies. These services include supplying facilities, investigators, patients, equipment, laboratory testing, protocol development, data collection, and statistical interpretation. Some large outfits supply the full range of services, while others are little more than brokers, bringing pharmaceutical companies in contact with investigators and institutions where the needed patients, facilities, and support are available.[16]

The most important of all these elements is the provision of patients. Huth's formal guidelines indicate that it is unethical to advertise the availability of one's patients. This can be done indirectly. Physician-scientists and/or their institutions are retained by CROs, which, in turn, advertise in medical journals. The most valuable product they advertise—albeit most often between the lines—is patient–subjects.

A more blatant example of trading in patients is the payment of finders' fees for enrolling patients in clinical studies. Stuart Lind has written that although the extent of this practice is not known, there are clear examples of it in many parts of the country.[17] We agree with his observation that finders fees are equivalent to fee splitting, which is clearly prohibited in the practice setting and is improper in the research setting as well. But are the particular CROs that essentially do nothing more than broker patients engaged in conduct less objectionable than paying finders' fees? Their activities are arguably worse because the brokers in CROs are isolated from patients; to them, patients are just commodities or statistics.

Representative of the erosion of borders between industry, academic, and government sectors, pharmaceutical companies can now enter into agreements—called "Clinical Trial Agreements"—with NIH whereby the latter essentially becomes a CRO. For a fee (denominated a "donation" since fees are not permissible), NIH subcontracts or grants to investigators—usually in large academic centers—the task of doing clinical studies necessary for the studied products' approval by the FDA. Alternatively, the NIH can perform some or all of the studies on its own campus.[18] (This would seem to be a particularly attractive arrangement when a product is somewhat controversial or has significant potential side effects. Here the mantle of government involvement and approval might shield companies from certain liability risks.)

In the past, there was a "separation of powers" among industry, academia, and government. Each stood as a potential check on the other. These possible checks ameliorated the risks of exploitation of patients and sacrifice of the public interest because each center of power had some incentive to police its "competitors."

Application of Models of the Physician-Patient Relationship to Conflicts Posed by the Research Setting

Even before the current coalescence of power among industry, academia, and government, Arnold Relman spoke of the dangers of a "medical–industrial complex."[19] Now we are faced with the reality of a medical–industrial monolith. One common need of each participant in this monolith is research subjects. In light of this situation, we will apply the models of the physician–patient role discussed in Chapter 3 to the research setting. The paternalistic model would seem to require that a physician not enroll a patient in an RCT unless that is the only way the patient may have access to a treatment that the physician thinks is the only one that may benefit the patient. Otherwise, the physician should either offer his preferred treatment(s) or suggest that nothing be done. The informative model would require the physician to disclose and emphasize the information that would most likely lead the paternalistic physician to argue against enrollment in an RCT.[20] The interpretive model would not add much, except in the rare case where it was evident that the patient placed a high value on helping society by volunteering to participate in a clinical study. Recall, however, that the deliberative model allows the physician as "friend or teacher to draw upon his own values in an attempt to influence the patients' choice and development of values." The Emanuels give the example of a physician encouraging a woman with breast cancer to enter an adjuvant chemotherapy clinical trial because it would allow her "to contribute something to women with breast cancer in the future who will face difficult choices." On the other hand, the interpretive physician might say to the same woman: "[Y]ou have too many new preoccupations to undergo months of chemotherapy for a questionable benefit."

What model should be embraced? We recommend the informative model *in the research setting*. In the practice setting, this model is too sterile and its definition of autonomy is crimped. In the research setting, however, the decision to do the study creates strong pressures in favor of enlisting patients. Even the interpretive model offers the physician some room to convince himself that enrolling is what the patient wants. The informative model restricts the physician to the role of technocrat; indeed, the research setting makes him that at best.

The dual agent and good citizen models illuminate the situation too. The physician is a dual agent because he is both a physician-agent of the patient and a scientist-representative of science and his sponsor, with whom he has a contractual relationship. Just as we argued in the practice setting, the first obligation is to the patient, but the physician's contractual obligations to others cannot be ignored. The good citizen model sheds light through recognition of its nonapplicability. The physician-scientist should *not* consider science or society when discussing with a patient whether to enroll or stay in a study. Once again, the conflict between the patients' and others' interests is too great.

Allocation of Scarce Resources and Conflicts of Interest

Entanglements among industry, academia, and government are more bewildering when one considers another issue that will assume increasing importance as health care budgets are more tightly controlled: allocation. To what extent should researchers consider the potential costs of their work if it is commercialized? To some extent, any rational firm will consider the potential profitability of a product before deciding to market it. However, the fixed or tightly constrained health care budgetary climate and the "moral hazard" inherent in any form of insurance make it likely that the availability of any expensive new health care technology will lead to less money for childhood immunization (or breast cancer or cervical cancer screening, or cataract or hip replacement surgery for the elderly, etc.).

It would appear that government has a unique interest in ensuring that such conflicting priorities be considered at the earliest stage possible, that is, when deciding whether to research and develop a new technology in the first place. Yet any such limitation on discovery is anathema to the entrepreneurial spirit of industry and the inquisitive tradition of academia, that is, it is counter to the interests of government's new partners in the medical–industrial monolith. This might partially explain why government largely ignores questions of allocation at the research stage. It is ironic, for example, that government encourages health care cost containment but, at the same time, prohibits IRBs from even considering the possibility that the development of new treatments will exacerbate problems of accessibility to or equity in the distribution of health care.[21] Just as most ethicists argue that physicians must not consider costs to society when prescribing treatments for individual patients, the IRB regulations prohibit reviewers from considering costs to society when determining whether to approve individual research projects. Many years ago, a National Academy of Sciences committee studying this issue urged coordination in the research and development of new and expensive technologies. The coordination was to expressly take into account problems of accessibility and equity.[22] Such coordination regarding the artificial heart and other technologies has not occurred.

The federal government has, however, made a substantial effort to judge the efficacy of medical interventions and to discard those without demonstrable benefit. The Agency for Health Care Policy and Research (AHCPR) has led the development of multidisciplinary Patient Outcome Research Teams (PORTs) as a mechanism for determining the most cost-effective means for managing costly or common medical problems.[23] PORTs are large multi-institutional and multidisciplinary teams of academic and clinical practitioners, epidemiologists, statisticians, economists, and other specialists convened to review the relevant literature; to collect and analyze data on treatment variations, outcomes, and costs; and to disseminate their findings. Their findings are likely to result in the formulation of practice guidelines and will likely affect reimbursement for drugs, devices, and procedures not favored by the teams' findings. PORTs represent an interesting hybrid of clinical practice and clinical research (outcomes research). Although we cannot examine them here, Donaldson and Capron[24] have identified several issues that raise concern about conflicts of interest in PORTs themselves.

Related to but distinct from issues raised by PORTS, concern by government and private payers over the efficacy and cost of medical interventions has led to a shift in pharmaceutical companies' advertising, detailing, and research efforts. Advertising and detailing are now more than ever focused on relative efficacy and cost. Moreover, research efforts are directed increasingly to cost-effectiveness studies. This has spawned a new set of concerns about conflicts of interest and the objectivity and competence of such studies. Hillman and his colleagues have concluded: "Because economic analysis is poorly understood and unsupervised by an external agency, existing university policies to protect academic integrity are less able to detect and prevent bias in such studies than in other forms of research. Although the supervision of all types of clinical research may need strengthening, additional explicit guidelines are especially needed for economic analysis."[25]

Conclusion

Kurt's chapter demonstrates that the clinical research field is quickly changing. While government and its scientists were once primarily disinterested referees, they are now both collaborators–participants in and regulators of the clinical research process. This change continues a process begun with the forging of research ties between private industry and academia. This coalescence of previously separate centers of power threatens traditional research norms and arguably exacerbates the risk of exploitation of patient–subjects and the public interest. In this milieu, awareness about and study of conflicts of interest are more important than ever before.

As Huth points out, the conflicts of interest presented by academic–industry ties must be systematically studied to foster development of specific guidelines that will reconcile the various interests of all the participants. As Brody points out, scholars and public policy analysts should not overlook the conflicts of interest presented by all incentives—not just equity interests or consulting arrangements—offered by both industry and government. Regulatory mechanisms beyond disclosure or prohibition of equity and consulting fees must be created. Policies should be created that ameliorate conflicts of interest presented by several distinct points of decision-making in the clinical research process.

It is appropriate that Francis has explored the IRB process because, for one thing, many of the guidelines studied by Huth suggest that the IRB can be used to address conflicts of interest presented in the clinical research process. The Canadian Royal College Guidelines suggest review by an independent committee. Francis's chapter raises the question of whether IRBs are independent. If not, it is difficult to justify extension of their jurisdiction to conflicts of interest.

Perhaps more radical changes are needed. NIH has recently added another national level of review (a "super" IRB) for clinical research judged to be sensitive for a variety of reasons, including financial conflicts of interest.[26] It has also been suggested that neutral physicians should monitor the entire research process. This would include not only the informed consent process, the general construction of the clinical protocol, and the delineation of the characteristics of eligible subjects, but also the choice of individual subjects.[27] We will not explore these initiatives and proposals. That they have been conceived, however, shows the degree of concern engendered by ever-increasing coalescence of power and emergence of conflicts of interest. The need is greater now more than ever for careful empirical study of the effects of conflicts of interest, and for creative development of mechanisms to bridle those conflicts so as to preserve the goal of discovery of truth and knowledge for the benefit of the public interest.

Notes

1. We have avoided the term "experimentation" for the reasons explained by Robert Levine in *Ethics and Regulation of Clinical Research* 8 (1981). *See* also his discussion of "innovative practice," "nonvalidated" "interventions", and "therapeutic" versus "non-therapeutic." *Id.*, at 3 to 9.
2. J. Palca, AIDS Drug Trials Enter New Age, 246 *Science* 19 (1989).
3. *Informed Consent: Legal Theory and Clinical Practice* 247 (P. Applebaum, C. Lidz, and A. Meisel, eds., 1987), citing L. L. Park and L. Covi, Nonblind Placebo Trial: An Exploration of Neurotic Patients' Responses to Placebo When Its Inert Content Is Disclosed, 12 *Arch. Gen. Psychiatry & Psychology* 336 (1965).
4. Don Marquis, Leaving Therapy to Chance, 13 *Hastings Cent. Rep.* 40 (1983).
5. *See, e.g.*, Robert Levine, Clinical Trials and Physicians as Double Agents, 65 *Yale J. Biol. Med.* 65 (1992).
6. Samuel Hellman and Deborah Hellman, Of Mice But Not Men: Problems of the Randomized Clinical Trial, 324 *N. Engl. J. Med.* 1585 (1991).
7. Eugene Passamani, Clinical Trials: Are They Ethical?, 324 *N. Engl. J. Med.* 1589 (1991).
8. Stanley Reiser and Paula Knudson, Protecting Research Subjects After Consent: The Case for the "Research Intermediary," 15 *IRB* 1 (1993).
9. *See* Buchanan's discussion of the use of such mechanisms in Chapter 5 of this volume.
10. R. Steinbrook, AIDS Trial Shortchange Minorities and Drug Users, *Los Angeles Times* A1 (September 25, 1989); E. L. Kinney et al., Underrepresentation of Women in New Drug Trials, 95 *Ann. Intern. Med.* 495–499 (1981); P. Cotton, Examples Abound of Gaps in

Medical Knowledge Because of Groups Excluded from Scientific Studies, 263 *JAMA* 1051, 1055 (1990); and C. Levine, Women and HIV/AIDS Research: The Barriers to Equity, 13 *IRB* 18–22 (1991).

11. Clair Maatz, University Physician-Researcher Conflicts of Interest: The Inadequacy of Current Controls and Proposed Reform, 7 *High Tech. L.J.* 137, 156-159 (1992).

12. David Shimm and Roy Spece, Jr., Industry Reimbursement for Entering Patients into Clinical Trials: Legal and Ethical Issues, 115 *Ann. Intern. Med.* 148 (1991); and David Shimm and Roy Spece, Jr., Conflict of Interest and Informed Consent in Industry-Sponsored Clinical Trials, 12 *J. Legal Med.* 477 (1991).

13. Tom Reynolds, House Subcommittee Scrutinizes Taxol Agreements, 83 *J. Natl. Cancer Inst.* 1134 (1991).

14. John Carey, NIH Is Not the Institution It Was, *Newsweek* 145, 148 (November 5, 1990).

15. Rebecca Eisenberg, Academic Freedom and Academic Values, 67 *Tex. L. R.* 1363, 1389, 1398 (1988).

16. Telephone interview, July 12, 1993, with Elton Fewell, Business Manager, Biomedical Research Group, Inc., 3200 Red River, Suite 300, Austin, Tex. 78705.

17. Stuart Lind, Finder's Fees for Research Subjects, 323 *N. Engl. J. Med.* 192 (1990).

18. Telephone interview, July 15, 1993, with Harold Safferstein, Ph.D., Corporate Venture Manager, National Institute of Allergy and Infectious Diseases.

19. Arnold Relman, The New Medical–Industrial Complex, 303 *N. Engl. J. Med.* 963 (1980).

20. *See* our discussion of the informative model in Chapter 3 of this volume, text at notes 28 and 29.

21. 21 C.F.R. § 56.111(2) (1992); and 45 C.F.R. § 46.111(2) (1991). *See also* 46 *Federal Register* 8969 (January 27, 1981).

22. National Academy of Sciences, Institute of Medicine, *Disease by Disease Toward National Health Insurance?* (June 1973).

23. *Patient Outcomes Research Teams: Managing Conflicts of Interest* (Molla Donaldson and Alexander Capron, eds., 1991).

24. *Id.* at 47–59.

25. Alan Hillman *et al.*, Avoiding Bias in the Conduct and Reporting of Cost-Effectiveness Research Sponsored by Pharmaceutical Companies, 324 *N. Engl. J. Med.* 1362 (1991).

26. Richard Stone, NIH Adds an Extra Lawyer of Review for Sensitive Grants, 259 *Science* 1820 (1993).

27. David Meyers, *The Human Body and the Law* 267 (1990).

16

Regulation of Government Scientists' Conflicts of Interest

Thomas L. Kurt

In this chapter the motivations, conflicting interests, and conflicts of interest of government scientists will be compared and contrasted to those of scientists in academia and private industry. In particular, regulation of government scientists under existing federal statutes and regulations will be compared with the regulation of nongovernmental scientists under the regulations adopted in 1995 by the Public Health Service (PHS) for funded extramural research.[1] While government scientists may be less subject to conflicts of interest, this is less likely due to altruism than to the relatively detailed statutes and regulations to which government scientists are subject.

This chapter will also describe the Cooperative Research and Development Agreement (CRADA),[2] whereby government laboratories and scientists are now allowed, in a limited sense, to enter into joint ventures with private companies. Critics argue that CRADAs threaten the traditional independence of government scientists. I argue, however, that CRADAs were created with sufficient accompanying restrictions to prevent corruption of government scientists' objectivity and that they are justified by the need to retain scientists within the public service and to spur scientific and economic development.

Comparison of the Motivation of Private Sector, Academic and Government Scientists

Top level pharmaceutical industry scientists are, on the average, the highest–paid scientists.[3] They often have conflicting obligations as scientists to the pursuit of the truth and the scientific method and as corporate employees to their corporations and stockholders. There are no ethical codes binding corporate scientists other than those of the professional groups to which they belong and the code of the Pharmaceutical Manufacturers' Association (PMA). Academic researchers are, on the average, less well compensated than pharmaceutical company scientists. Although tenure is becoming more difficult to attain, academic researchers with tenure have greater security than corporate researchers. Most government scientists have civil service tenure, but they are even less well compensated than academic scientists.[4]

Academic scientists' compensation and prestige depend significantly on obtaining extramural grant funding. As Huth points out in Chapter 17, academic scientists are increasingly involved as consultants in institutional–business joint ventures or other financial arrangements with private companies. These arrangements raise the possibility of decreased scientific objectivity, compromised teaching, and inhibition of the traditional open exchange of information among academic scientists. This led the PHS in 1995 to adopt regulations addressing conflicts of interest in government–funded extramural research.[5]

The motivations, priorities, and expectations of government scientists arguably differ from those of other scientists in several ways:
1. Government scientists share responsibility for the public trust of more than 240 million U.S. citizens, not just that of an individual patient, client, customer, or institution;
2. In the competition for survival, reputation and glory are more important to private sector and academic scientists than to government scientists; and
3. Government scientists, as civil servants, function under rules that are extensions of federal law, are enforced by federal courts and magistrates, and involve major penalties.

Regulation of Government Scientists

Most government scientists with health-related tasks are employed by agencies of the executive branch, such as the National Institutes of Health (NIH), the Food and Drug Administration (FDA), and the Centers for Disease Control and Prevention (CDC). While these fall within the Department of Health and Human Services (DHHS), others are located in the Department of Agriculture, the Environmental Protection Agency, and elsewhere. They are governed by various federal laws and the Standards of Ethical Conduct for Employees of the Executive Branch.[6] The scope of the Standards is demonstrated in Table 16-1, the Standards' Table of Contents. The Standards are supplemented by individual agency rules and interpretations, all of which must be consistent with the Standards.[7] The Standards state that no scientist or employee is subject to disciplinary action if he acts in good faith in relying on the advice of an agency official given after full disclosure of all relevant circumstances.[8] To a certain extent, therefore, disclosure and obedience are reassuring to government scientists.

Although this chapter will not survey the Standards, it is helpful to consider the possible sources of conflicts of interest for government scientists and the basic regulatory approaches included in the Standards. Government scientists might skew their decision-making out of deference, fear, or loyalty to former employers; to those who give them gifts; to political officials with powers of appointment, removal, and influence; to strongly held ideological viewpoints; or to companies in which they have an investment or other monetary relationship. The Standards deal with these risks by prohibiting gift giving (with strict exceptions covered in guidelines), financial interests, payments from former employers, seeking certain other employment, and misuse of position (such as misuse of information); and by limiting permitted "outside activities."[9] The limited exceptions to these restrictions may not be used so frequently as to cause others to believe that the government scientist is using his official position for private gain.

No government employee can engage in outside employment activity where it conflicts with his official duties.[10] For any other outside government employment, like consultation (Table 16-2), prior permission must be obtained. No compensation is allowed for teaching, speaking, or writing that relates to the government employee's official duties.

If a government employee is subpoenaed to appear as a witness on a matter involving government business, or interpretation of a matter based on knowledge of government work, this must be approved by his superiors, usually with the discussion and consent of the general counsel for the government branch; otherwise, the general counsel will initiate proceedings to quash the subpoena.

Disclosure is required where potential financial conflicts of interest might arise. Each DHHS employee must annually file Form HHS-473 (Rev 1/82), "Confidential Statement of Employment and Financial Interests" (Table 16-3), as required by Section 402 of Executive Order 11222, dated May 8, 1965.[11] The items listed include, under "Employment and Financial Interests," all companies with which the government employee is connected as a consultant (contracting employee), regular employee, officer (such as the member of a board of directors or officer of a corporation), owner, or other relationship, or in which he has a continuing financial interest, such as a retirement plan (Table 16-3).[12] In

Table 16.1. Part 2635: Standards for Ethical Conduct for Employees of the Executive Branch

Subpart A	**General Provision**
Section	
2635.101	Basic obligation of public service.
2635.102	Definition.
2635.103	Applicability to members of the uniformed services.
2635.104	Applicability to employees on detail.
2635.105	Supplemental agency regulations.
2635.106	Disciplinary and corrective action.
2635.107	Ethics advice.
Subpart B	**Gifts from Outside Sources**
2635.201	Overview.
2635.202	General standards.
2635.203	Definitions.
2635.204	Exceptions.
2635.205	Proper disposition of prohibited gifts.
Subpart C	**Gifts Between Employees**
2635.301	Overview.
2635.302	General standards.
2635.303	Definitions.
2635.304	Exceptions.
Subpart D	**Conflicting Financial Interests**
2635.401	Overview.
2635.402	Disqualifying financial interests
2635.403	Prohibited financial interests.
Subpart E	**Impartiality in Performing Official Duties**
2635.501	Overview.
2635.502	Personal and business relationships.
2635.503	Extraordinary payments from former employers.
Subpart F	**Seeking Other Employment**
2635.601	Overview.
2635.602	Applicability and related considerations.
2635.603	Definitions.
2635.604	Disqualification when seeking employment.
2635.605	Waiver or authorization permitting participation whil seeking employment.
2635.606	Disqualification based on an arrangement concerning prospective employment or otherwise after negotiations.
Subpart G	**Misuse of Position**
2635.701	Overview.
2635.702	Use of public office for private gain.
2635.703	Use of nonpublic information.
2635.704	Use of government property.
2635.705	Use of official time.
Subpart H	**Outside Activities**
2635.801	Overview.
2635.802	Conflicting outside employment and activities.
2635.803	Prior approval for outside employment and activities.
2635.804	Outside earned income limitations applicable to certain Presidential appointees and othe noncareer employees.
2635.805	Service as an expert witness.
2635.806	Participation in professional associations (Reserved).
2635.807	Teaching, speaking, and writing.
2635.808	Fund raising activities.
2635.809	Just financial obligations

Table 16.2. Brief Contrast of Consulting with Collaboration

	Consultant	**Collaborator**
References	"Outside Work" NIH Manual Chapter 2300-735-4; date: 9/1/88	"Official Duty" Joint Ventures Information and Information Memorandum OD-84-2
	(ADAMHA) Administrative Management Instruction 12-6-1; date: 10/16/95	FTTA 1986
Time	On "own" time, i.e., evenings, weekends, or on annual leave	On government time
Compensation	Up to $12,500 per annum for one company, $25,000 total	As share of government; collect license fees and royalty income up to $100,000 per annum (unless President approves more)
Equity position	No stock ownership is permitted	No stock ownership is permitted
Service on board of directors	No	No
Service on scietnific advisory committee?	Yes, if not more than one-third of members are from NIH	No
Agreement utilized	Consulting agreement	CRADA

Table 16.3. HHS-473 (Rev. 1/82) Confidential Statement of Employment and Financial Interests.

Ask NIH and FDA staff for:

Part I: *Employment and Financial Interests:* List the names of all corporations, companies, firms, or other business enterprises, partnerships, nonprofit organizations and educational or other institutions (a) with which you are connected as an employee, officer, owner, director, member, trustee, partner, advisor or consultant, or (b) in which you have any continuing financial interests, through a pension or retirement plan, shared income or other arrangements as a result of any current or prior employment of business or professional association, or (c) in which you have any financial interests from the ownership of stock, stock options, bonds, securities, or other arrangements including trusts.

Part II: *Creditors:* List the names of your creditors *other than those* to whom you may be indebted by reason of a mortgage or property which you occupy as a personal residence or to whom you are indebted for...other expenses.

Part III: *Interests in Real Property:* List your interests in real property or rights in lands, other than property which you occupy as a personal residence.

Part IV: *Information Requested of Other Persons*

addition, creditors and interests in real property other than one's primary residence must be listed. These financial interests include the interests of "a spouse, minor child or other member of your immediate household...as [equivalent to] your [own] interest."[13]

The Historical Backdrop to Entrepreneurial Activities of Academic and Government Scientists

In the 1970s, many academic scientists joined with private industry to research and develop biotechnologies. Federal and state governments welcomed these joint ventures. Concerns raised by these activities—skewing of scientific priorities and judgment, interfering with training of new scientists, appropriating public resources, and stopping the flow of information within the scientific community—continue today. On the whole, however, policy makers have considered industry–academic interaction to be beneficial and have encouraged it.[14]

Many believe that one explanation for our failure to keep pace with Japan and Germany in certain endeavors was their greater cooperation among industry, academia, *and government*. For example, discoveries made in the United States were converted into useful products overseas, while only 5 percent of federal government patents were being licensed.[15] With this in mind, Congress passed the Stevenson-Wydler Technology Innovation Act of 1980, aimed at "stimulating improved utilization of federally funded technology developments by state and local governments and the private sector."[16] This legislation was complemented by the Bayh-Dole amendments to the U.S. patent laws, which changed the general rule that inventions developed with federal funds belonged to the federal government, so that ownership of most inventions developed by small businesses and nonprofit organizations belonged to those entities.[17]

Cooperative Research and Development Agreements (CRADAs)

Confusion over the authority of government laboratories to enter into cooperative agreements with private companies and uncertainty over rights to inventions resulting from such joint ventures continued to impede technology transfer from federal government laboratories to the marketplace. Moreover, lack of funding led to the problem of retaining qualified scientists within government service. The gap between government and private sector compensation packages was a substantial problem. This led to passage of the Federal Technology Transfer Act of 1986.[18] The Act permits the director of any government-operated federal laboratory to enter into CRADAs with academic and industry representatives in the private sector. CRADAs[19] have revolutionized the collaboration between government scientists and outside joint venturists.

Government laboratories can contribute information, personnel, services, facilities, equipment, or other resources to these joint ventures. Additionally, they can provide private sector partners with options, assignments, or licenses on any inventions that result from the venture. The private sector venturists can provide information, personnel, services, facilities, equipment, and operating funds.[20] The act also requires that (1) agencies operating large laboratories establish a program of cash awards for scientists who contribute in an exemplary manner to technology transfer, and that (2) royalties received by a federal agency under a CRADA be shared at a rate of at least 15 percent with the employee-inventor.

Certain aspects of CRADAs violate a strict reading of the federal conflict-of-interest statutes and regulations mentioned above. CRADAs have been encouraged, nevertheless, to retain government scientists and to spur scientific development. For example, under current law, an NIH scientist may not receive a "financial interest" that would result from a "particular matter" in which the scientist is engaged.[21] A literal reading would prohibit the same royalty payments that are *required* by the Technology Transfer Act. The justification behind the prohibition of certain financial interests is to prevent NIH scientists from being enticed away from their fundamental research mission by undue focus on commercial rewards and to discourage them from improperly favoring the subjects of the financial interests. The Office of Government Ethics has issued an advisory opinion that royalty payments under a CRADA do not constitute prohibited financial interests.[22]

This advisory opinion reconciles the Technology Transfer Act and conflict–of–interest rules in light of Congress's policies of fostering technology transfer and retaining government scientists. Yet, royalty payments do present conflicts of interest. Indeed, a specific federal statute prohibits any supplemental salary from being paid by an outside entity for the very reason that such additional compensation is thought to represent an intolerable conflict of interest.[23] But royalty payments are arguably *more likely* to present a conflict of interest than are supplemental salaries. Royalty payments are potentially very large and will occur only if the venture succeeds, while supplemental salary is fixed and likely a moderate sum. Royalty payments therefore would seem more likely to lure a government scientist into undue devotion to a commercial joint venture.

Optimum CRADA regulation might require amending the conflict–of–interest statutes and regulations to better balance the competing costs and benefits of CRADAs. For example, suppose it were determined that a supplemental salary would be likely to help retain scientists in government service and to encourage technology transfer, without much risk of encouraging neglect of the overall research mission, appropriating government resources and talent, losing objectivity, or restricting the free flow of scientific information. Assume further that

(1) because of their speculative and relatively infrequent nature, royalty payments were no better, or possibly worse, than supplemental salary at encouraging scientists to remain in government service, and (2) because of their potential size, royalty payments posed a substantial risk of luring government scientists into neglect of duty, secrecy, fixation on commercial gain, and even slanting data to enhance the likelihood of profit. If all this were true—and it *might* be in some instances—the law should be changed to allow supplemental salary and to limit royalty payments. One commentator has suggested that "the NIH might lawfully be permitted without legislative action to establish a pool of funds from collaborating companies and use it to supplement the salaries of scientists participating in a CRADA."[24]

This chapter will not suggest how the costs and benefits of CRADAs can be optimally balanced. The point is that scientists, policy makers, and academicians should constantly strive for better ways to limit the costs and maximize the benefits of CRADAs. CRADAs have increased rapidly, from 200 in 1990 to over 500 in 1992, spreading from NIH to other DHHS branches such as FDA and CDC.[25] The concept of allowing government scientists to collaborate (Table 16-2), especially on government time, offends many.[26]

Critics have pointed out that the usual openness of government scientists is disappearing, and that reporting of discoveries at scientific meetings and in journals is being delayed, due to the time necessary for discoveries to be patented by the CRADA joint ventures. This arguably betrays the public trust and diverts scientific or regulatory missions.[27] Furthermore, formerly harmoniously functioning teams of scientists could be diverted in many directions by multiple CRADAs. CRADAs have the potential to create confusion among and weaken the allegiance of government scientists. Originally their responsibility was to their own government agency and the public (quasi–stockholders). Now government scientists are arguably being torn from this traditional role by CRADAs.

On the other hand, CRADAs may help retain government scientists who would otherwise be tempted away by private industry. Also, advances in biotechnology are so rapid that collaboration is needed to compete with countries such as Japan, where government, industry, and academia cooperate. Similar cooperation in the United States might accelerate development, reduce government laboratory budgetary costs, provide collaborative funding, and spur global competition.[28]

PHS Regulations

Prior to 1995, guidelines in the PHS Grants Policy Statement on Standards of Conduct for Employees (of Grantee Organizations) were very simple.[29] They stated: "Recipient organizations must establish safeguards to prevent employees, consultants, or members of governing bodies from using their positions for purposes that are, or give the appearance of being, motivated by a desire for financial gain for themselves or others such as those with whom they have family, business, or other ties."[30] The intent of these simple guidelines was to ensure objective research not influenced by financial gain. On September 15, 1989, NIH proposed additional conflict–of–interest guidelines for extramural institutions receiving NIH and Alcohol, Drug Abuse and Mental Health Administration (ADAMHA) grants,[31] which provided for considerable responsibility and initiative within each institution. These were guidelines, not rules, and did not have exacting implications. Nevertheless, furious scientists and their supporters responded with over 700 letters within the ninety days allotted for comments.[32] Dr. Janet Newburgh, the Deputy Director of Extramural Affairs at NIH, indicated at that time that the first stage of rule making would apply only to "already commercially available" products, not to new inventions or investigational drugs.[33]

The next significant step in an ongoing process of revision was the Department of Health and Human Services (DHHS) 1991 publication of proposed regulations to ensure that PHS funded research would not be compromised by financial interests of investigators.[34] One hundred and two comments were received during the six-month comment period that followed.[35] Finally, in July 1995, PHS published its final regulations regarding Responsibility of Applicants for Promoting Objectivity In Research for Which PHS Funding is Sought.[36] Although these are binding regulations, as opposed to the NIH Guidelines proposed in 1989, the 1995 rules do not contain specific prohibitions as did the 1989 proposals, and they require disclosure of fewer financial interests.

Specifically, the 1995 regulations require that each grantee institution: (1) maintain and educate investigators about a written, enforced conflict of interest policy complying with certain criteria; (2) designate officials to solicit and review investigator financial disclosure statements; (3) require investigators to disclose "significant financial interests" that either would reasonably appear to be affected by the research for which PHS funding is sought or in entities whose financial interests would reasonably appear to be affected by the research; (4) provide guidelines to identify conflicts of interest and to allow them to be managed, reduced, or eliminated; (5) certify in each application for funding that (1) to (4) are complied with; and (6) report conflicting interests and how they will be handled prior to any grant expenditures.[37]

Significant financial interest is defined as "anything of monetary value, including but not limited to, salary or other payments for services (e.g., consulting fees or honoraria); equity interests (e.g., stocks, stock options or other ownership interests); and intellectual property rights (e.g., patents, copyrights and royalties from such rights)." Salary and intellectual property rights are excluded from the definition unless they exceed $10,000 aggregating each investigator's interests with those of his spouse or dependent children. Equity interests are excluded until they either exceed $10,000 or comprise greater than a five percent interest in a single entity, once again aggregating investigator, spouse, and dependent children's interests.[38]

The grantee official(s) designated to administer the institution's policies must:

> Review all financial disclosures; and determine whether a conflict of interest exists and, if so, determine what actions should be taken by the institution to manage, reduce or eliminate such conflict of interest. A conflict of interest exists when the designated official(s) reasonably determines that a Significant Financial Interest could directly and significantly affect the design, conduct, or reporting of the PHS-funded research. Examples of conditions or restrictions that might be imposed to manage conflicts of interest include, but are not limited to: (1) Public disclosure of significant financial interests; (2) Monitoring of research by independent reviews; (3) Modification of the research plan; (4) Disqualification from participation in all or a portion of the research funded by the PHS; (5) Divestiture of significant financial interests; or (6) Severance of relationships that create actual or potential conflicts.[39]

The institution must report investigators' failures to comply that have biased the design, conduct or reporting of PHS funded research and how the dereliction has or will be handled. The PHS then can "take appropriate action," direct the institution to take further action, or invite the institution to take further action. The PHS can audit institutions for compliance and identify conflicts that have been overlooked or improperly managed, and this can even lead to suspension of funding to the offending grantee. Finally, "[i]n any case in which the HHS determines that a PHS-funded project of clinical research whose purpose is to evaluate the safety or effectiveness of a drug, medical device, or treatment has been designed, conducted, or reported by an Investigator with a conflicting interest that was not disclosed or managed as required by this subpart, the Institution must require the Investigator(s) involved to disclose the conflicting interest in each public presentation of the results of the research."[40]

Conclusions

This chapter has compared and contrasted the motivations and conflicting interests of government scientists with those in academia and industry. While government scientists function under stringent rules with court-enforced penalties, there are minimal, primarily institutionally monitored regulations governing extramural PHS research. While government scientists function under explicitly detailed regulations with serious penalties, academic and industry scientists often complain (or their employers complain) about the minimal additional primarily self-enforced regulations adopted by PHS. An important issue for continuing debate is whether the regulations of academic and industry scientists should be brought closer to the stringent rules applied to government scientists.

In addition, this chapter has examined the new CRADA mechanism whereby government scientists can become cooperative venture capitalists with the private sector. With this concept expanding from NIH to other DHHS agencies such as FDA and CDC, hundreds of CRADAs now allow government to collaborate with private industry and academia. Disclosure is a key ingredient in these endeavors. While CRADAs may divert a government scientist's attention from his agency's mission, divide investigating teams, and delay reporting of scientific studies, they do appear to help retain government scientists and boost U.S. global competitiveness in biotechnology. On the other hand, CRADAs allow a kind of profit sharing that seems contradictory to the spirit of ethics regulation, even though it is allowed. Ongoing scrutiny and surveillance for conflict of interest are therefore mandatory.

Notes

1. 60 *Fed. Reg.* 35810-01, July 11, 1995, to be codified at 42 CFR Parts 50 and 94, effective October 1, 1995.
2. NIH/ADAMHA Patent Policy Board, *NIH Policy Statement on Cooperative Research and Development Agreements and Intellectual Property Licensing*, March 27, 1989, and April 24, 1989.
3. P. Coggeshall, et al., Changing Post-Doctoral Career Patterns for Biomedical Scientists, 202 *Science* 487, 493 (1979).
4. Thomas Bulleit, Public–Private Partnerships in Biomedical Research: Resolving Conflicts of Interest Arising Under the Federal Technology Transfer Act of 1986, 4 *J. Law & Health* 1, 2 (1989–90).
5. 60 *Fed. Reg.* 35810-01, July 11, 1995, to be codified at 42 CFR Parts 50 and 94, effective October 1, 1995.
6. Office of Government Ethics, Standards for Ethical Conduct for Employees of the Executive Branch, Final Rule, 5 CFR Part 2635, Part II, 57 *Fed. Reg.* 35006-35067, August 7, 1992, at 35006-35067.
7. Bulleit, note 4 *supra*, at 4; and Note, Regulating Conflicts of Interest in the Technology Transfer Age: Promoting Public Trust or Defeating Public Interests?, 40 *Drake L. Rev.* 385, 399–400 (1991).
8. *See* note 6 *supra*.
9. *Id.*
10. *Id.*
11. See Thomas Kurt, FDA Issues Concerning Conflicts of Interest, 12 *IRB* 6 (Sept/Oct.1990).
12. *Id.*
13. *Id.* and note 6 *supra*.
14. Bulleit, note 4 *supra*, at 4.
15. *Drake L. R.*, note 7 *supra*, at 400.
16. Public Law N. 96-480 (Codified at 15 U.S.C. § 3702(3) (1982)).

17. Bayh-Dole Amendments, Public Law No. 96-517, § 6(A) (1980) (codified at 35 U.S.C. §§ 201 (a)-(i) (1982)); Bulleit, note 4 *supra*, at 5.

18. *Id.* at 6–7.

19. *See* note 2 *supra*.

20. Bulleit, note 4 *supra*, at 7.

21. *Id.* at 11.

22. *Id.* at 13.

23. *Id.* at 10-11.

24. *Id.* at 17.

25. NIH/ADAMHA; *Industry Collaborative Directory*, NIH/ADAMHA, October, 1989; and Barbara Culliton, NIH, Inc.: The CRADA Boom, 245 *Science* 1034-1036 (1989).

26. Philip Chen, Jr., Perceptions of Impropriety or Conflict, NIH Office of Intramural Affairs.

27. *See* Bulleit note 4 *supra* and *Drake L. Rev.*, note 7 *supra*.

28. *See* notes 2 and 6.

29. Katherine Bick, Request for Comment on Proposed Guidelines for Policies on Conflict of Interest (Developed by the National Institutes of Health and the Alcohol, Drug Abuse, and Mental Health Administration), 18 *NIH Guide for Grants and Contracts* 1 (1989); and Thomas Kurt, FDA Issues Concerning Conflicts of Interest, 12 *IRB* page 6 (Sept/Oct 1990).

30. *Id.*

31. Joseph Palca, NIH Conflict-of-Interest Guidelines Shot Down, 247 *Science* 154-155 (1990); H.E. Bythman, Conflicts of Interest, 258 *Science* 1717 (1992) (letters); Eliot Marshall, When Commerce and Academe Collide, 248 *Science* 152-156 (1990); and Daniel Koshland, Conflict of Interest (editorial), 249 *Science* 109 (1990).

32. *See* note 31 *supra*.

33. M. Janet Newburg, Personal communication, June 20, 1990.

34. 59 *Fed. Reg.* 33242, June 28, 1994. At the same time, the National Science Foundation (NSF) published its Policy. The Policy was very similar to the regulations proposed by DHHS.

35. 60 *Fed. Reg.* 35810-01, July 11, 1995, to be codified at 42 CFR Parts 50 and 94, effective October 1, 1995. At the same time, NSF published revisions to its Investigator Financial Disclosure Policy to make it almost identical to PHS's regulations.

36. *Id.*

37. 42 CFR Section 50.604

38. 42 CFR Section 50.603.

39. 42 CFR Section 50.605.

40. 42 CFR Section 50.606.

17

Conflicts of Interest in Industry-Funded Clinical Research

For over a century, medical research has been growing in importance for the public's health. Why, then, has clinical research become a subject of intense public concern and governmental scrutiny only recently? Until World War II, medical research was largely laboratory based, only a small fraction involving clinical studies. Funded via medical school budgets, philanthropic foundations, or private sources, most clinical research was inexpensive and consisted largely of case studies relying on observation and simple laboratory investigations. However, the success of government-funded, war-related research led to increased government funding for basic and clinical research. This funding allowed many medical schools to become, in effect, medical universities, devoting only a small proportion of their effort to medical education leading to the MD degree. As expansion outpaced government funding, industrial sources of research funding made up the difference as pharmaceutical, biotechnology, and equipment firms recognized in medical schools the expertise, both basic and clinical, that could serve their needs.

The Food and Drug Administration's (FDA) requirements for documentation of the safety and efficacy of new drugs for which pharmaceutical firms seek FDA approval have been a second stimulus to clinical research. Although manufacturers can perform preclinical *in vitro* and animal studies, clinical studies of pharmacokinetics, toxicity, and efficacy require physician-investigators as collaborators to gain access to patients.

Emergence of Potential Conflicts of Interest in Clinical Research

Concerns about the scientific integrity of commercially supported academic research appeared as commercial support became more visible, coming into sharp focus in 1981[1] with a congressional hearing on commercial sponsorship of academic biomedical research. Academic physicians have worried that commercial support is intended to buy legitimacy for research that may or may not be honest and competent. A related concern has been that the academic tradition of open reporting of research findings might be abandoned to protect commercially valuable research findings.

Parties with Potentially Conflicting Interests

Conflicts of interest in clinical research resemble those in medical practice.[2] Both investigators and practicing physicians may be tempted to favor their financial (or other) interests over those of other parties whose interests should be paramount—especially patients and potential patients.

Erde argues in Chapter 2 that, in analyzing conflicts of interest, one should focus on structures as well as desires. In analyzing structures, one must consider all the agents who play a part in each structure. Each might embrace improper motives or act inappropriately, and each might be amenable to incentives to alter behavior.

The investigator serves at least six parties with interests, however remote, in the research. The investigator serves *personal professional and financial interests*. The investigator belongs to the *scientific community*, which needs reliable information and public respectability. The *investigator's institution* is served by the investigator's productivity, the reputation attached to good scientific studies, and financial support. The *patient* participates in a clinical trial hoping for benefit from the research or, at least, no harm. The fifth party is the commercial *sponsor* of the research. Such sources have been willing to fund reputable academic units to conduct the research needed to legitimize their products. Because nonprofit institutional or governmental funding sources generally have not held a vested interest in a particular outcome, few concerns have arisen over how the noncommercially funded investigator conducted research. The growth in commercial sponsorship, and the sponsors' vested interests in a favorable result, have raised concern about conflicts of interest. The final interested party is the *public*, whose tax support has been responsible for the vitality of academic medicine. Each of these parties—the investigator, the scientific community, the host institution, the commercial sponsors, patients, and the public—and its interests should be kept in mind as one considers possible responses to conflicts of interest in clinical research.

Issues Represented by "Conflict of Interest"

Congressional hearings and published commentaries in the 1980s identified five concerns relating to academic–industrial collaborations:

1. What are the risks that research might violate scientific standards? What might lead to a flawed study serving a commercial interest at the expense of reliable research?
2. Will industry collaboration shift university research away from basic questions and toward applied and market-oriented research?
3. Will such collaboration reduce the quality of graduate scientific education by minimizing educational objectives and using graduate students as cheap labor?
4. Will industry sponsors limit scientific communication to protect proprietary information?
5. How can an academic institution prevent exploitation of its resources through diversion of faculty effort and laboratory space to the industrial sponsor's interests? How will the federal government prevent diversion of its support for research to proprietary commercial interests at the expense of broader societal interests?

While some of these questions may be tangential to clinical research, together they imply that conflicts may arise among any of the six parties identified above.

Potential Guidelines for Clinical Research

Parties interested in clinical research want to safeguard their own interests and evaluate how the conduct of the other parties might affect their interests. Useful guidelines must be based on clear analysis of each party's desires and risks and a clear hierarchy of the desired outcomes for each party. Without such explicit grounding, the guidelines would appear *ex cathedra* and to be arbitrary.

One analytic approach is to apply Occam's razor to the interests of individual parties with a stake in clinical research. First, the interests of each of the six parties are listed in descending order of importance to each party. After weighing different parties' interests according to the parties' relative sizes and the ethical importance of their interests, the ordered array of interests can be examined for common themes, which can be used to establish a hierarchy of interests by giving priority to the most widely shared interests. Table 17-1 represents an unweighted array of the parties and their interests in clinical research.[3]

Table 17-1. Parties with Interests in Clinical Research.[a]

Party	Interest
The investigator	Gain in reputation through effective and properly published research
	Valid answers via properly designed trials
	Fair compensation for skills, effort, and time invested in research
The Patient	Effective treatment or accurate diagnosis
	Low risk of harm
	Investigator putting the patient's interests ahead of other interests
The Public[b]	Effective, safe, and inexpensive diagnostic methods and treatments
Minimal delay in applications of research	
	Least costly research
	Trust in scientific community
The Commercial Sponsor	Research relevant to marketing needs
	Prompt research findings
	Minimal cost
	Protection of allied financial interests such as patent opportunities
The Host Institution	Academic reputation
	Industrial financial subsidy of research compatible with other interests
	Protection of investment in plan and staff
	Marketing advantage due to enhanced reputation
The Scientific Community[c]	Good reputation of science in general
	Access to products of specific research efforts

NOTE: a) The hierarchies are those judged to be the probable interests, in descending order of priority. These are intended to illustrate an analytical technique for designing guidelines on conflicts of interest for interested parties. b) This includes government, since government mainly represents public interests. c) Scholarly journals have interests akin to those of the rest of the scientific community.

Using the above approach, the following hierarchy of all interests emerges:

1. Research leading to safe, effective, and inexpensive diagnostic methods and treatments.
2. Information available to enable all interested parties to judge how effectively their interests are protected.
3. Low risk/benefit ratio to patients or other research subjects.
4. Adequate information for decisions by the sponsor on further development or marketing.

5. Fair compensation to the investigator and the host institution for their participation.
6. Minimal cost to the sponsor.
7. Time-efficient conduct of research.
8. Protection of the scientific community's need for respect by the public and government.
9. Rapid dissemination of new information resulting from the research.

The leading interest for the group is that clinical research yield effective, safe, and inexpensive diagnostic methods and treatments. Such results can come only from research designed and conducted to yield relevant and reliable results.

This raises the question of which guidelines will reduce the risk of flawed research and will foster sound research. I suggest seven metaprinciples to guide the development of these guidelines.

1. Guidelines should encourage meeting technical and ethical standards for clinical research. This encouragement should be prescriptive, with guidance for the parties involved, rather than focusing on punishment.
2. All parties' expectations should be addressed, with attention to each party's benefits and risks.
3. Responsibility for supporting the highest–priority interests should devolve to those parties most able to act accordingly. For example, a host academic institution might be expected to be a surrogate for the public interest.
4. Standards and guidelines should be as explicit as possible, stated either in a document or by reference to externally published documents. The researcher should understand the standards by which he or she is expected to work.
5. Parties other than the researchers themselves should share responsibility for the scientific soundness and ethical integrity of the research. These include the commercial sponsor and the host institution.
6. The contract between the researcher and the sponsor should be explicit and should include the host institution as a partner or a fiduciary. This requirement, like that immediately above, spreads responsibility to all parties with high–ranking interests in the outcome of the work.
7. The guidelines should serve the highest–priority interests first.

Organizational Responses to Congressional and Other Public Concerns with Conflicts of Interest and Their Potential Undesirable Effects

Many professional societies responded to public concern over conflicts of interest by drafting guidelines addressing this issue. Although potential mischief due to conflicts of interest is great, the extent of actual bias is unknown.

Suspicion that the few well-known episodes represent the tip of the iceberg has probably arisen because of the increasing dependence of academic physicians on industrial support for clinical trials. Nevertheless, guidelines and policies developed by academic institutions, medical and scientific societies, and medical journals seem to affirm their belief that the risk of such conflicts of interest merits defenses.[4] I will now consider guidelines proposed by a number of prominent organizations. I will apply the metaprinciples described above to these guidelines in order to develop an ideal set of guidelines to protect the various interests of the affected parties listed above.

American College of Cardiology

The American College of Cardiology (ACC) convened a group of physicians, investigators, government administrators, and ethicists to consider ethics in clinical practice and research, which issued its report[5] in July 1990. The analysis concentrated on research where the investigator had, or appeared to have, financial interests hinging on the outcome of the research. These interests included "holding or receiving stock, stock options or other equity positions (other than remotely as through mutual funds)," repeated compensation for sponsored research, consultation, or lecture fees from a single company, royalties personally received or paid to family members, and lesser kinds of income such as entertainment, travel, and hospitality.

Three recommendations followed. First, the investigator must decide whether the arrangements and support for the research might lead to real or possible financial gains of the suspect types or even to the appearance of such possible gain. Second, if the investigator cannot avoid a financial gain or its appearance, the proposed research should be reviewed by the institution accommodating the research, with the review conducted "by disinterested persons who are mindful of the interests of science and the public as well as the responsibilities of the investigator and the institution." Third, the investigator must identify "a real or apparent conflict" in publications and presentations resulting from the research, in consultations, and in reviews (presumably of others' research proposals and of papers undergoing peer review for journals).

Several points about this analysis merit comment. First, the task force distinguishes between commercial and academic settings: "a role that may be considered acceptable for a scientist identified and recognized as an employee of a commercial firm may be considered unacceptable for one identified and recognized as a faculty member of an academic institution." Although this implies that the commercially employed investigator has responsibilities to the public and science as a discipline that differ from those of the academically based investigator, the task force does not indicate on what basis it makes this distinction.

The report represents its recommendations not as proscriptions but as "affirmative responsibilities." Second, the report emphasizes the investigator's decisions and leaves the host institution with only a fallback responsibility.

Compared to the metaprinciples, the ACC guidelines support research standards only in a hortatory sense, without any explicit standards. That good science should be the leading interest is only implicit. The expectations and responsibilities of the various agents are unclear. The guidelines are sensitive to the appearance of investigators' financial conflict of interest; however, they involve the host institution in the financial arrangements only with clear investigator conflict of interest. That the host institution should share responsibility for proper design and conduct of the research and for financial arrangements does not represent a major emphasis of these guidelines.

American College of Physicians

Although the American College of Physicians' (ACP) Ethics Manual[6] focuses mainly on conflicts of interest in practice, it does raise several relevant points in its section on research. The first is that "the basic principle underlying all research is honesty," a premise that can be taken to imply that conflicts of interest in research should be resolved to put a priority on maintaining honest research. Honesty is ensured by having "institutional protocols...in place." The standard of honesty is joined a few sentences later by the need to maintain "integrity...in all stages of research." This section also recommends that "the sources of funding for the research project must be disclosed to potential collaborators in the research and in publications."

These conclusions stand *ex cathedra*, do not stem from explicit principles, and are not supported by analysis. Consideration of the need for honesty is not paralleled, for example, by consideration of the dependence of the public and of the host academic institution for valid experimental design to ensure that research findings are reliable. Research can be incompetent but honest, and this violates the public's expectation for reliable scientific data. Like the ACC guidelines, the ACP guidelines are largely hortatory, with little explicit guidance. Further, like the ACC guidelines, there is little emphasis on shared responsibility for scientific and financial oversight.

American Medical Association

The Councils on Scientific Affairs and on Ethical and Judicial Affairs of the American Medical Association (AMA) analyze the relationships among investigators, medical centers, and commercial enterprises in their paper "Conflicts of Interest in Medical Center/Industry Research Relationships".[7] The analysis is largely concerned with the possibility that potential financial gains may lead to distortion of the scientific process and loss of integrity, but it also calls attention to other issues, for example, obstruction to the free flow of scientific information. These guidelines distinguish between real and perceived conflicts. The question of appearances leads to the need for accountability (presumably to external parties—the public, government, and professional societies) on the part of the host institution and the investigator.

This analysis' recommendations can be paraphrased as follows:

1. Professional societies should inform their members of real and apparent risks and benefits in medical center–industry joint ventures; presumably these ventures include those arranged by investigators themselves.
2. Medical centers should develop guidelines on conflicts of interest for their staff.
3. An investigator should not buy or sell a company's stock from the time the joint venture begins until the time the results are known by the public, either directly or through scientific publication of a report.
4. Remuneration of the investigator by the commercial sponsor "must be commensurate with the efforts" of the investigator in its behalf.
5. Material ties to companies must be disclosed to the host institution, to other sponsors, and in published reports.
6. Medical centers should form review committees to examine staff's "financial associations" with commercial sponsors.

The AMA guidelines fall short of the proposed metaprinciples. Material suggestions appear only in recommendations 3–5 above; experiment design and execution are not addressed. The proposed review committees (recommendation 6) are to oversee protection of human subjects, observance of governmental rules and regulations, and adherence to financial constraints. Sharing of responsibility with the host institution is addressed only in the development of explicit guidelines (recommendation 6).

American Psychological Association

Many sections of the American Psychological Association's (APA) guidelines[8] relate to conflict of interest and can be used to develop specific guidelines, as illustrated:

> When undertaking research, [psychologists] strive to advance human welfare and the science of psychology. [Principle F]

> Psychologists...take reasonable steps to ensure the competence of their work and to protect patients, clients,...research participants, and others from harm. [1.04 Boundaries of Competence]

> Psychologists recognize that their personal...conflicts may interfere with their effectiveness. Accordingly, they refrain from undertaking an activity when they know or should know that their personal problems are likely to lead to harm to a

patient, client, colleague, student, research participant or other person to whom they may owe a professional or scientific obligation. [1.13 Personal Problems and Conflicts]

Psychologists take reasonable steps to avoid harming their patients or clients, [and] research participants,...and to minimize harm where it is foreseeable and unavoidable. [1.14 Avoiding Harm]

A psychologist refrains from entering [into a]...scientific, professional, or financial...relationship...if it appears likely that such a relationship might reasonably impair the psychologist's objectivity or otherwise interfere with...effectively performing his or her functions as a psychologist. [1.17 Multiple Relationships] Psychologists appropriately document their professional and scientific work...to ensure accountability, and to meet other requirements of institutions or the law. [1.23 Documentation of Professional and Scientific Work]

Psychologists design, conduct, and report research in accordance with recognized standards of scientific competence and ethical research. [6.06 Planning Research]

Psychologists obtain from host institutions or organizations appropriate approval prior to conducting research, and they provide accurate information about their research proposals. They conduct the research in accordance with the approved research protocol. [6.09 Institutional Approval]

These standards and procedures comport with the metaprinciples proposed. However, they lack recommendations on modes of compensation. Clearly, these elements could be readily placed in a procedural framework of practical value.

Royal College of Physicians

A paper prepared by a Working Party of the British Royal College of Physicians (RCP)[9] considered the influence of pharmaceutical firms on physicians' practices, while two additional documents[10] proposed more detail on experimental design. The RCP recommended:

1. Formal arrangements should be made directly with the firm.
2. Financial processing should be through the host institution.
3. Compensation can be used for legitimate clinical and educational programs of the host institution.
4. The research physician should not "have any personal financial interest in studies carried out on patients under his care," and it is "reprehensible to advertise the availability of his own or his colleagues' patients for use as research subjects."
5. The research physician has a responsibility to ensure the scientific integrity of the research:
   a. To ensure their scientific merit and competent planning;

b. To get the approval for the research of an independent committee on ethical research that is fully informed of the financial arrangements.

6. The physician must be free to report the research in a journal of his or her choice and without influence from the company on publication of the report. Reasonable requests for delay of publication for protection of patent rights may be acceded to.

The RCP guidelines generally comport with the proposed metaprinciples by involving the host institution in the financial arrangements and by specifically addressing experimental design.

US National Academy of Sciences

In 1992, the U.S. National Academy of Sciences (NAS) issued, *Responsible Science: Ensuring the Integrity of the Research Process.*[11] It considers potential threats to scientific integrity arising from university–industry cooperation; discusses conflicts of interest, including those that may arise from researchers' desire for personal profit or temptations to influence competing researchers' positions in the peer review and publication processes; and recommends that "disclosure, either public or institutional, is essential," disclosure being the responsibility of the scientist. This NAS report closes with twelve formal recommendations, one of which suggests what academic institutions might do in response to faculty conflicts of interest that might impair the quality of their research: "Adoption of formal guidelines for the conduct of research, which can provide a valuable opportunity for faculty and research institutions to clarify the nature of responsible research practices, should be an option, not a requirement, for research institutions."

The discussion that follows does not indicate why adoption of guidelines should be "an option, not a requirement." A recommendation that "formal guidelines...should be adopted...and take into account local situations" would have greater force. Who might "require" guidelines is not stated—institutional governing bodies, state or federal governing bodies?

The minimal attention in the report devoted to conflicts of interest prompted a "Minority Statement" that "conflicts of interest directly related to research can be more complex, potentially more serious and perhaps more numerous than the examples of fabrication, falsification, and plagiarism, and therefore need to be addressed in this report."

These guidelines are largely hortatory and do not specifically address the metaprinciples. In particular, there is no significant involvement by the host institution in financial or scientific oversight, and no guidance regarding acceptable versus unacceptable financial or scientific practices.

The Institute of Medicine

At the request of the Veterans Administration (VA), in 1989 the Institute of Medicine convened a workshop[12] charged with identifying and considering problems that might arise when VA researchers collaborate with industry. The workshop also considered how such problems were being handled in other government agencies. It concluded that such collaborations might be fruitful but that more time was needed for assessment of the possibilities. No specific guidelines for research collaboration with industry were developed, but the workshop sketched out five central issues that needed further addressing:

1. Clarification of the values, missions, and relationships of collaborative institutions, including government agencies, industrial organizations, and academic institutions
2. The nature of guidelines on conflicts of interest that might guide researchers in government agencies, and how the guidelines might relate to legal and ethical precedents and deal with questions of real and apparent of conflicts
3. Continuing education and communication among all the parties in existing and potential collaborations
4. Differences in practices and standards among collaborative parties
5. Questions of disclosure and disqualification requirements and their possible effects.

The previous year, the Institute had convened a workshop with a much broader scope—"Responsible Conduct of Research in the Health Sciences." Its report[13] is useful for its review of preceding academic, professional, and governmental efforts to identify and handle issues related to the proper conduct of research. The breadth of the charge to the workshop precluded its examining issues of conflict of interest in detail, but some of the recommendations developed are relevant:

1. The National Institutes of Health should develop and monitor high standards for research in grantee and applicant institutions, with an NIH office charged with this and related duties
2. Universities, medical schools, and other research organizations should develop guidelines indicating the standards of research conduct to be followed by their investigators
3. These organizations should designate specific individuals, and perhaps committees, to promote responsible research and to guide investigators
4. Professional and scientific societies should support studies to identify and encourage responsible practices in research.

How these recommendations might be specifically applied in settings of conflicts of interest was not developed, but they are in accordance with the metaprinciples calling for host institutions to share responsibilities with investigators.

Public Health Service (PHS) and National Science Foundation (NSF)

In 1994, NSF published its Investigator Financial Disclosure Policy at the same time the PHS issued proposed regulations on the same topic. PHS adopted regulations in July of 1995, while, at the same time, NSF revised its policy to conform almost completely to the new PHS regulations. The history and content of these regulations is described in Chapter 16 by Thomas Kurt. The PHS regulations meet some, but not all, of the metacriteria described above. First, although they do not attend to technical requirements of research and ignore ethical issues such as informed consent and disclosure to subjects, they do focus on the ethical issue of conflicts of interest. Second, the regulations, both in the process that generated them and in their content, seem to represent an attempt to accommodate certain interests of all the relevant parties. Third, the regulations place responsibility for suggesting the highest-priority interests with the parties most able to act accordingly. For example, responsibility for protecting research subjects is primarily placed with investigators, while the general public interest in objective research is the principal responsibility of grantees' institutions. Fourth, the regulations require explicit local guidelines that are made known to investigators. Fifth, the host institution and PHS share responsibility for the objectivity of the research, e.g., the host institution must enforce its guidelines with sanctions and PHS can audit the hosts' compliance and even suspend funding. However, the regulations do not specifically address the responsibilities of sponsors. Sixth, the regulations do not directly address the contract between the researcher and sponsor. Seventh, the regulations seem to focus on lower priority items such as protection of the scientific community's need for respect by the public and government and rapid dissemination of new information, paying little attention to high priority items such as the need for safe, effective, and inexpensive diagnostic methods and treatments and assuring availability of information to enable all interested parties to judge how effectively their interests are being protected.

National Council on Bioethics in Human Research

The National Council on Bioethics in Human Research, established by the Medical Research Council of Canada and the Royal College of Physicians and Surgeons of Canada, organized a workshop to consider a range of issues in clinical trials and issued a draft paper[14] addressing conflicts of interest. A research ethics board prepared to review proposed trials and monitor ongoing trials is vital to many of the recommendations.

1. Clinical trials should be undertaken only if they will be scientifically valid.
2. Physicians and other professionals engaged in clinical trials must have the scientific competence needed to conduct and interpret them.

3. The board judging the scientific and ethical validity of a trial must be independent of the investigators and the industrial sponsor.

4. Methods should be established for monitoring the accuracy of the clinical data and reporting to all interested parties (subjects, investigators, sponsors, regulatory authorities) any fraudulent or erroneous data already published.

5. Investigators and review boards must agree on how to monitor adherence to the approved protocol.

The draft has detailed recommendations on financial arrangements of collaboration.

1. The investigator should support trust in his or her work by not owning equity in the sponsoring firm during the trial. This should apply to associates who might influence the conduct of the trial or get trial results. Conflicts of interest must be disclosed to the review board and may be the basis for its disapproving a trial.

2. Financial arrangements must be available and acceptable to the review board. Disclosure to subjects can be included in the consent form.

3. Financial compensation to the investigator should be consistent with norms for the work and should not include a salary, gifts, or benefits that indirectly represent excessive compensation.

4. Payments should generally not be based on the number of subjects enrolled.

5. Incremental costs should be borne by the industrial sponsor rather than the academic institution.

6. Compensation to subjects for untoward events must be explicitly addressed.

7. Payments to subjects should not be so large as to serve as a major inducement to participate.

These recommendations give detailed guidance on how to minimize bias in research design and execution and how to minimize the possibility of financial conflicts of interest. They do not, however, spread responsibility for financial arrangements beyond noting that the host institution should approve the compensation for the investigator. Insisting that payment for the investigator be channeled through the host institution would be more consistent with the metaprinciples.

Responses of Medical Journals

Journals should ensure, to the extent possible, that they publish research designed, conducted, analyzed, and reported in accordance with generally accepted standards for scientific evidence, through peer review and editorial discretion and judgment. Journals generally have tried to deal with investigator conflicts of interest via disclosure. Representative of such efforts are the positions taken by the *Journal of the American Medical Association*[15] and *Science*.[16] Authors are expected to indicate "potential conflicts-of-interest" to the editors. These journals do not indicate how their editors will use this information. External reviewers might be alerted to the authors' financial interests, perhaps to suggest that such reports be scrutinized more closely than otherwise.

A Proposal for Ideal Guidelines

All the reviewed guidelines address conflicts of interest to some extent, and the Canadian guidelines closely approach an ideal set. Using the array of interested parties and their hierarchy of interests as outlined in Table 16-1, and choosing elements from the above sets of guidelines, I propose the following guidelines, arranged in the order in which they should be applied.

1. The research sponsor should provide the investigator with all available information, in written form, that might be relevant to the interests of the investigator, of patients, of the public, and of the host institution.

2. The sponsor should provide the potential investigator with a detailed written description of the research it desires; of its expectations of the investigator before the research is begun, during, and after completion; of the investigator's right to modify the proposed research; of the investigator's right to disseminate and publish the results of the research; and of the compensation to the investigator and to the host institution. The proposal should also indicate how liability will be managed, including compensation to subjects for injury from the research.

   The detailed research proposal should include justification for the research, a specific protocol for research design and methods, a clear estimate of possible risks and benefits to research subjects, a description of the procedures for seeking the informed consent of subjects, a description of methods for maintaining research records, and a description of the proposed relations among the investigator, the host institution, and the sponsor during and after the research. The proposal should also include itemized budgets describing compensation by the sponsor to the investigator, to the host institution, or to both for the research; this section should stipulate compensation for incomplete as well as completed research. The sponsor should not compensate the investigator directly but rather via the host institution.

3. The written proposal acceptable to both the sponsor and the investigator should be presented to the host institution for review. The review should be carried out formally by an institutional standing body, with members equipped by education, training, and experience to judge the proposal critically with regard to both ethical and scientific questions. This review should cover the potential importance of the proposed research to patients

and the public, the potential risks for subjects, the adequacy of information to be made available to subjects (and, if necessary, to their families or guardians), the likelihood that the experimental design will answer the questions posed, and the right of the host institution to be informed of the progress (including protocol changes) and results of the research, and how that information will be made available to it and the other interested parties. The reviewing body should be free to query both the investigator and the sponsor at any point during the review with regard to any aspect of the proposal, and to receive written as well as oral replies.

The reviewing body should develop guidelines for the institution and its investigators on both procedure and documentation, especially if it has circumstances that make external guidelines not entirely suitable.

If the host institution cannot review the proposed research for scientific, fiscal, and ethical issues, it should seek such expertise from another institution with the needed competence and experience for such reviews.

4. The reviewing body should prepare a written account of its conclusions, including an opinion on the acceptability of the compensation proposed by the sponsor. This document should be reviewed by both the sponsor and the investigator as a basis for further negotiation or for signed acceptance by them.

5. Once the sponsor, investigator, and host institution have agreed on a written proposal, the research can proceed.

6. As the research proceeds, the investigator should maintain written records of the procedure and its findings, including the information given to potential subjects during informed consent, and the proportions of subjects consenting to and refusing the proposed study.

7. During the research, the investigator, the commercial sponsor, and the host institution should keep each other informed of any events that might bear on departure from the agreed-on proposal or on unanticipated risks to subjects.

8. On completing the research, the investigator should submit to the sponsor and to the host institution a written report of all research findings, anticipated or not, whether or not they favor the interests of the sponsor.

9. Unless an exception has been agreed on, the investigator will be free to, and should, report the research findings via customary means to the scientific community. Results that cannot be published because of length restrictions imposed by journals should be made available on request to interested parties unless the research agreement explicitly excluded this— for example, for protection of patent rights.

10. All records of the research—including the proposal, informed consent procedure and results, research findings, and communications among the

investigator, the sponsor, and the host institution—should be retrievable for at least five years.

In summary, these guidelines emphasize procedures and methods to prevent any lapses from scientific and ethical standards due to conflicts of interest. Principal responsibility is borne by sponsors, investigators, and host institutions, the last serving as surrogates for the public and government (which could be brought into the process only with difficulty while preserving the process). The main requirements are that the process be deliberate, systematic, and thorough and that documentation of the participation and opinions of each party be kept. These ideal guidelines satisfy the metaprinciples proposed above by providing explicit description of each party's scientific and financial obligations, and by closely involving the host institution in oversight of the scientific and financial arrangements between the investigator and the sponsor. Note that issues of fair compensation are shared with the sponsor as well as with the host institution, which has more to lose from faulty or fraudulent research. These guidelines do not explicitly address equity interests of the host institution, because they are not necessarily germane to the intent of the guidelines—valid and unbiased scientific research. A large profit for the host institution for well-conducted and important research is more defensible ethically than a small profit for the investigator for biased or fraudulent research. Many institutions may wish, however, to prohibit equity interests for themselves as well as for investigators for appearance.

Issues for the Future

In planning for the future, we are hampered by ignorance about how often and how severely investigators yield to desires for financial (and other) gain by abandoning scientific standards. How many IRBs have explicit standards for evaluating research and adequate monitoring procedures? Since most clinical research in the United States is conducted in medical school–affiliated hospitals, the one organization setting national standards for academic medicine, the American Association of Medical Colleges, could collaborate with organizations representing other major parties (such as the American Federation for Clinical Research and the Pharmaceutical Manufacturers Association) in drafting guidelines and standards.

Attention to conflicts of interest on the part of the public and the scientific community[17] is likely to increase. On one side, the economic pressures on medical institutions, medical schools, and their hospitals, will increase; these establishments will continue to seek commercial support consistent with their academic aims and standards. The public and government will increasingly demand research of adequate quality at low cost. This is the central issue, not whether investigators may profit (e.g., through equity interests in the sponsoring firm). Some commentators' preoccupation with equity interests appears based on the premise that "a man can always be bought at some price."[18] As Brody points out in Chapter 18, the control of investigator conflicts of interest should be designed to ensure good science. For the public at large, the income of the individual investigator is not likely to be an important and central interest; the quality of medical care is a central issue, and that quality will depend in part on competent and honest research, regardless of the investigator's earnings. The high costs of medical care in the United States have brought pharmaceutical firms and hospitals under close and hostile scrutiny, and this hostility could spill over to medical research. Keeping medical research honest by requiring that it meet high standards[19] is necessary to ensure ongoing public faith in, and funding for, biomedical research.

Notes

1. Kathi Hanna, Biomedicine: Resolving Conflicts, Collaborative Research, in *Government and Industry collaboration in Biomedical Research and Education* (1989).
2. Sanford Teplitzky, Physician Ownership and Patient Interests: Where Are the Boundaries?, 30 *Internist* 6 (August 1989).
3. These judgments are necessarily personal and have been deduced from pieces of evidence too numerous and informal for documentation here. They are not based on any published consensus assessments, although they and their hierarchies might be deduced from some of the guidelines reviewed later in this chapter. They might differ from arrays developed by formal inquiry, as in a delphic process.
4. While some of these actions may be due to influential members of the relevant groups having personal knowledge of such violations, they also might be simply the result of wanting to appear to be against sin.
5. American College of Cardiology, 21st Bethesda Conference: Ethics in Cardiovascular Medicine, October 5–6, 1989, 16 J. *Am. Coll. Cardiol.* 1 (1990).
6. Ethics Committee, American College of Physicians, *American College of Physicians Ethics Manual* (3d ed., 1992).
7. Council on Scientific Affairs and Council on Ethical and Judicial Affairs, American Medical Association, Conflicts of Interest in Medical Center/Industry Research Relationships, 263 *JAMA* 2790 (1990).
8. American Psychological Association, Ethical Principles of Psychologists and Code of Conduct, 47 *Am. Psychologist* 1597 (1992).
9. Working Party, Royal College of Physicians, The Relationship between Physicians and the Pharmaceutical Industry, 20 *J. Roy. Coll. Physicians* 235 (1986).
10. Working Party on Research Involving Patients, Royal College of Physicians, *Research Involving Patients*, (1990); and College Committee on Ethical Issues in Medicine, Royal College of Physicians, *Guidelines on the Practice of Ethics Committees in Medical Research Involving Human Subjects* (2d ed., 1990)

11. Panel on Scientific Responsibility and the Conduct of Research, National Academy of Sciences, *Responsible Science: Ensuring the Integrity of the Research Process* (1992). A number of papers in Volume II of the report are especially relevant to conflict of interest—a survey by Mark S. Frankel, "Professional Societies and Responsible Research Conduct" (which includes a list of scientific societies that have issued guidelines on ethical conduct and related matters), and guidelines on diverse aspects of research conduct issued by the NIH, the Harvard University Faculty of Medicine, the Johns Hopkins School of Medicine, the University of Michigan School of Medicine, and the Massachusetts Institute of Technology.

12. Committee on Government and Industry Collaboration in Biomedical Research and Education, Institute of Medicine, *Government and Industry Collaboration in Biomedical Research and Education* (1989).

13. Committee on the Responsible Conduct of Research, Division of Health Sciences Policy, Institute of Medicine, *The Responsible Conduct of Research in the Health Sciences* (1989).

14. Gerald Klassen, Bioethics When Undertaking Clinical Trials, 2 *National Commission on Bioethics in Human Research Communique* 19 (1991).

15. George Lundberg and Annette Flanagin, New Requirements for Authors: Signed Statements of Authorship Responsibility and Financial Disclosure, 262 *JAMA* 2003 (1989); and Drummond Rennie, Annette Flanagin and Richard Glass, Conflicts of Interest in the Publication of Science, 266 *JAMA* 266 (1991).

16. Daniel Koshland, Jr., Conflict of Interest Policy, 257 *Science* 595 (1992).

17. Marcia Barinaga, Confusion on the Cutting Edge, 257 *Science* 616 (1992).

18. Edward Huth, Conflict-of-Interest Rules as They Relate to Clinical Investigation: What Should They Be?, 45 *Food, Drug, Cosmetic L. J.* 511 (1990).

19. Curtis Meinert, *Clinical Trials: Design, Conduct, and Analysis* (1986); and Bert Spilker, *Guide to Clinical Trials* (1991).

18

Conflicts of Interests and the Validity of Clinical Trials

Baruch A. Brody

This chapter deals with the structuring of clinical trials to avoid potential conflicts of interest between the economic interests of the investigators and the interest of society at large in obtaining scientifically valid results from clinical trials. This problem has received extensive discussion in the last few years, a discussion greatly stimulated by the revelations in 1987–88 of the stockholding by some clinical investigators of tPA, a thrombolytic agent, at Genentech, the company that manufactured tPA. Some have looked into the licitness of the behavior of particular investigators in the tPA trials; my concern, however, is not with particular individuals but rather with the broader policy issue. This observation is particularly important, for, as I shall shortly show, many have been led, by excessive attention to the details of stockholding at Genentech, to miss the broader issues and to propose solutions that are incomplete.

I will first examine the reasons for being concerned with conflicts of interest, arguing that they are very different from the concerns about scientific fraud and misconduct that have also attracted much interest recently. The real reasons for concern will then be illustrated by examples drawn from the trials of various thrombolytic agents. Then I will argue that the conflict-of-interest issue is far broader than the stockholding question, and that the various proposals have surfaced (which focus on stockholding and other relations with drug companies) are therefore inadequate. I will end by putting forward some proposals of my own for dealing with this set of problems.

Conflict of Interest versus Fraud

The original *Newsday* article that called attention to the stockholding in Genentech[1] discussed the possibility that this type of conflict of interest might lead to fraud in research, that is, to the publication of incorrect data. The report of Congressman Ted Weiss's subcommittee at the end of its hearings, which combined investigations into fraudulent misconduct with investigations into conflicts of interest, was entitled "Are Scientific Misconduct and Conflicts of Interest Hazardous to our Health?",[2] and may also have encouraged the view that conflicts of interest are troubling because they will lead to publication of fraudulent data. But I want to argue that this concern with fraudulent data is not central precisely because the design of contemporary clinical trials makes it difficult to perpetrate frauds. Instead, the concern should be with how conflicts of interest may lead investigators, perhaps unconsciously, to make inappropriate decisions about the design and conduct of clinical trials. Let me explain.

Many standard features of modern clinical trials are designed, at least in part, to protect against fraud. The fact that patients are randomly assigned to the various treatment arms in a clinical trial means that the investigators cannot assign more favorable cases to their favorite treatment. The fact that neither the subjects nor the investigators know which treatment the patient is getting (i.e., that the trial is double-blinded) makes it difficult (although not always impossible, since you can sometimes know from other clinical data which treatment a subject is getting) for the investigators to improve the data on patients getting their favorite treatment. The fact that the clinical data are often gathered and analyzed by an independent group (a central lab and/or data analysis group) prevents investigators from perpetrating fraud in the manipulation of the data. I do not want to suggest that these measures are foolproof. What I do want to say is that if fraud were our real concern, we would do best to focus on improving these features of modern clinical trials to make fraud highly unlikely.

What then are the concerns with conflicts of interest? It seems to me that the concerns grow out of the recognition that many decisions have to be made about both the design and implementation of a clinical trial, and that these decisions provide ample opportunity for those with a conflict of interest to make decisions that promote their favored treatment. This may be a conscious process, in which case we are dealing with personal guilt, or it may be an unconscious process, in which case we are not. In either situation, the social problem of how to minimize these inappropriate decisions remains.

Some of these decisions have to do with the design of the clinical trials. The issues include the following: (1) Which treatments will be tested in the proposed trial, and which ones will not be tested?; (2) Will there be a placebo control group as well, or will the treatments be tested against each other or against some active control group?; (3) What will be taken as the favorable endpoint (the result constituting the evidence of efficacy of the treatment), and what will be taken as the adverse endpoint (the result constituting the evidence of the dangerousness of the treatment)?; (4) What will be the condition for inclusion or exclusion of subjects from the trial?; (5) What provisions will be made for informed consent, and what information will be provided as part of the informed consent? Some of these decisions have to do with the actual conduct of the clinical trial. They include the following: (6) Under what conditions will the trial be stopped or modified because there have been too many adverse endpoints in one or more arm of the trial or because the preliminary data have shown that one of the treatments is clearly the most efficacious treatment? (7) Under what conditions will the trial be stopped or modified because of the newly available results of other trials? (8) Which patients who meet the criteria will actually be enrolled, and which ones will not?

These are only some of the many questions that inevitably will arise in the design and conduct of clinical trials. The answers will profoundly influence the results of the trial, with some answers being more favorable to one treatment than to another. In some cases, the answers to these questions will be straightforward, so the opportunity for biased, flawed decision-making will be modest. In other cases, the answers will be far from obvious, with great potential for conflicts of interest leading, consciously or unconsciously, to flawed decision-making. In either case, however, the actual data are not fraudulent. Therefore, flaws in design, rather than fraudulent data, are the reason we need to be concerned with conflicts of interest.

Illustration of the Conflict of Interest Issue

These are not merely theoretical concerns. In fact, many of these decisions, made in the design and conduct of the clinical trials of the thrombolytic agents, were quite controversial, so the potential for flawed decisions resulting (consciously or unconsciously) from conflicts of interest was real. I will now illustrate the existence of that potential by listing a series of highly controversial decisions involving all of the trials of thrombolytic agents. I am not claiming that any of these decisions was a flawed decision produced by a conflict of interest. All I am claiming is that these types of decisions create the possibility of conflicts of interest leading to flawed decision-making, and that these examples illustrate why we need to be concerned about conflicts of interest.

To enable the reader to follow the illustration of the problem, I will briefly summarize the recent history of the development of thrombolytic therapy.[3] In 1980, Marcus DeWood published a study showing that clots (thrombi) in the coronary arteries are usually the immediate cause of myocardial infarctions. This led to a renewal of interest in the treatment of patients undergoing a myocardial infarction with clot-busting (thrombolytic) agents. These included streptokinase (SK), which had been available for many years, and tissue plasminogen activator (tPA), which was purified in 1981 and produced by genetic engineering in 1982.

The National Institutes of Health therefore planned a series of trials (the Thrombolysis in Myocardial Infarction [TIMI] trials) designed to test the efficacy of these drugs. After considerable planning, the strategy adopted was to test SK against tPA in the TIMI-trial, using clot lysis as the endpoint that measured comparative efficacy (as opposed to improved left ventricular ejection fraction or increased survival). The winner was to be tested in a TIMI-2 trial against a placebo to demonstrate absolute efficacy. The TIMI-1 trial was stopped in 1985 because of early impressive results, and tPA was declared the winner. The originally planned TIMI-2 trial of tPA against a placebo was not run because of the evidence of the absolute efficacy of thrombolytic agents in reducing mortality derived from other trials (primarily trials of SK).

The two major trials of SK against a placebo demonstrated significant efficacy as measured by improved survival. These were the Gruppo Italiano per lo Studio della Sopravvivenza nell' Infarcto Miocardio (GISSI) trial (whose results were published in 1986 and were part of the reason for the cancellation of the planned TIMI-2 trial) and the International Study of Infarct Survival-2 (ISIS-2) trial (its impressive preliminary results were published in 1987; the trial continued anyway). The GISSI trial did not attempt to obtain informed consent from participants because of the emergency nature of the situation, while the ISIS-2 trial allowed for considerable latitude in obtaining informed consent.

Placebo-controlled trials with mortality as the endpoint were also run for tPA and for a third thrombolytic agent, anoisylated plasminogen streptokinases activating complex (APSAC), and these trials also demonstrated efficacy. The most important of these trials were the Anglo-Scandinavian Study of Early Thrombolysis (ASSET) trial of tPA (1986–1988) and the APSAC Intervention Mortality Study (AIMS) trial of anoisylated plasminogen streptokinases activating complex (1987–87).

Keeping this history in mind, I will now review the eight types of questions listed above. Questions of type 1 involve deciding which treatments to test and which treatments not to test. The TIMI trials provide good examples of these controversial decisions. The initial decision to take tPA as a serious candidate for study so soon after its synthesis, the decision to run a preliminary TIMI-1 trial and then to run all the rest of the studies involving only the winner of TIMI-1, and the decision to not study APSAC are all good examples of controversial decisions of type 1. Questions of type 2 involve deciding whether or not to use placebo control groups. Nearly all of the trials provide good examples of such controversial decisions, ranging from TIMI's decision not to run any placebo-controlled trials after the results of GISSI were published in 1986 to those (including ISIS-2 itself, AIMS, and ASSET) that continued such trials after the publication of the GISSI and the ISIS-2 preliminary data. Questions of type 3 involve deciding what to take as favorable and adverse endpoints. In the thrombolytic trials, the choice of the favorable endpoint was quite controversial, with some trials using survival and others surrogates. Of particular significance was the controversial decision of TIMI-1 to use reperfusion (clot lysis) as the favorable end-point rather than other surrogates such as ejection fraction. Questions of type 4 involve decisions about inclusion and exclusion criteria and are closely related to questions of type 3. Investigators who want large trials, like the European trials (GISSI, ISIS-2, AIMS, and ASSET), must include nearly everyone, but if they are running smaller trials with surrogate endpoints (like TIMI-1), they can employ stricter inclusion and exclusion criteria, and these can be quite controversial. Questions of type 5 involve decisions about informed consent. Nearly all of the trials involved controversial decisions of this type. The GISSI and ISIS-2 investigators made the controversial decision to modify the standard informed consent process. But the investigators' decision in the other trials to proceed in the emergency setting with a normal consent process is equally controversial. Questions of type 6 involve decisions about the early stopping of trials in light of their own data. The decision to stop TIMI-1 because of its reperfusion data and the decision not to stop ISIS-2 in spite of its own very impressive survival data are good examples of controversial decisions of this type. Questions of type 7 involve decisions about trial abandonment or modification in light of new data from other trials. The decisions to continue ISIS-2, AIMS, and ASSET even after receiving the GISSI and preliminary ISIS-2 data are good examples of controversial decisions of this type, as is, of course, the decision not to run the originally planned placebo-controlled TIMI-2 trial in light of the GISSI data. Questions of type 8 are raised in day-to-day decision-making by clinicians on which patients should participate in the clinical trials.

The thrombolytic trials illustrate how many controversial decisions have to be made in the design and conduct of clinical studies. There is clearly great potential for conflicts of interest to lead, consciously or unconsciously, to flawed decision-making. Therefore, the conflict-of-interest problem is how to develop policies that will minimize that potential.

Two Flawed Proposals

Two approaches have emerged. The first is the disclosure approach, as found, for example, in the following policy of the *New England Journal of Medicine*:[4]

> The Journal expects authors to disclose any commercial associations that might pose a conflict of interest in connection with the submitted article. All funding sources supporting the work should be routinely acknowledged on the title page, as should all institutional or corporate affiliations of the authors. Other kinds of associations, such as consultancies, stock ownership or other equity interests, or patent-licensing arrangements, should be disclosed to the Editor in a covering letter at the time of submission. Such information will be held in confidence while the paper is under review and will not influence the editorial decision. If the manuscript is accepted, the Editor will discuss with the authors how best to disclose the relevant information.

This policy covers a wide variety of potential conflicts of interest. It attempts to deal with them by requiring disclosure, presumably in the expectation that those who read the resulting publications will be alerted to the potential conflict of interest and will adopt an appropriately cautious attitude to the resulting publication.

The second, very different approach was described in an influential article published at the same time as the disclosure policies were being promulgated. The authors of the article were the leading investigators in a multicenter trial funded by the NIH. Their approach, the elimination approach, rests on the claim that the best way to deal with conflicts of interest is to ban the commercial relations that generate the conflicts. The policy is formulated as follows:[5]

> Investigators involved in the post-CABG study will not buy, sell, or hold stock or stock options in any of the companies providing or distributing medication under study . . . for the following periods: from the time the recruitment of patients for the trial begins until funding for the study in the investigator's unit ends and the results are made public; or . . . until the investigator's active and personal involvement in the study or the involvement of the institution conducting the study (or both) ends. Each investigator will agree not to serve as a paid consultant to the companies during these same periods. . . Certain other activities are not viewed as constituting conflicts of interest but must be reported annually to the coordinating center: the participation of investigators in educational activities supported by the companies; the participation of investigators in other research projects supported by the companies; occasional scientific consulting to the companies on issues not related to the products in the trial and for which there is not financial payment or other compensation; and financial interests in the companies over which the investigator has no control, such as mutual funds and blind trusts.

This approach has attracted much attention, in part because of its obvious merits and in part because Dr. Healy was subsequently appointed to head the NIH, which developed final regulations on this matter under a successor. In September 1989, the NIH[6] proposed a policy on this issue that was an expansion of the elimination approach. In addition to banning equity holdings and paid consultancies, it required that companies sharing the costs of research with the NIH not to be in a position to influence the research plan or get access to the information in advance. After much controversy those policies were put on hold, and less draconian PHS regulations—described in chapter sixteen—that borrow from both approaches were adopted.

Much needs to be said about the details of these approaches, about their respective merits and demerits, and about ways of combining aspects of both of them. But that will not be my concern in the remainder of this chapter, although I heartily endorse some combination of these approaches. What I want to do instead is to identify a fundamental presupposition of both approaches and to suggest some broader policies that will need to be adopted since the presupposition in question is almost certainly incorrect.

This presupposition is that the conflict-of-interest problem arises primarily out of the commercial relation between clinical investigators and drug companies whose products they are investigating. The disclosure policy of the *New England Journal of Medicine*, for example, is concerned with the "commercial associations" of the investigators, and emphasizes disclosures of equity interests, consulting fees, and so on. The NIH proposal and Dr. Healy's earlier policies are primarily concerned with prohibiting stockholding, consultancy fees, and so on. This is understandable when one remembers that the attention to this issue grew out of particular allegations about the relation between certain investigators and Genentech. But as understandable as it may be, the conflict-of-interest problem extends beyond these commercial relations. Let me explain why I think so.

I have argued that the conflict-of-interest problem arises when (1) there are controversial decisions that must be made in the design and conduct of clinical trials, and (2) these decisions may be biased by the investigators' financial interests. It is obvious that condition 1 will be satisfied in many clinical trials whether or not the investigators have commercial relations with any drug companies. But it seems to me that condition 2 may also be satisfied even when these commercial relations are not present, because of problems growing out of grant funding. If this is correct, both approaches are at best incomplete solutions because their fundamental common presupposition is false.

To explain why condition 2 may be satisfied even if the investigators have no equity interests, consultancies, or other commercial relations with any drug company, we need to reflect on the grants funding the trial in question. The clinical centers receive substantial support from the funding source, support that pays the salaries of the staff and investigators, helps cover the administrative expenses of the center, and even offers the possibility of a profit (especially if one considers the marginal, as opposed to the average, cost of running the trial). If that support is cut off, there can be substantial financial losses to the center, as well as career losses to the investigators. This certainly has the potential for influencing decisions involving questions of type 6 or 7—questions of stopping trials. Similarly, investigators may be influenced in their decisions about patient eligibility, decisions involving questions of type 8, since failure to enroll enough patients may lead to a lessening of support or even to elimination of the center from the trial. Clearly, there is a potential for biased decisions due to conflicts of interest in the conduct of a trial because of the benefits of grant funding, even if the investigators have no commercial relations with the relevant drug companies. The same point is true, in a different and slightly more subtle fashion, when it comes to decisions involving the design of trials. Different trial designs, involving different decisions concerning questions of types 1 to 5, are likely to have more or less appeal to the crucial decision-makers in, and advisers to, the drug company or the public agency, and those who seek grants may be influenced in their decisions by the desire to maximize the chances of funding. I see no reason to believe, then, that condition (b) is only, or even primarily, satisfied when the investigators have close commercial connections to the companies whose products are being tested.

An Alternative Approach

I suggest, as an alternative to the common presupposition, the following view about conflicts of interest. Conflicts of interest are a matter of concern whenever conditions (a) and (b) are satisfied. Both of these conditions can be satisfied when the investigators have stocks in, or receive consulting fees from, a drug company whose product is being tested, but they can also be satisfied when the trial in question is being funded by a grant either from a drug company or from some public agency. We need to develop policies that are sensitive to all of these possibilities. The current proposals, disclosure and/or elimination of commercial relations, are therefore incomplete even if meritorious.

One discussion that has focused on these broader concerns is the discussion in the policies of the Royal College of Physicians in an important statement on research involving patients.[7] I now turn then to a careful examination of those policies.

The main thrust of those policies is to avoid situations in which researchers are induced by financial considerations to pressure patients to participate in clinical trials. That is why the Royal College would totally ban per capita payments to physicians (payments in proportion to the number of subjects recruited). That is also why the Royal College would allow research grants conditional on recruiting a minimum number of patients only if the independent committee reviewing the research protocol determines that it is reasonable to assume that the clinic in question can get that number of volunteers in light of the nature of its patient load and the nature of the research.

All of these are quite reasonable policies, and their adoption would go some way toward minimizing the potential for conflicts of interest in questions of type 8, questions about subject eligibility and subject enrollment. Moreover, these policies have the virtue of focusing on what I have identified as a neglected topic: the shaping of decisions so as to maximize financial gain from grants. Nevertheless, they are far from complete solutions, since they really focus only on question 8. This is understandable in the context of the report from the Royal College, since its report is devoted to protecting the interests of patients who are also research subjects. But can we learn from its recommendations about steps that can be used more generally? I think we can.

At a crucial point in its discussion, when considering payments to institutions as opposed to physicians, it has the following to say:[8]

> Payment for recruitment should not exceed a reasonable estimate of the cost of studying the patient together with any legitimate expenses. There should be no element of profit to the institution or department related to the number of patients recruited.

This is a crucial point. As noted above, grants often cover more than the marginal costs of research, so they constitute a source of additional revenue to institutions. This is part of the way in which grants (as well as equity holdings and consultancies) are the source of potential conflicts of interest.

We need better information about income from grants if we really want to minimize the potential for conflicts of interest. In an important recent study, Shimm and Spece[9] estimated that at their institution an investigator can harvest a profit of $75,000–$225,000 from a drug company study involving fifty patients. Their analysis is not entirely convincing, since they derived their estimate by simply subtracting the salary of a data coordinator ($25,000) from the income derived from the drug company (fifty patients at $2000–$5000 per patient), not considering other marginal expenses. They themselves point out that the calculation will be different if these other marginal expenses are counted. Moreover, I am not convinced that they are right in their claim (unsupported by data) that there is no similar potential in federally funded research. This skepticism is related to the recent controversies about indirect costs. Nevertheless, Shim and Spece have done a great service by beginning to identify the true institutional gains from grant income.

The development of detailed guidelines for avoiding conflicts of interest resulting from grant income lies beyond the scope of this chapter, since one can only develop them in response to a detailed examination of a wide variety of fundamental accounting issues about individual and institutional profits from grants. The crucial philosophical point is, however, clear. Profits to individuals or institutions from grants can be just as much a source of conflicts of interest as equity holdings or consultancy fees, and the former should be avoided as much as the latter.

One needs to be realistic about how much such guidelines could accomplish. Even if they resulted in grants producing no direct financial profit to institutions or individuals, securing grants and implementing research under them would still be in the professional and/or financial interest of both individual researchers and their institutions. That is both inevitable and probably desirable. But guidelines of the sort I am advocating would at least minimize the extent to which controversial decisions about the design and implementation of research are influenced, consciously or unconsciously, by the prospect of direct financial gain.

Let me add one other observation. If one reviews questions 1–8 in response to which, I have argued, conflicts of interest might induce biased inappropriate decisions, one sees that many of these questions deserve independent discussion and policy formulation. To the extent that society adopts some well-designed policies about them (e.g., about when placebo controlled trials are justified) and incorporates them into appropriate regulations and/or guidelines, it will limit the extent of discretion about these matters, thereby also limiting the possibility of conflicts of interest.

In summary, I have argued that conflicts of interest are to be avoided not because they lead to fraud but because they can be the source of biased inappropriate decisions when there are controversial questions about the design and implementation of research protocols. I have also argued that grant support can be just as much a source of conflicts of interest as equity holdings, so that the current emphasis on equity holdings and paid consultancies is misleading. Finally, I have suggested that what is required is a ban on individual and institutional direct profits from grants, whether from industry or from the government, as well as the more familiar bans on equity holding and paid consultancies and the requirement of full disclosure.

Notes

1. Doctors as Stockholders, *Newsday* 1 (Discovery Section (September 29, 1987)).
2. Committee on Government Operations, *Are Scientific Misconduct and Conflicts of Interest Hazardous to our Health?*, 101st Congress, 2nd Session (1990).
3. The details of this account are based on chapter 1 of my forthcoming book, *The Clot Busters.* Until it appears, readers can consult G. T. Taylor, *Thrombolytic Therapy for Acute Myocardial Infarction* (1992).
4. Information for Authors, 320 *N. Engl. J. Med.* 952 (1989).
5. Bernadine Healy, *et. al.,* Conflict of Interest Guidelines for a Multi-Center Trial of Treatment after Coronary-Artery Bypass-Graft Surgery, 320 *N. Engl. J. Med.* 949–951 (1989).
6. Requests for Comments in *N.I.H. Guide for Grants and Contracts*, vol. 18 (September 15, 1989).
7. Royal College of Physicians, *Research Involving Patients* (1990).
8. *Id.* at Sect. 7.86–7.87.
9. David Shimm and Roy Spece, Industry Reimbursement for Entering Patients into Clinical Trials, 115 *Ann. Intern. Med.* 148–151 (1991).

19

IRBs and Conflicts of Interest

Leslie Francis

Institutional Review Boards—IRBs—review research on human subjects. Their aim is to ensure that research subjects are treated ethically. Structured by federal regulations, IRBs have become significantly standardized and institutionalized. Some commentators charge that conflicts of interest lie at the very heart of the notion of an *institutional* review board. George Annas, for example, writes that the term "*institutional* review board" seems "just right, because the primary function of the committee has become to protect the institution, and its membership is almost exclusively made up of researchers (not potential subjects) from the particular institution."[1] Others view IRBs as involved in a desirable effort to harmonize the interests of clinical researchers and research subjects—and perhaps the interests of others as well, such as patients—to the extent that conflicts can be limited.[2]

This chapter addresses problems of conflicts of interest related to IRBs. How are IRBs constituted, and how are their tasks defined? What kinds of conflicts can be anticipated for IRBs, and why are they of concern? Are any data available about the epidemiology of IRB conflicts of interest? That is, how frequently do they arise, in what forms, and in what settings? What mechanisms can best identify and minimize conflicts of interest for IRBs? The chapter begins with a description of IRB membership and functions as they are laid out in the federal regulations. It then surveys the broad range of conflicts of interest that seem possible for IRBs to encounter and presents the little available data on the actual incidence of conflicts of interest in IRB decision-making. Particularly given the limited data, the survey of likely kinds of conflicts may seem unduly broad. More has been written, however, about some of the conflicts that arise in two related enterprises: hospital ethics committees and institutional investigations of scientific fraud. The chapter concludes, therefore, by calling on what is known about conflicts in these two areas for the light it can shed on the identification and minimization of conflicts for IRBs. The overall perspective of the chapter is that the most obvious conflicts—such as investigators participating in reviews of their own research—are not the most problematic ones for IRBs. These conflicts are comparatively easy to identify and avoid. More subtle pressures, however, such as loyalty to colleagues or concern for the institution's reputation, are far more troublesome, both to recognize and to control.

The Functions and Structure of IRBs

IRBs were developed in the wake of several highly publicized and quite shocking examples of deceit or coercion of human subjects in research. From 1932 to 1972, a study in Tuskegee, Alabama, followed the natural history of untreated syphilis in 400 black males. The men were included in the study without even knowing that it was taking place. Procedures used to monitor the progress of their disease were misrepresented as free, beneficial medical care. When penicillin became available as a treatment for syphilis in the 1940s, the men were not told that it was an option; the study continued to describe the progress of their disease until 1972, when it was halted in response to publicity. In another much-criticized example, at Willowbrook State School, a New York facility for the mentally disabled, patients were inoculated with the hepatitis virus in order to test the efficacy of various therapies. Because the school was overcrowded, parents were frequently able to secure places for their children only by agreeing to their participation in the study.[3] These and several other incidents led to the initial publication in 1973, by the Department of Health, Education, and Welfare, of regulations governing research with human subjects. In 1974, Congress established a national commission to review research with human subjects; the Belmont Report,[4] issued by the commission in 1978, contained a number of recommendations about IRBs. These recommendations were the basis for the current IRB regulations, now issued in common form by both the Food and Drug Administration and the Department of Health and Human Services.[5] Thus, by the early 1990s, IRBs had a nearly twenty-year history of development within the regulatory process.

IRB Functions

The federal regulations specify what research must be reviewed by IRBs and set out explicitly the terms of that review.[6] The purpose of IRBs is to protect the "rights and welfare" of human subjects.[7] To protect subjects' rights, IRBs must ensure that research subjects (or, when appropriate, their legally authorized representatives) do not participate in studies without giving informed consent.[8] The FDA regulations add an exception to the requirement for consent when a new drug or device is used in an emergency situation and no ordinary therapy gives the patient an equal or greater likelihood of survival than the use of that drug or device.[9]

To protect subjects' welfare, IRBs must assess the risks and benefits of proposed research. The standard to be applied is whether the risks to research subjects are "reasonable in relation to anticipated benefits, if any, to subjects, and the importance of the knowledge that may reasonably be expected to result." "Importance" is not further explained; in the context of this paragraph of the regulations, it is perhaps best understood as "importance to other patients of this or a similar kind, or to the development of medical knowledge more generally." In their assessment of research, IRBs are explicitly prohibited from considering possible longer-range risks of research, including impacts on public policy.[10] Thus, the possibility that research would result in the development of a new, highly effective form of therapy would be within the IRB's purview as a benefit, but not the additional observation that the therapy would most likely be highly expensive and impose significant financial burdens on third-party payers. Also off limits as a risk for IRBs to consider is the possibility that knowledge gained from a study might later be used in a discriminatory fashion, such as concerns about the potential for genetic discrimination in employment or insurance.[11]

IRB Membership

Several IRB membership requirements are specified by the federal regulations.[12] IRBs must have at least five members—a number, it might be noted, that is one fewer than the constitutional minimum for a jury, set by the Supreme Court with the aims of promoting effective deliberation, providing a check on the arbitrary exercise of state power, and reflecting an adequate cross section of the community.[13] Guidelines for selecting IRB members attempt to further several different goals. One goal is expertise in assessing the research; IRBs must include members with the relevant scientific competence, or they may invite the help of nonvoting members when special knowledge is required. Another goal is knowledge of relevant legal and professional norms; IRBs must include members who can interpret applicable law and professional codes of ethics. IRBs must also include members who are capable of understanding the character of the institution engaged in the research: as the regulations put it, "ascertain[ing] the

acceptability of research in terms of institutional commitments and regulations."
A further goal of IRBs is inclusion of a diversity of perspectives. The regulations
require that every IRB have at least one scientist and at least one non-scientist
member, and that no IRB may be made up solely of members of one profession.
They also require membership to be sensitive to issues of race, gender, and culture. However, although "every nondiscriminatory effort" is to be made to ensure
that no IRB is composed entirely of men or of women, no selection to the IRB is
to be based on gender. A final goal is an outside perspective; IRBs are to be sensitive to community attitudes. In support of this general concern about community feelings, as well as perhaps in the effort to provide some outside oversight,
every IRB is required to include at least one member who is not affiliated with
the institution (and does not have a family member affiliated with the institution). The regulations do not define affiliation but are construed quite broadly by
DHHS to cover anyone with an association with the institution, even a noneconomic, honorific tie.[14] These goals of IRB membership may not always be consistent; some of the most important kinds of conflicts considered below illustrate
the tensions involved when the goals conflict.

IRB Procedures

IRB procedures are designed, at least in part, to prevent or identify conflicts of
interest. IRBs are not permitted to allow members to participate in reviewing
their own research.[15] Thus, IRB members, in their official capacity, may not be
present at meetings when their own research is under discussion. This does not
preclude clinical investigators who are also IRB members from providing the
IRB with information about their research, just as other clinical investigators
do.[16] Anecdotal evidence suggests that the line between providing helpful information and functioning as an IRB member is not always strictly drawn. The
opportunity for ready interchange between IRBs and member-investigators raises possibilities of conflicts that are discussed below. In part as a control against
IRB members participating in decisions about their own research, IRBs are
required to keep minutes in sufficient detail to show attendance at meetings,
votes and abstentions.[17] The minutes must also describe controversial issues and
their resolution.[18]

To guarantee diversity of perspectives, the regulations require that at least one
nonscientist be present for a quorum in IRB meetings. But in other respects, the
regulations make relatively weak efforts to guarantee diversity in practice. They
do not mandate the presence at IRB meetings of a member who is not affiliated
with the sponsoring institution.[19] Information sheets provided to IRBs by the
FDA indicate, moreover, that IRB members may be paid consultant fees for their
work.[20] Indeed, some IRBs function on a for-profit basis, reviewing studies for
investigators who do not have access to an IRB where they are located, perhaps

because of the size of their institutions or because using an outside IRB is more convenient. The regulations are silent on the possibility of malpractice or other tort liability on the part of IRB members for decisions they have made in reviewing research. They are also silent about institutional policies on potential tort liability for IRB members, such as decisions about legal defense or indemnification.[21]

In order to monitor IRB compliance with the regulations, the FDA performs on-site audits of IRBs on a regular schedule. DHHS, on the other hand, reviews IRB assurances and investigates only in response to complaints or other information about difficulties; DHHS has only three compliance officers for the 1000 or more IRBs that now function in the United States.

Conflicts of Interest for IRBs: The Possibilities

As the chapter by E. L. Erde[22] in this volume admirably illustrates, conflict of interest is a complex concept. On the level of motivation, a conflict of interest occurs whenever an IRB member—or the IRB itself—has interests that affect the independent review of research involving human subjects. A potential conflict of interest occurs when the IRB or its members have interests that might reasonably be thought likely to affect independent review. Many possible kinds of motivational conflicts fall under this broad characterization: economic interests; interests in job security; interests in the prestige or research reputation of the institution in which the IRB is located; commitments to scientific colleagues or to the advancement of technological medicine; or deep and overriding allegiance to other values that are specifically excluded from IRB consideration, such as opposition to abortion. In short, the possibility of a conflict is raised by any concern that does (or, for a potential conflict, could) cause an IRB member to place it in the balance alongside the factors IRBs are supposed to consider or to give it more (or less) weight than it is supposed to bear.

Given the breadth of this working characterization of a conflict, several initial caveats are in order. This section does not contend that all of these conflicts are of equal frequency or seriousness, or that they all can or should be regulated. The delineation of possible conflicts presented in this section is speculative. It makes no claims about the actual occurrence or frequency of these conflicts, or about whether they are likely to affect particular members of IRBs or IRBs in general. What little is known about the epidemiology of IRB conflicts is presented in the next section. The claim here is only that it is important to begin by exploring the kinds of conflicts that IRB members might at some time face, and that therefore should be the subject of inquiry.

The most direct, and most easily identified, conflict of interest for an IRB involves members' own research. The member presumably has an interest in conducting the research and thus in seeing the research approved. When approval of the research is necessary for a grant application, the researcher may also have a direct financial as well as professional stake in IRB approval. The federal regulations prohibit this kind of conflict, and both FDA and DHHS inspections cite IRBs that allow researchers to participate in reviews of their own work.

Indirect versions of the investigator–reviewer conflict, however, are also possible and are not prohibited by the federal regulations. IRBs design formal procedures for the review of research; for example, particular IRBs may have rules governing payment or recruitment of subjects for participation in research. Or they may apply informally agreed-on methods for dealing with recurrent problems—for example, requesting researchers to provide the IRB office with copies of any advertisements used to recruit subjects. As these procedures are developed, IRB members who are themselves actively involved in clinical research may be acutely aware of the possible implications for their own research, and their judgment may be affected by this awareness.[23]

The conflict between IRB membership and research involvement is not the only economic conflict IRBs may encounter. Even when IRBs function within nonprofit institutions such as academic medical centers, many economic pressures are possible.[24] When grant applications include overhead reimbursement, payments to defray the costs of patient care, or other resources of the institution, both the institution itself and IRB members who are colleagues of the researcher may have significant financial stakes in the success of the research proposal. Affiliated IRB members may be salaried or otherwise compensated by the sponsoring institution; this compensation relationship gives them an indirect interest in how the institution fares generally. They may have laboratories or research assistants who are supported by institutional research overhead funds. These are quite general interests in the institution, but it is not impossible for IRB members to find that their compensation could be affected much more directly—for example, if they are involved in reviewing protocols submitted by department chairs or others with the authority to fix their compensation. Tenure status or other job responsibilities or important institutional resources, like funds or personnel to support their own work, may also be at issue if IRB members are involved in reviewing protocols from their superiors.

When IRBs function in a for-profit institution, economic conflicts may be shaped by the economic incentives of the institution. For-profit health care facilities have interests in their overall rates of return; IRBs may be indirectly or even directly aware of the profit potential of particular research protocols or their potential to attract other profitable business to the facility. Discrete services within the facility may be aware of their profitability—or their more marginal economic status—and members of these services might, while on the IRB, watch out for studies that may affect their own economic profiles, either absolutely or comparatively within the institution. IRB members may even know that their own jobs, or the continuation of their programs or services, depend directly on their profitability for the institution; this knowledge may not be easy to set aside in the review of research with possible consequences for profitability.

Free-standing IRBs, particularly those that are themselves profit-making, may face further economic conflicts. For-profit IRBs, if their earnings depend on the frequency with which they review studies, have interests in steady business. These interests quite innocuously may encourage them to review studies efficiently and properly. But they also create the incentive for for-profit IRBs to take into account the interests of the institutions for which studies are being reviewed. Consistently unfriendly reviews might be thought to threaten ongoing relationships between IRBs and the institution with which they contract. Even when a for-profit IRB reviews studies for many individual investigators, rather than establishing a contractual relationship with one or more research institutions, concerns about its reputation in the research community and its desirability as a reviewer might create incentives that affect the consideration of protocols.

Another significant economic conflict for IRBs is the potential for legal liability, both for IRB members and for the institutions they serve. While threats of legal liability might seem most likely to encourage especially careful scrutiny of research that is risky for subjects, these incentives do not always protect research subjects. Under the federal regulations, the process of informed consent may not be used to relieve researchers from liability for negligence or allow them to waive subjects' rights.[25] Yet there may be pressures to draft consent forms to reduce as much as possible the institution's exposure to legal liability. If the institution's lawyer is a member of its IRB, which is not prohibited under the federal regulations, there may be direct conflicts between the lawyer's professional obligation to serve as advocate for his or her client and the obligation as an IRB member to give independent scrutiny to proposed research.[26] In discussions, it may be unclear whether the lawyer is acting as an advocate or as an independent reviewer; and the lawyer's comments may greatly influence other IRB members. In addition, IRB members may be concerned about their own legal liability for participation in the review process. Institutional practices may vary in the extent to which IRB members are offered legal counsel or indemnification. While subjects who believe they have been injured in a research study are certainly one source of potential litigation against IRB members, researchers who believe they have been defamed or subjected to discrimination are surely another source.

Economic conflicts are only part of the picture for IRBs, however. IRB members may also find themselves facing conflicts between their responsibilities to the IRB and their other responsibilities. One obvious issue here is time. If IRB members are selected for their expertise, they may be already overworked members of an institution. While the lack of time does not by itself suggest either a favorable or an unfavorable bias toward research, it may well result in less careful review of protocols and a tendency toward more or less automatic approval.

IRB members may also be friends, colleagues, mentors, or superiors of researchers whose protocols they review. They may want to see their colleagues do well and wish to support them. They may want to further the careers of younger scientists working with them. They may have personal knowledge of the study, or of the researcher, that leads them to judge it more favorably than is warranted by the actual submission made to the IRB for its review. Or they may rely on what they believe about the researcher from what they have heard from other friends or colleagues. These motives of friendship or mentoring may be principally altruistic. They may also be intermingled with the IRB member's own reputation: as a helpful colleague, a successful mentor, or a member of a high-powered team of research colleagues. On the darker side, IRB members may be professional rivals of those whose research they review and may therefore be inclined to hypercritical scrutiny.

Another potential conflict may arise for IRB members between their IRB roles and their roles on other institutional ethics committees. Particularly in smaller institutions, where relatively few studies are reviewed, some members of ethics committees—or even the entire committee—may be pressed into doing double duty as IRB members. The roles of hospital ethics committees are ill-defined; they may range from education to policy formulation, case consultation, or case review.[27] Knowledge gained from work on the IRB, or on these other committees, is one potential source of conflicts. IRB members may acquire information, for example, about researcher-clinicians' reputations, or about drugs or devices under study, that would be relevant to ethics committee activities such as policy formulation or case review. In some cases, this information may be confidential under IRB rules or administrative law, but there may be temptations to reveal it or use it in other committee settings. On the other side, in their roles on other ethics committees, IRB members may acquire knowledge of the conduct of particular clinicians, or of incidents with particular patients, that is relevant to the IRB, such as experimentation involving human subjects that has not been approved by the IRB. This knowledge may be useful to the IRB, but IRB members with a duty of confidentiality to other committees might not be willing to use it in the way that would best protect human subjects. In addition to information, commitment to policies is another likely area of conflicts for IRB members with multiple committee roles. As ethics committee members, IRB members may find themselves involved in drafting institutional policies that are problematic from the perspective of the IRB. For example, institutional policies about confidentiality of patient records or about reimbursement for patient injuries may not be entirely consistent with IRB policies, yet IRB members who have participated in formulating these policies may not question them from the point of view of the IRB. Finally, experience with and loyalty to the norms of other ethics committees, such as a reluctance to reach decisions in certain cases or a desire to include more general social issues in ethical deliberations, may conflict with IRB requirements. The extent to which these conflicts are likely to occur may itself be affected by the institutional roles played by the other ethics committees and the types of pressures to which they, too, are subject.

Another source of potential conflicts for the IRB is its own needs for effective functioning. For much of what they do, IRBs need access to information: to review protocols well, to ensure that the process of informed consent is taking place as represented, and to determine whether the research taking place in the institution is brought to the IRB for its scrutiny. Yet, commentators suggest, if the IRB is seen as a representative of outside interests—the community, the police, or the federal government in the person of the FDA or DHHS—it will have great difficulty in gaining access to the information it needs to function successfully.[28] The IRB may then need to see itself as an agent of its own institution; the obligations of loyalty involved in this role may result in less than fully independent scrutiny of research.

Issues of institutional loyalty may also be important to individual IRB members. Departmental or institutional prestige may be a factor with the capacity to affect the independence of judgment of IRB members. IRB disapproval may stand in the way of major federal or foundational support and reduce the visibility that receipt of a multi-million-dollar grant may bring. IRB action may delay or block the introduction of a major new program at an institution—for example, a new transplant program-if some of the crucial work is experimental. Ease of IRB approval may also be a factor in attracting well-known researchers or clinicians to an institution. Departmental or institutional loyalties may not always push in the direction of approval, however; interdepartmental rivalries, exacerbated by scarce resources, may drive IRB criticism of proposals.

Another possible source of conflicts is the commitment to a particular set of scientific norms. To be sure, intellectual perspectives and disagreements do not by themselves signal conflicts of interest; in some views of science, all judgments of scientific merit are theory dependent. But conflicts are involved if the commitment to a scientific paradigm is linked to other advantages for the IRB member, such as his or her own advancement in the field. These linked commitments might dispose IRB members to deny approval to studies that, although meeting the federal criteria for the scrutiny of risks,[29] nonetheless are judged to be of limited merit in terms of one of several rival scientific paradigms. Judgments of disapproval in terms of scientific paradigms may also be linked to conflicts that occur elsewhere in health care institutions. Disputes between nurses and physicians, for example, about models of patient care or health care research may be replayed in the IRB if some kinds of protocols are viewed as having little scientific benefit in terms of medical management but are viewed more favorably from a nursing care perspective. The trend in some large research institutions toward highly specialized IRBs, composed of scientists with shared expertise to review studies with limited subject matter, has the potential to reduce the diversity of scientific perspectives on review boards. This may lessen conflict on particular IRBs but may at the same time weaken IRB scrutiny.

Still other conflicts may arise because of IRB members' commitments to patient care. That the clinician's commitment to the interests of individual patients may conflict with the optimal scientific design of a randomized clinical trial has been much discussed.[30] But IRB members themselves may have interests on one side or another of this debate. Some IRB members, clinicians who treat particular subgroups of patients, or advocates for patients with particular conditions, may wish to see the rapid dissemination of potentially promising therapies and may let this interest distort the weight given to the risks and benefits of the research.

Indeed, for some IRB members, representation of outside interests is built into their selection. The most obvious example is the requirement for IRBs that review research with prisoners to include at least one prisoner or prisoner advocate.[31] This role definition is designed to ensure particularly protective scrutiny of research involving prisoners based on knowledge of prison conditions and the special vulnerability of prisoners to coercion within the institution. But the role of this IRB member is to advocate prisoners' interests, a role that is at apparent odds with the more general, nonadvocacy concept of IRB membership.

Community representatives on IRBs face similar ambiguity about whether they are to be advocates for interested parties. If community representatives are seen as representatives of community interests generally, then they may embody multiple conflicts. If they are seen as advocates of particular community concerns—abortion rights or rights to life, genetic knowledge or opposition to the genome project, Act-Up or the identification of homosexuality with immorality—the IRB may become significantly politicized. As one experienced community representative on an IRB wrote:

> I did not represent anyone other than myself. I believe very strongly that a Human Subjects Committee would make a catastrophic mistake to see a community person as representing the community's interests. This stance would immediately occasion appeals, lobbying, and manipulative efforts from well-organized, vocal, and powerful groups within any community that their opinions be represented by a person congenial to their interests. The subsequent politicization of the process would likely destroy the HSC, which functions best insulated from those kinds of pressures.[32]

IRBs thus may face a wide range of conflicts. Direct professional affiliations and economic interests are the simplest to identify and eliminate. But indirect economic interests, collegial and institutional loyalties, and political or scientific allegiances all have the potential to affect the judgment of IRB members when they review research proposals.

Conflicts of Interest for IRBs: What Is Known and What Is Unknown

Commentators critical of IRBs allege that many kinds of conflicts are endemic in the functioning of IRBs. As evidence, critics cite anecdotes such as approval by the Loma Linda IRB of the Baby Fae experiment with transplantation of a baboon heart or approval by the University of Utah IRB of the implantation of the artificial heart.[33] But there is almost no systematic information about IRB membership, procedures, or decision-making that is relevant to the assessment of the significance of these anecdotes. The extent to which IRBs actually experience or are swayed by conflicts of interest is largely unknown. A major study of how IRBs are functioning, funded by DHHS as of the fall of 1992, has the potential to identify the types and frequency of conflicts experienced by IRBs.[34]

As of the fall of 1992, it appears that no systematic data on IRBs or their membership have been assembled. Neither the FDA nor the Office For Protection From Research Risks (OPRR) apparently keeps even an ongoing total of how many IRBs there are, and how they are distributed among types of institutions—for example, university medical schools or for-profit hospitals. There are no systematic studies of the percentages of IRB members who are physicians, nurses, other scientists, or non-scientists. Nor are there studies of the frequency with which IRB members are engaged in extensive clinical research. No studies track whether IRBs pay their members. None tracks whether institutional authorities such as lawyers, risk managers, or hospital members sit on IRBs. No American studies track the frequency with which IRB members sit on other institutional ethics committees, although a recent study in the Netherlands showed that only 2.5 percent of hospitals distinguished between exclusive activities of IRBs and activities of institutional ethics committees.[35] No studies track the methods by which IRB members are selected or the frequency with which they are removed. And since there are no systematic data, there is also no way to know whether there are differences in membership patterns among different kinds of IRBs: for example, in universities, in non-university-affiliated health care facilities, or in unaffiliated IRBs reviewing proposals on contract.

There is one systematic study of a subgroup of IRB members: Joan P. Porter's work on unaffiliated, nonscientist ("lay") members.[36] This study showed that lay members are most frequently clergy (46/189) or lawyers (36/189). They tend to report that they were appointed by relatively high-level institutional officials, often through friendship with (46/127) or at the suggestion of (33/127) the appointing official; at least in 1985, there appeared to be little or no effort on the part of IRBs to recruit outside members from community or patient advocacy groups. A low percentage (16 percent) reported being given expenses or paid for their IRB work. Three-quarters served on IRBs that included at least one other lay member. Over 80 percent reported that they had received no training for their service on the IRB; no lay members reported that they had been specifically told that one of their roles was to watch for conflicts of interest. Over half (56 percent), however, strongly agreed that watching for conflicts was an important part of their role, along with representing community values (53 percent), reviewing informed consent documents (173/198), acting as an advocate for human subjects (164/198), and speaking up (181/198). Dr. Porter describes this finding:

> This response represents underlying concern about the research goals becoming more important than the patient's or subject's welfare and concern that the physician can have motivations that color or override the best interests of the subject. The theme of ensuring accountability of the researcher in the best interest of the subject (patient) is reflected. Some commentators on the questionnaire did note, however, that medical personnel or those in the institutions were probably in a better position to evaluate if there was a possible conflict of interest in each research protocol, and they were therefore reluctant to report this as their role.[37]

Two lay members volunteered the additional role of watching out for vulnerable patient populations. Lay members who were women strongly agreed more frequently than would have been expected by chance with the role expectations of representing community attitudes and acting as an advocate for human subjects; unemployed (but not retired) members more frequently saw their role as watching out for conflicts of interest. Based on her data, Dr. Porter recommends more training of lay members and more attention to setting standards for their selection; she also recommends raising their numbers and increasing their sensitivity to concerns of the disadvantaged.

Anecdotal evidence suggests that IRB memberships are heavily weighted toward physicians involved in clinical research. According to one published description, Yale University's IRB in 1986 had twenty-six members, including over half (fifteen) who were full-time medical school faculty and eleven who were tenured. The other members included four medical students, a grants administrator, the hospital's medical director of quality assurance, a staff nurse, a clinical pharmacist, and a consultant for minority affairs. There was one outside member, a psychological counselor with no ties to Yale; the counselor was, however, paid for service on the IRB at a rate equivalent to that paid by NIH for advisory committee service. No data were provided about the demographic variables of the Yale IRB members, such as age, sex, or race.[38] At present, my own IRB at the University of Utah has twenty members, ten of whom are physicians. Of the remainder, two are nurses, two are pharmacists, two are philosophers, one is a librarian, one is a clergyman not affiliated with the university, one is a prisoner advocate not affiliated with the university, and one is a member of the faculty in the College of Health.[39] But the Yale and Utah IRBs are isolated examples, both at academic medical centers. It would be useful to know whether other IRBs parallel these distributions of membership, and whether there are characteristic differences between IRBs at different kinds of institutions. It would also be useful to know more about how IRB members are selected or—perhaps even more significantly—deselected. At present, we do not even know the frequency with which IRB members are removed for conflicts of interest.

By contrast, a recent British study has obtained comprehensive evidence about research ethics committee membership and functioning.[40] It found that over half (52 percent) of the members of research ethics committees were hospital doctors and just under one-fifth (19 percent) were lay members. Many committees had a general practitioner member, but the 15 percent of committees that did not were viewed with concern because of the role of the British general practitioner as a patient advocate. Nearly half (49.5 percent) of the committees had two lay members, the number required under National Health Service guidelines effective February 1992.[41] About one-third of the committees had lay chairs; National Health Service guidelines now require either a lay chair or a lay vice chair of the committee.[42]

Epidemiology of Conflicts

The FDA tracks the frequency with which IRBs are cited for various deficiencies during site visits. These data indicate that the absence of a member with knowledge of the community, the lack of a nonscientist or nonaffiliated member, and the presence of a member whose study is under review continue to be matters of concern for a persistent but comparatively small number of IRBs. These violations of the regulations tend to be more frequent in IRBs that do not have multiple project assurances approved by the FDA.[43] The FDA site visit data, however, are quite limited. The FDA makes site visits to IRBs on a rotating basis; its workload is heavy, and the site visits consist largely of inspecting the paper records. Unless the information comes to light in some other way—for example, by a complaint—FDA site visits check for recorded violations of formal requirements but do not observe the more subtle institutional pressures that may be at work in IRB decision-making.[44] The FDA's counterpart in DHHS, OPRR, has only three compliance officers. OPRR monitors IRBs largely through their submitted assurances, checking them for compliance with the regulations, and makes site visits only in response to complaints or to extraordinary incidents such as an unusual number of patient deaths.[45]

Very little is known about the processes or outcomes of IRB decision-making. The description of the Yale IRB suggested that there were no significant differences among the voting patterns of various kinds of IRB members. Yale IRB procedures originally gave groups of IRB members, arranged by perspective (all scientists, chaplain, students, etc.), each one vote. Because differences of opinion were not correlated with the members' groupings, this procedure was abandoned in 1979.[46] There are apparently no other studies of patterns of opinion among IRB members. Nor is much known about the rates with which protocols are tabled or disapproved by IRBs, about what kinds of protocols tend to meet with disapproval, or about why members vote to disapprove protocols. Two published reports from single IRBs show relatively low rates of disapproval and relatively higher rates of required amendment. Yale reported in 1984–85 (number of protocols = 145) immediate approval of twenty-four, withdrawal of sixteen, and approval of the remainder pending revisions.[47] UCLA in 1982–83 reported 27.9 percent of protocols (*n* = 168) approved at first review, 64.4 percent approved "with comment," 7.7 percent deferred, and one disapproved.[48] Without further knowledge of IRB decision-making, it is hard to interpret these numbers. Low rejection rates may mean that most submitted research proposals protect human subjects quite well. On the other hand, low rates may indicate that many significant problems remain unrecognized by IRBs. Reasons for dissenting votes need not be recorded by IRBs; although cumbersome, the practice of recording reasons for dissents would be a useful source of information about sources of disagreement within IRBs. Receiving similar criticism, the comprehensive British study described earlier observes the potential for personal knowledge of researchers to bias committee review. The study also notes critically that British committees are not very open about their decision-making practices.[49]

A final impressive lacuna in our knowledge about IRB functioning concerns IRB monitoring of studies that have been approved. Anecdotal evidence suggests that IRBs require reports of adverse occurrences or protocol amendments, but they do not delve further into ongoing assessments of the risk/benefit ratio of experiments with human subjects or of how the process of informed consent works in practice. A recent study by Shimm and Spece reports fragmentary data on refusal rates by patients asked to participate in clinical trials; suggests that more systematic data be collected for various kinds of trials; and recommends that IRBs require investigators to keep records of patient refusals to enter into their studies.[50]

Two Analogies

Two areas of recent ethical investigation may provide helpful analogies to IRB decision-making. First, although they play differing roles,[51] hospital ethics committees may face problems that parallel those of IRBs. One study of lawyers on hospital ethics committees found that most committees had lawyer members, and that in over half of the cases the lawyer member was the lawyer for the institution.[52] Another study attempted to assess patients' attitudes toward the hospital ethics committee; it found that patients preferred to have the committee play a consultative role and to have final decisions about care be made by patients themselves.[53] There is an ongoing debate about the actual and desirable roles for ethics committees, and the extent to which they should follow a model of legal due process that gives patients notice and an opportunity to be heard when their cases are the subject of committee discussions.[54] To be sure, these studies are fragmentary. But they do suggest concern about the extent to which institutional interests may influence ethics committee proceedings, and about whether ethics committees are structured in ways that make these pressures easy to resist. Institutional pressures are certainly a possible source of conflicts for IRBs, and it would be useful to have far more systematic information about whether and how they affect the decision-making of both ethics committees and IRBs.

A second suggestive analogy for IRBs may be scientific fraud investigations. Several notorious recent examples[55] have led to efforts to assess how frequently research fraud occurs and how it can best be prevented or detected. Studies of fraud cases suggest that scientific misconduct is the result of a complex interplay of individual pathology and environmental factors. Career pressures, as well as inadequate institutional oversight and training, have been implicated in scientific fraud cases.[56] There are allegations that scrambles for federal and corporate research dollars play a major role in scientific fraud, as well as in institutional failures to identify and control it.[57] Another suggestion about why scientific fraud may be difficult to uncover is that mentors and colleagues are reluctant to believe that persons they know well and have come to respect could be deceitful.[58] These data, too, are fragmentary; although some estimates indicate that scientific fraud is rare, even these frequency data may well suffer from under-reporting.[59] However, what information there is about scientific fraud suggests the importance of personal loyalties, of funding pressures, and of institutional interests in complicating adequate surveillance of scientific honesty.

Conclusion

The possible scope of conflicts of interest for IRBs is wide indeed. Yet very little is known about the extent to which these conflicts occur or about the capacity of IRBs to resist them. Current monitoring efforts focus on formal compliance with the federal regulations governing the composition of IRB membership and the participation of investigators in reviews of their own studies. Yet the examples of hospital ethics committees and scientific fraud reviews suggest that more serious conflicts may lie in the institutional pressures that affect IRBs and their members. Hopefully, empirical studies may remedy some of the informational gaps about IRB membership and decision-making.

In the meantime, IRBs would do well to educate their members about the possibilities for conflicts of interest that extend beyond formal participation in reviews of their own studies. Institutions would do well to broaden their lay membership and to expand the orbit of selection. IRBs might also experiment with keeping records of dissents from protocol approvals and their reasons, an addition to the current requirement that they must note controversial issues and their resolution. Finally, the British guidelines adopted in 1991 may provide a salutary corrective example for members of IRBs in the United States: "Any member of the [research ethics committee] who has an interest which may affect their consideration of a particular research proposal should be asked to declare that interest, and if necessary should temporarily withdraw from the committee."[60]

Notes

1. George Annas, Ethics Committees: From Ethical Comfort to Ethical Cover, 21 *Hastings Cent. Rep.* 18 (1991).
2. Robert Levine, *Ethics and Regulation of Clinical Research* 327 (2d ed., 1986).
3. A good description of this history of the development of IRBs is Levine, *supra* note 2, especially chapter 4.
4. The National Commission for the Protection of Human Subjects of Biomedical and Behavioral Research, *The Belmont Report: Ethical Principles and Guidelines for the Protection of Human Subjects of Research* (1978).
5. The FDA regulations are at 21 C.F.R. Part 56 (1992); the DHHS regulations are at 45 C.F.R. Part 46 (1991). The two sets of regulations have been brought into common form after many years of effort.
6. In general, FDA regulations require IRB scrutiny of clinical investigations with human subjects submitted in support of applications to test or market new medical devices or drugs. 21 C.F.R. § 56.101(a) (1992). IRBs also must review any research with human subjects that is supported, conducted, or regulated by federal agencies. 45 C.F.R. § 46.101(a) (1991). At many institutions, IRB review of research with human subjects extends well beyond the federal mandate.
7. 21 C.F.R. § 56.101(a) (1992).
8. 21 C.F.R. § 56.111(a)(4) (1992); 45 C.F.R. § 46.111(4) (1991). The elements of informed consent include a full description of the study, its risks and benefits. 21 C.F.R. § 50.25(a),(b) (1992); 45 C.F.R. § 46.116(a) (1991). Consent must be given under circumstances that do not permit undue influence or coercion. 21 C.F.R. § 50.20 (1992); 45 C.F.R. § 46.116 (1991). Researchers must be careful to reassure subjects that benefits they have enjoyed—such as their medical care—will not be affected by the decision to refuse to participate in a study, and that they are free to withdraw from the research at any point. 21 C.F.R. § 50.25(a)(8) (1992);

45 C.F.R. § 46.116(a)(8) (1991). This reassurance is complicated, however, by the dual goals of research and treatment. In some cases, such as chemotherapy trials, new drugs may not be available without participation in the study; although the study is designed to test whether the new therapy is any better than current standard therapy, there may be some suspicions that the new therapy is preferable and some incentives to enter the trial on that accord. Randomized clinical trials in general present role conflicts for the clinical investigator between the role of a treating physician, in which the best interests of the patient are paramount, and the role of the clinical researcher, in which the integrity of the study takes first priority. The significance of this conflict for IRBs is discussed later in the chapter.

9. 21 C.F.R. § 56.104(e) (1992). This exception is carefully circumscribed by reporting requirements.
10. 21 C.F.R. § 56.111(2) (1992); 45 C.F.R. § 46.111(2) (1991); *see also* 46 *Fed. Reg.* 8969 (January 27, 1981).
11. Dennis Karjala, A Legal Research Agenda for the Human Genome Initiative, 32 *Jurimetrics* 121, 172–192 (1992).
12. 21 C.F.R. § 56.107 (1992); 45 C.F.R. § 46.107 (1991).
13. Ballew v. Georgia, 435 U.S. 223 (1978).
14. Telephone conversation with Dr. Edward Allan, OPRR (September 18, 1992).
15. 21 C.F.R. § 56.107(e) (1992); 45 C.F.R. § 46.107(e) (1991).
16. Food and Drug Administration, IRB Information Sheets (1989).
17. 21 C.F.R. § 56.115(a)(2) (1992); 45 C.F.R. § 45.115(a)(2) (1991).
18. *Id.*
19. 21 C.F.R. § 56.108(c) (1992); 45 C.F.R. § 46.108(c) (1991).
20. Food and Drug Administration, IRB Information Sheets (1989).
21. *Id.*
22. Chapter 2.
23. *See, e.g.*, Leonard Glantz, Contrasting Institutional Review Boards with Institutional Ethics Committees, in *Institutional Ethics Committees and Health Care Decision Making* 129 (Ronald Cranford and Edward Doudera, eds., 1984).
24. For a discussion of some of the similarities between for-profit and nonprofit health care facilities, see Paul Starr, *The Social Transformation of American Medicine* (1982).
25. 21 C.F.R. § 50.20(1992); 45. C.F.R. § 46.116 (1991).
26. For a discussion of the analogous conflicts that may arise for lawyer-members of hospital ethics committees, see D. A. Buehler, R. M. DiVita, & J. J. Yium, Hospital Ethics Committees: The Hospital Attorney's Role, 1 *HEC Forum* 183 (1989).
27. *See, e.g.*, Susan Wolf, Ethics Committees and Due Process: Nesting Rights in a Community of Caring, 50 *Maryland L. Rev.* 798 (1991); John Robertson, Committees as Decision-Makers: Alternative Structures and Responsibilities, in *Institutional Ethics Committees and Health Care Decision Making, supra* note 23, at 85.
28. Levine, *supra* note 2, at 342.
29. 21 C.F.R. § 56.111(a)(1) (1992), (2); 45 C.F.R. § 46.111(a)(1), (2) (1991).
30. *See, e.g.*, Fred Gifford, The Conflict Between Randomized Clinical Trials and the Therapeutic Obligation, 11 *J. Med. Philosophy* 347 (1986).
31. 21 C.F.R. § 50.46(a) (1992); 45 C.F.R. § 46.304(a) (1991).
32. Kenneth Roseman, Man-Child in a Promised Land: A Layman Serves on the Human Subjects Committee, 9 *IRB* 8 (March-April 1987).
33. Annas, *supra* note 1, at 18.
34. Telephone conversation with Judith Swazey, September 30, 1992.
35. H. H. van deer Kloot Meijburg, 1992 data on institutional ethics committees in the

Netherlands (meeting of the International Association of Bioethics, Amsterdam, October 5–7, 1992).

36. Joan Porter, How Unaffiliated/Nonscientist Members of Institutional Review Boards See Their Roles, 9 *IRB* 1 (November-December 1987); Joan Porter, What are the Ideal Characteristics of Unaffiliated/Nonscientist IRB Members?, 8 *IRB* 1 (May-June 1986); Joan Porter, The Lay Member on the Institutional Review Board: An Exploratory Study of Roles (Ph.D. dissertation, University of Southern California School of Public Administration, 1985), esp. Chapter 6. Dr. Porter surveyed 198 outside members of 200 IRBs with multiple project assurances (a response rate of just under 50 percent). I am grateful to Dr. Porter for sharing her data with me; the data reported in this paragraph are hers.

37. Porter, *supra* note 36, at 1, 6.

38. Levine, *supra* note 2.

39. University of Utah Assurance Number M1082, on file with the FDA.

40. Julia Neuberger, King's Fund Institute Research Report 13, *Ethics and Health Care: The Role of Research Ethics Committees in the United Kingdom* (1992).

41. Health Service Guidelines(91)5 § 2.5 (Aug. 19, 1991).

42. *Id.* § 2.8.

43. In 1991, 112 IRBs were given letters of deficiency by the FDA; these included (with possible overlaps) 9 non-MPA IRBs for lack of a member with community knowledge; 3 MPA and 8 non-MPA for lack of a non-affiliated member; 1 MPA and 5 non-MPA for conflict-of-interest violations. In 1992, 119 letters of deficiency were issued, with 1 MPA and 7 non-MPA for lack of community knowledge; 1 MPA and 10 non-MPA for lack of a non-affiliated member; and 1 MPA and 11 non-MPA for conflict-of-interest violations. FDA, *Deficiency Summary, FY 91, FY 92* (1992).

44. Telephone conversation with Paul Goebel, FDA, Sept. 29, 1992.

45. Telephone conversation with Dr. Edward Allan, OPRR, Sept. 22, 1992.

46. *Id.*, p. 331.

47. *Id.*, at 334.

48. R. T. Chlebowski, How Many Protocols Are Deferred? One IRB's Experience, 6 *IRB* 9, 10 (Sept./Oct. 1984).

49. *Supra* note 40, at 25.

50. David Shimm and Roy Spece, Jr., Rate of Refusal to Participate in Clinical Trials, 14 *IRB* 7 (March-April 1992).

51. *See, e.g.*, Leonard Glantz, Contrasting Institutional Review Boards with Institutional Ethics Committees, in *Institutional Ethics Committees and Health Care Decision-Making, supra* note 23 at 129.

52. Stewart Spicker and Thomasine Kushner, Editors' Introduction, 1 *HEC Forum* 179, 180 (1989).

53. Stuart Youngner, Claudia Coulton, Barbara Juknialis, and David Jackson, Patients' Attitudes toward Hospital Ethics Committees, in *Institutional Ethics Committees and Health Care Decision-Making, supra* note 23, at 73. Ironically, the authors of this study encountered difficulty in obtaining IRB approval, in their judgment because the IRB chair opposed involvement of patients in health care decision-making. *Id.* at 76.

54. *Supra* note 57.

55. *See, e.g.*, William Broad and Nicholas Wade, *Betrayers of the Truth* (1982).

56. National Academy of Sciences, *Responsible Science: Ensuring the Integrity of the Research Process* 30 (1992); H. K. Bechtel, Jr., and W. Pearson, Jr., Deviant Scientists and Scientific Deviance, 6 *Deviant Behavior* 237 (1985).

57. Robert Bell, *Impure Science* (1992).
58. *E.g.*, Eugene Braunwald, Cardiology: The John Darsee Experience, in *Research Fraud in the Behavioral and Biomedical Sciences* 55 (David Miller and Michael Hersen, eds., 1992).
59. *Supra* note 56.
60. Health Service Guidelines(91)5 § 3.23 (August 19, 1991).

Index